WHEN THE HEART SPEAKS

WHEN THE HEART SPEAKS

Memoirs of a Cardiologist

DR UPENDRA KAUL

KONARK

Konark Publishers Pvt Ltd

New Delhi

Konark Publishers Pvt Ltd
206, First Floor,
Peacock Lane, Shahpur Jat,
New Delhi - 110 049
Tel : +91-11-4105 5065
e-mail : india@konarkpublishers.com, us@konarkpublishers.com
website : www.konarkpublishers.com

The photographs used in this book are from the author's collection.

ISBN: 978-81-949286-5-2

Edited by Ranjana Narayan
Cover jacket by Sanjeev Mathpal
Back cover painting by Syeda Afshana
Printed and bound at Thomson Press (India) Ltd

This book is dedicated to
the memory of
my immortal mother
Gauri Kaul

Contents

Foreword

I can state with near certainty that few of you would know that the princely state of Jammu and Kashmir was bought for a mere Rs 75 lakh. Such nuggets, and many more, are hidden in this lucid, conversational narrative of Padma Shri Dr Upendra Kaul, a gold medallist in surgery and the first qualified cardiologist of Kashmiri origin. It is difficult to discern distinctly which is his first love—Kashmir or cardiology. The dice, however, rolls in favour of Kashmir where, despite his academic and research commitments, he goes regularly to conduct camps in pursuance of his mission of 'No More Heart Attacks by 2025' under the banner of an NGO set up as a tribute to his late mother.

In this book, the author has not only traced the history of Kashmir from the late 14th/early 15th century but also laid bare the wrangles and challenges during the past five decades in the medical profession in general and cardiology in particular. He is brutally frank, demonstrates a phenomenal memory for events, names, places and narrates the incidents as if they had transpired yesterday. He uses the scalpel as skilfully on some of the ills of his profession as he does on the operating table. But the book is eminently readable, resplendent with brilliant anecdotes and difficult to put down.

Dr Kaul's poetic description of tranquillity and nature's bountiful beauty of Srinagar and its environs and the vivid elucidation on details of constructed houses are admirable. He recollects how education came to Srinagar. Though most of his education was at Delhi, he offers resonating reflections and poignant accounts of his annual holidays in Srinagar, his childhood friends, the games and pranks they used to play. Those memories are etched in his mind. The historical facts on Kashmir are well researched and richly supplemented and embellished by first-hand accounts, including the traumatic events of the 1990s and the possible reasons thereof.

A large part of the book is devoted to his more than 50 years in the medical profession, generously interlaced with amusing anecdotes replete with saucy details. From the use of mnemonics to remember the names of all 206 bones in an adult during medical education to a payment of only Rs 250 a month for a 'house job', now termed as 'junior residency', after more than two years as an MBBS, it's all there. He laments that 'the art of bedside clinical sense and reaching a diagnosis has remarkably come down'. Up to the middle of the 1990s, the author says, things were reasonably in order and the medical fraternity was held in very high esteem. But then the menace of kickbacks for referrals spread its tentacles over the medical field leading to unnecessary tests, unnecessary drugs and vitamin supplements. In the first decade of the 21st century, he says, the increasing need for specialists resulted in mushrooming of cardiology clinics and associated laboratories, with the downside that there was no auditing, no appropriateness criteria stipulated by authorities, and unnecessary, uncalled for procedures were performed.

Dr Kaul has very eloquently brought out that we have 4,000 registered cardiologists with a paltry figure of one per 300,000 population, as compared to 23,000 in the USA, giving a figure of 43.8 per 100,000. Stents, he says, came into the forefront in 1986 but AIIMS started using them in 1992. The first cardiac transplantation in India was done on 3rd August 1994, and the author was one of the cardiologists taking care of the person who survived for 14 years post-surgery. In 2014, the issue of exorbitant prices of stents came up since the number of patients needing angioplasty was 500,000 per year with an annual increase of 30 per cent. A person filed a case in the Delhi High Court, but it took three years before the government handed it to the National List of Essential Medicines to fix a price. It was discovered that the cost was being escalated by 1,000 to 2,000 times and there was no MRP on the boxes.

The above are only a few glimpses of this book by my three-decades-old dear friend who puts his work and relationships ahead of himself. I have watched him tirelessly serving the community, even putting his life at risk during the pandemic. Dr Kaul is a Dr B.C. Roy Award winner and an author of innumerable studies acclaimed worldwide. He has travelled across the globe to deliver lectures on his professional expertise, and has always been involved in academics and research alongside clinical and interventional cardiology.

This book is truly straight from the heart from one who knows the human heart like we know the palm of our hand.

M.A. Pathan
Former Chairman, Indian Oil Corporation &
Former Resident Director, Tata Group

Pre-Publication Reviews

"

Dr Upendra Kaul has spent much of the last few years flying in to Srinagar every week to meet and treat patients unable to afford to fly to Delhi for expensive cardiac treatments. His journey, as he has outlined in his own words, is an inspiration and a lesson to all of us.

Omar Abdullah

Former Chief Minister, Jammu and Kashmir

The first time Dr U. Kaul told me that he desires to pen down his memoirs, I immediately thought that a book is waiting to be written. While congratulating him I said that it must be comprehensive—covering his entire life and career. Soon we started to mull over his notes written randomly and, over a period of time, it started to take the shape of a book. I am personally delighted to have been associated with this noble project from day one. The book covers all important aspects of him: the rich life he has lived, excellent credentials he has earned as a cardiologist and now as a social architect serving the people of J&K through the Gauri Heart Foundation. The autobiography truly lives up to the title—*When The Heart Speaks*—and makes for an engrossing read.

Prof. Ashok Ogra

Media professional and currently Advisor (MC), Apeejay Education Society

Three people from Kashmir have strongly influenced me in the last three decades: Two 'Pandits' – Prof. Agha Ashraf Ali and Mir Mohammad Farooq Nazki, and one 'Muslim' – Prof. (Dr) U. Kaul. Dr Kaul lives and writes from his heart like that old-school enthusiast, believer, and makes us feel our world is simple, just, fair, beautiful. As a reader I'm tempted to agree, too.

Ajaz Rashid

Social Scientist and CEO, Gauri Kaul Foundation

Dr Kaul, or *Upipapa* as he is called by all of us, takes us on an exciting voyage through different parts of Kashmir and also different parts of the world with a special mention of his culinary experiences. The story when Sathya Sai Baba gave him the ring with precious stones was very exciting for me as a child. My dad never misses to wear that ring every day. He is a wonderful human being, always so generous, ready to help whoever approaches him. He is misunderstood by many as he has a strong mind and strong opinions, but he is a child at heart wanting love and to be cared for.

Amita Kaul

HOD Paediatrics, Surya Hospital for Child and Mother Care, Pune

Prof. Upendra Kaul's love for Kashmir runs in his blood as well as in his genes. I have personally witnessed many occasions when he would go to any level to help patients from Kashmir who came to see him. I was amazed to see that this love was not one-sided. It was reciprocal. During my association with him and seeing his vast experience throughout his life, I persuaded him to write his memoirs. He took it with reluctance but I am glad that the book *When The Heart Speaks* is finally ready. It is going to be a very useful and entertaining reading.

Dr Abid Hussain Hakim

Consultant Cardiologist, Gauri Heart Centre, Srinagar, Kashmir

Over the decades, I have come to know Upendra Kaul not so much as a doctor but as a Kashmiri man whose knowledge about the history of Kashmir is unusual. His story takes you into not only descriptions of the valley but the emotions of the valley too and grips you because of his passion. I strongly recommend this book for those who truly want to understand Kashmir and the Kashmiris.

Devaki Jain
Indian Feminist, Economist and Writer

A personality difficult to define in words as he is rarest of the rare. A child-like soul who doesn't understand the intricacies of life as he understands only loving and caring for people and working hard till his last breath. An excellent cardiologist, academician, researcher, writer and a wonderful person by nature. His book clearly will take you on a simple yet magnificent journey of his life.

Priyadarshini Arambam
General Manager–Academics and Research
Batra Hospital and Medical Research Centre, New Delhi

Medical biographies have a special significance as they penetrate into the art and science of Medicine. *When The Heart Speaks* is one such biography written very lucidly, in which the author has projected himself more as a storyteller than as a biographer.

Prof. G. Q. Allaqaband
Former HOD Medicine & Principal, Govt. Medical College and SMHS Hospital, Srinagar, Kashmir

It should be read by all those who are interested to know about the past and present culture of Kashmir. It is an eye-opener for those who are pursuing to excel in their careers and want to get a feel of passion, dedication, zest to learn and serve the motherland. For those patients and their families who have benefitted from his service, the book tells what Upendra Kaul stands for. Of course, to the medical fraternity at all levels, the book teaches how to serve and balance your career despite fame, glory, and success. For those who want to serve their motherland, including the NGOs, the book shows a way of how to walk and tread on the right path of service.

Prof. (Dr) M. S. Khuroo
Former Dean and Director, and
HOD, Dept. of Gastroenterology, SKIMS, Srinagar

Professor Kaul represents the acme of a professional cardiologist. In *When The Heart Speaks*, he traces the journey of a simple village boy from interior Kashmir through the travails of a middle-class urban Delhi, to an exceptional Padma Shri-awarded professional cardiologist. In his inimitable direct style, he narrates numerous anecdotes that engage, entertain, and educate the readers in many ways. His vast experience in different medical setups may serve as useful tips to many in the profession. The dry humour in many accounts actually hides the sensitive persona of the author who has been a teacher, a healer and a friend to many people, including the commoners and the royals. In *When The Heart Speaks* you get a glimpse of it.

Prof. (Dr) S. S. Kothari
HOD, Cardiology, AIIMS, New Delhi

Roots never desert.... This perhaps sums up the entire life journey of a person who has dedicated himself to humanity.

Original, ingenious and a brilliant masterpiece that not only engages but also informs and entertains the reader. An interesting personal narrative with an incisive story and information that conveys the essence of experience and wisdom. The author tries to deeply explore his life—what life really means to him, and his vision of serving mankind. And importantly, Kashmir, underpins his life story— that comes full circle by the author's repeated return to his roots.

There is a combination of lucid emotional narrative and descriptive writing style. The book also provides thrilling adventures of various places in the form of a travelogue. Indeed, one of the most exciting memoirs that I have glanced through cursorily. Will be a great read.

Prof. Syeda Afshana

Media Education Research Centre, University of Kashmir, India and Visiting Fellow, Centre of International Studies, Cambridge University, United Kingdom

To Dr Upendra Kaul I owe my life when a heart attack at the age of 58 almost ended it. The 22 years Dr Kaul has given me since that event have been the best years of my life, personally and professionally. I have a deep respect and affection for Upendra who has dedicated his tireless life to the service of his patients and to the people of Kashmir. This fascinating story of his life is told 'straight from the heart', and does not miss a beat.

Roshan Seth

British Indian Actor, Writer and Theatre Director

In this book, Dr Upendra Kaul, one of India's top cardiologists, whom I have had the privilege to know as a close family friend, details his remarkable journey of public service. Perhaps the most fascinating aspect of his personal and professional arc is his decades-long engagement with Kashmir, all the more notable given that he belongs to the minority Kashmiri Pandit community which left the valley in droves during the years of militancy. Instead, 'U Kaul', as he is known in Kashmir, returned to the valley again and again, becoming a sort of healer to the troubled region, treating thousands of ordinary Kashmiris irrespective of their religious beliefs, social status, etc., as he details in

his book. All of this makes *When the Heart Speaks* a must-read for all.
Sreenivasan Jain
Journalist and Group Editor, NDTV

Prof. Kaul describes his childhood and the family pattern at his native village Hawal, Pulwama, and becomes very nostalgic about his childhood. He is above religious prejudices. As Chairman Ethics Committee at Fortis Escorts Hospital, New Delhi, I found him very sound professionally and apt ethically, always speaking 'straight from the heart'. His memoir is full of the realistic facts of his life.
Prof. Abdul Hamid Zargar
Former Director of SKIMS, Srinagar

”

Preface

My desire to return to the green meadows and the snow-capped mountains of the Kashmir Valley burns like a wildfire within me. I dream and long of a day when I can finally settle there and spend my remaining life in its beauteous lap. As a prerequisite to make that desire materialize, I have already built a house there. My mother always had a desire to return to the valley and have a place of our own. She did not live long enough to see it but I wanted to fulfil this desire of hers. My friends are always delighted when I go and spend my time for a few days or a week there at least once a month. Travelling to all parts of the valley and giving public talks on prevention of heart disease and building awareness about high blood pressure and diabetes bring joy to my life. I try to make the people of the valley realize that managing these problems early can reduce the chances of heart attacks, strokes and kidney failures which are major public health problems. I have many colleagues and friends to help me in carrying out this mission. I am a regular writer of educative articles on preventive medicine in the most popular daily, *Greater Kashmir*.

Kashmir, my birthplace, even though most of my education has been in Delhi, has always enamoured me and given me the strength to become what little I have achieved today. In my younger days, the magnetic pull to go there for spending my vacations always made me perform better. Hence, my parents would willingly allow me to go as often as I could. My love for the people there has always been reciprocated by them. Despite the ill feelings of Kashmiri Pandits towards the majority community after the happenings of 1990, my affection for my people never changed. This has often led to criticism by many people, especially on social media, who have repeatedly questioned my integrity. My reaction has always been that we need to stand together and not be polarized. The very small Pandit community needs to realize this and move forward if we have to preserve our culture—which cannot be centric to just one religion. This preservation can only come by being in Kashmir as often as possible and not by imagining the serene valley and trying to replicate the valley elsewhere—in other parts of the world.

The Kashmiri heritage in me continues to thrive and my visits to the valley are becoming very frequent. On my every visit, I go to see places which I had missed around the city and the valley. I have developed friendship and intimacy with the young and old, poor and rich, and always tried to learn something about the valley and its people.

New Delhi **Dr Upendra Kaul**

Acknowledgements

The idea that I should write a book of my experiences in life was first given to me several years ago by Dr Abid Hussain Hakim, my student who later became a friend and a colleague. I never thought I would be able to do it since my experience of writing was only confined to medical literature.

Reluctantly, I started scribbling it, when another friend Prof. Ashok Ogra, noted media professional and currently Advisor (MC) of Apeejay Educational Society, supported the idea and helped me throughout the process of writing. The title of the book *When the Heart Speaks* was given by him. He also suggested the name of Shreya Chakrobarti, who contributed by way of her suggestions of putting in anecdotes and improving my style which otherwise was like a Cardiology Professor's.

A lot of this writing was done on long overseas flights till Covid-19 arrived on the scene; and then on my weekly travels to Srinagar, my colleague Ajaz Rashid would give his critical but constructive comments on my notes.

Finally, I am grateful to Mr K.P.R. Nair, Managing Director of Konark Publishers, for facilitating it through his team, especially Ranjana Narayan and Jiza Joy, who gave me the confidence that this memoir would make an interesting reading.

1

From Khans to Kauls

I was born of parents who had grown up in completely diverse environments and dissimilar upbringings in the early years of their lives. My father Prem Nath, or Papa as we call him, was born in the village of Hawal. It is a hamlet situated about 45 km away from the city of Srinagar on the Pulwama–Shopian Highway, which is now known as the Mughal Road. A picturesque village, Hawal is almost idyllic with a majestic view of the snow-clad Himalayas, surrounded by several streams where the water is so clear that it reflects the cerulean sky. Heavy snowfall always used to make the village inaccessible during winters. In the summers, when the rivulets got flooded and washed away the bridges, Hawal was cut off from the world.

Remote as it was, Hawal had no medical facility. People didn't know the feeling of having toilets and electricity at home. The village was inhabited mainly by 40 families of Pandits, who were primarily agriculturists. Their Muslim neighbours—not more than 20-odd families—were either artisans or landless agricultural peasants who worked on the Pandits' land. Some of them also worked as servants for the well-off Pandits. *Dadaji*, Papa's father, was Prasad Joo Khan, who worked as a *patwari* (land records officer), a profession he had inherited from his ancestors. He eventually gave up this job as he did not like it. He started a general store, which catered to the local needs of the village—all the daily necessities were available there. *Dadaji* was married to a girl from the village and lived at his in-laws' house. My grandmother—*Dadi*—was a very graceful lady, though she was quite stern. She was very affectionate but, at the same time, was a hard taskmaster. She would rule the kitchen with an iron fist and all my aunts were careful while dealing with her. The marriage brought 12 siblings—eight sons and four daughters. Papa was the seventh child.

Hawal had only one primary school with only one teacher. Papa went to this school for his initial education. He further pursued his middle-level education in the tehsil town of Pulwama, which had the only middle school in the tehsil those days. This school was nearly 10 km away from Hawal. Every day, Papa and a few other boys from the village would walk to the school and return home in the evening, covering almost 20 km daily with a heavy load of books on their shoulders and with no midday meal. While the boys could easily buy bread from Pulwama, it was a forbidden food for the 'high caste' Brahmins of the valley as Muslim bakers made them.

Our house in Hawal was five-storied, the tallest and the largest building of the village. The architecture was a typical Kashmiri one with slanting ceilings studded with wooden conical pieces called shingles. This was later replaced by tin. The walls were made of a mixture of clay and cement, and several layers of bricks to give it strength. The house had wooden windows. The outer walls were made of bricks, clay and rubble along with wooden frames and bracings for the windows. The sitting room (*baithak*) had a beautiful false ceiling of wooden *khatmband* (intricately carved) panels with interlocking geometric shapes. These were made of walnut wood and are known for their invisible joints. The top floor of our building had wooden extensions protruding out for the summers. These structures are called *dubs* and are typical to the Kashmiri houses of that era. A cool breeze would welcome anyone sitting there in the mornings and after the day's work in the evenings. One could often find people sipping *kahwa* or *noon* chai (salted tea) while having a relaxing time.

There were two more small shacks in the compound. One was meant for keeping firewood and fodder for the cows. The other one housed the cows and a horse of superior breed that the family owned. It was a prized possession of the Khans. These shacks had clay plaster on the outer walls. Our family also owned huge tracts of land for paddy.

Dadaji left his business when he was 50 and handed over the shop to his eldest son Shyam Lal, while he took to prayers and entertaining sadhus coming on pilgrims to the Amarnath Temple or the temples of the Shopian area. Papa was the only brother who went to college; the others joined the family business with only two younger brothers passing high school. Shyam Lal, who was eight years older than Papa and treated Papa as his son, made him go to college because he was forward looking and knew the value of education. He was, unfortunately, a very miserly person. Hence, Papa faced financial crunches and had to endure struggles.

After Papa finished middle school, he stayed with his eldest sister Durga Mal, affectionately called Benidyad, in Srinagar for matriculation. It was due to this reason that he always considered her like his mother. Benidyad was 10 years older than my father, which made her very affectionate towards her younger brother. After high school, he graduated in arts from Sri Pratap College and then Amar Singh College in Srinagar, both of which were affiliated to Punjab University, Lahore. Both these colleges were built during Maharaja Hari Singh's reign and were named after his father Pratap Singh and uncle Amar Singh, respectively.

After his graduation, Papa went to Lucknow to study further and earned his Bachelor's degrees in commerce and law before returning to Kashmir in June 1947. This was two months before India gained independence. He got married to my mother Gauri during his studies in Lucknow, in October 1946. Papa started his law practice in Kashmir around August-September 1947, but within a few weeks, the valley was raided by tribesmen backed by the Pakistan Army in October. This threw everything out of gear and he was forced to leave the valley for Delhi where he finally secured a position in a general insurance company named New Asiatic Insurance Company run by the Birlas. The salary agreed upon was a meagre Rs 100 a month.

My Mother

My mother Gauri, though raised in Srinagar, was born in 1926 at Sopore, a town in North Kashmir. Her mother was from Sopore and she had gone to her parents' home for the delivery. Traditionally, in those days, women used to go to their parents' place for their deliveries. Her father, Vishna Joo Hakeem, came from a family of renowned *hakims* (physicians using traditional remedies). They lived in Rainawari, a suburb of Srinagar, but did not show any interest in *hikmat* (prescribing treatment by hakims) and treating patients. *Nanaji* had very little formal education but was an ace swimmer, athlete and mountaineer. One day, Tyndale Biscoe, a British missionary who brought modern education to the valley, heard about him from an acquaintance and called him for an interview. The position was for one of his schools in downtown Srinagar. Meeting a white man could have been intimidating in those times, especially for a man whose English was restricted to a few customary salutations. But *Nanaji* was made of stronger mettle and was quite unfazed.

On the day of the interview, Biscoe asked him, 'Tell me, what classes have you crossed?'

Nanaji confidently replied, 'Wular Cross!'

Wular Lake is one of the largest freshwater lakes of Asia. Biscoe couldn't stop laughing and *Nanaji* got the job. These abilities immediately made him the headmaster of a missionary school run by Biscoe near Fateh *Kadal* (meaning bridge)—the third bridge built over River Jhelum by Sultan Fateh Shah in 1499.

I had always considered my grandmother Radhamal a wise woman. She could recite Persian verses and the history of Kashmir and its beauty. According to her, this beauty was inviting aggression from other countries. She would also advise her children to be diplomatic and never be blunt in speaking. 'Never call a person with one eye *kana* (blind). It will hurt him,' she would say. The atmosphere at my grandparents' home was pro-British as my grandfather was working at a missionary school. He liked to have a glass of Scotch, and the Christmas week always called for celebration. This was not at all common in the neighbourhood. He ran the school for a decade and was in good health till he developed diabetes. Nanaji, unfortunately, succumbed to a complication of this disease—a big boil on his back called carbuncle at an early age. He was hospitalised but the infection developed further and started to spread. He passed away because of the infection in 1930. Ironically, this happened after a few years of the discovery of insulin by Banting and Best in 1921, but was not widely available in India when he passed away. This was one of my mother's biggest regrets as she knew that she could have saved *Nanaji* from the deadly diabetes had he lived a few years more.

My mother had three brothers—Prithvi Nath, Brij Lal and Makhan Lal—and one sister Janak Rani, who was the eldest sibling. The eldest brother, Prithvi, was affectionately called *Tathya* (meaning dear one). He was an intelligent man and was academically bright. He started his career as a college teacher teaching economics in Peshawar and then in Delhi at Hindu College. Eventually, he became a noted economist. He was one of the founders of the Delhi School of Economics and the director of the Institute of Economic Growth, University of Delhi, before joining the Prime Minister's Secretariat (now called the PMO) in 1970. During his later years, he became the Principal Secretary of Mrs Indira Gandhi. He also served as United Nations Assistant Secretary-General, Research and Policy Analysis. In 2008, the Government of India awarded him with the Padma Vibhushan.

As the eldest son, *Tathya* looked after the entire family and took care of his brothers' education. As their father had passed away early, *Tathya* was always a father figure to my mother, though the age difference between the siblings was only a few years. My mother had little formal education as girls were not encouraged to go to school during her time. Further, an embarrassing incident in Srinagar had discouraged girls' education. The incident was that a girl attending a local school was found missing one day. It turned out that she had a friendship that, over time, had transformed into something deeper with a young man who was a teacher in the school. She had eloped with this man after her parents had vehemently refused to accept their marriage. Eventually, they were found in Bombay, now Mumbai. This incident created panic among the locals and parents promptly pulled out their daughters from schools to avoid any untoward incident.

My mother, who had just started school and was in the second grade, became one of the unwitting victims of this paranoia. Her father was alive at that time, and had to agree with the community despite being a logical man. She took the blow in her stride and was determined to not let this affect her. She educated herself through books and newspapers available at home and had an excellent grasp of general knowledge and current affairs; she was also quite politically aware. She could describe in detail Sheikh Abdullah's movement and how he marshalled Kashmiris to fight for their rights. One of her grievances till she breathed her last was that she did not have a formal education.

The Khan Surname

The question that often arises is why our surname is Khan. Admittedly, this is an odd surname for a Brahmin family. For that, allow me to dig deeper and explain to you the genesis of this surname, which is carefully embedded in the history of Kashmir.

The Shah Mir dynasty ruled Kashmir from 1339 till 1561. It was founded by Shams-ud-Din Shah Mir in 1339 who succeeded the last ruler of the Hindu Lohara dynasty, Kota Rani, whom he had proposed for marriage but was turned down. This is the period when Islam was firmly established in Kashmir. One of the rulers of this dynasty was Sikandar Shah Mir, also known as Sikandar Butshikan, who is known to have destroyed several ancient temples of Kashmir, including the Martand Sun Temple and the Shiva temples at Avantipora. This dynasty also had many able and popular rulers like Zain-ul-Abdin, known by his subjects as 'Bod Shah', who reigned over Kashmir from 1420 to 1470. This was a very peaceful and well-governed period for the people of Kashmir. During his rule, he recalled the Pandits from various parts of India, resettled them and taught them Persian so that they could get employment. He banned the killing of cows by poisoning and regulated the consumption of beef.

Zain-ul-Abdin abolished the *jizya*, a discriminatory tax levied on non-Muslims, built new cities and several bridges on River Jhelum, and reintroduced stipends for learned Brahmins. After his death, he was succeeded by his son Haji Khan, better known as Haider Khan, who was a tyrant and resorted to cruelties like chopping off limbs and killing innocent Hindus. This was followed by a tumultuous period between 1561 and 1587 till the Mughals emerged as a dominating force. The Mughals seized Kashmir and their rule lasted from 1587 to 1752. This period too is considered a peaceful period. During this time, most of the beautiful gardens and picturesque spots that the valley is acclaimed for were developed by Emperor Akbar, his son Jahangir and grandson Shah Jahan. The rule, however, disintegrated after the death of Aurangzeb when corrupt governors started a despotic reign.

The Afghans under Ahmad Shah Abdali, the founder of Durrani Empire, who was ruling Afghanistan and North-West India, were invited by the representatives of the people of Kashmir. They responded and Abdali fought a fierce battle against the Mughals and conquered Kashmir in 1752 and ruled till 1819. It was during this period my forefathers worked under the Afghans as a *patwari* and our family got the surname Khan. This name is still retained in the revenue records as 'Pandit Khan'. The Afghans ruled with a lot of hard rules and were against idol worship and temples. The Afghan rule, which lasted till 1819, is known as the darkest period of the valley. The Afghans unleashed a reign of terror, especially on the Pandits and the Shias. Forced conversion to Islam resulted in a large population migrating to other places in India and it is said only 11 families of Pandits survived death. The atrocious rule came to an end when three Pandits led by Birbal Dhar quietly fled to Maharaja Ranjit Singh's Durbar in Lahore and narrated the plight of the people of Kashmir, especially the Pandits. The Maharaja got moved and immediately ordered his generals to invade Kashmir. Thus, the Sikhs arrived to take advantage of the weakened Afghan forces and seized control.

The Sikh rulers were generally tolerant towards different faiths but some decisions alienated the majority Muslim population in the valley. For instance, the first governor under the Sikh rule, Diwan Moti Ram, incidentally a Hindu, called for putting an end to public *azan* and Friday prayers at the Jama Masjid. The Sikhs were also very hard on the Muslim peasantry, imposing high taxation on agricultural land and forcing them to cultivate only a small portion of available land. Towards the end of their rule, they seemed to have realised their mistake when a massive famine hit the valley.

The Sikhs otherwise ensured there was adequate representation of all the major religions—Hindus, Muslims and Sikhs—in the administration. However, Ranjit Singh, the first Maharaja of the Sikh Empire, never visited the valley.

Ranjit Deo was the Raja of Jammu from 1728 to 1780. His death was followed by a number of successors and killings. Finally, Maharaja Ranjit Singh came on the scene and allotted it to his son Kharak Singh, who made a hash of it. Ranjit Singh was forced to take it away from Kharak Singh and gave it to Kishore Singh, a distant kinsman of Ranjit Singh. After Kishore Singh, his son Gulab Singh, who subsequently sought service at the court of Ranjit Singh, became the ruler. Gulab Singh became a distinguished figure due to his later campaigns, especially the annexation of the Kashmir Valley. For his services, he was appointed the governor of Jammu in 1820. With the help of his officer Zorawar Singh, he soon captured the lands of Ladakh and Baltistan to the east and north-east of Jammu, respectively.

Maharaja Ranjit Singh had maintained a cautious alliance with the British. However, there was infighting amongst the dynasty following his death in 1839. The British took advantage of this instability and assumed partial control over the Sikh territories. Kashmir was one of them. Under the Treaty of Amritsar, the British sold Kashmir to Raja Gulab Singh for just Rs 75 lakh, thus, establishing the princely state of Jammu and Kashmir. The Dogras ruled over the entire state till Maharaja Hari Singh was ousted by the popular movement of Sheikh Mohammad Abdullah, supported by Pandit Jawaharlal Nehru, in 1947. After India's independence, an attack on Kashmir by Pashtun tribals, backed covertly by Pakistan in October 1947, led to Hari Singh signing the Instrument of Accession with India against his will but there was no other option left for him. This accession formed the root cause of the Kashmir dispute with Pakistan. Nehru, the first prime minister of India, took the case to the United Nations on 1 January 1948 upon the advice of Lord Mountbatten, the last Viceroy of India, and suggested a referendum that never saw the light of the day.

Our family continued to use the surname Khan before Papa. However, in order to avoid the embarrassment of having a Muslim surname, he changed his surname from Khan to Kaul before matriculation. Kaul is a very common Kashmiri Pandit surname.

The suffix Joo, used by both my grandfathers, Prasad Joo and Vishna Joo, is rather interesting. Joo, the genesis of which is debatable, still is frequently used as a suffix for both Pandits and Muslims. Some say it is because of our Jewish ancestry, which has never been proven historically. Francis Edward Younghusband in his book *Kashmir* has imagined that Kashmiris might be the lost tribes of Israel. However, most believe it is a Hindi honorific of *ji*, which means life or soul. The change of surname was accepted by the family very well. A few other brothers changed to Bhat, another common Pandit surname. However, those who remained in the village preferred Khan as it was their identity not only in their village but also in the entire neighbourhood.

2

My Parents' Marriage and My Birth

When my mother turned 20, the family got anxious to find a suitor for her. Tathya was entrusted with this grave responsibility. He met my father through a few acquaintances. When he met the young, strapping man, he decided that Prem Nath, my father, who was 19 then, would be a good match for Gauri, though she was a year older than him. He knew that Papa was pursuing his graduation in commerce and law in Lucknow and that would help him get a reasonable job in the city; the couple could settle down in Srinagar. Shyam Lal, Papa's eldest brother, was also seeking a match for his younger brother from Srinagar. This would be the first time in the Khan's family that a girl from the city would join the clan. This was considered a matter of pride. The marriage was quickly finalised.

As narrated by Papa, the *barat* (celebratory wedding procession of the groom) went from the village to Srinagar in a bus. From the bus terminal, a car had been arranged which took them to Kanikadal,

Srinagar. The whole lane had been decorated and people of the neighbourhood of all religions were there to receive the *baratis* with garlands. The marriage ceremony followed typical Hindu customs and took place in a neighbour's house. This was followed by a grand vegetarian feast. Following the ceremony, Papa, along with my mother, her brother Brij Lal and the *barat,* went to Habba Kadal to Benidyad's (Papa's eldest sister) place. There they were taken to the kitchen and fed a delicacy made of rice and *Anna Pravesh* (yogurt) prepared by her. This was followed by returning to Kanikadal, where they changed and then went to Hawal in the evening. The village was waiting for their arrival, with women welcoming them by singing and sprinkling fragrant seeds, *mishri* (sugar candy) and almonds till they entered the premises. A grand non-vegetarian feast with several very well-cooked dishes was served to the whole village. The Muslims were served food after the Pandits had finished eating their vegetarian meals. The wedding was on the day of Ram Navami in 1946. The next morning, the newlyweds along with Brij Lal went back to Kanikadal.

Another non-vegetarian delicacy was awaiting them. Following this, my eldest *mama* (mother's brother) Prithvi Nath took them to the Dussehra mela at Chandmari ground, where the crowd had gathered to see Maharaja Hari Singh, the last Dogra ruler of Jammu and Kashmir, who had come with a huge procession. The venue was full of people of all religions, watching the grand show with the beating of drums and loud music that signified the victory of good over evil. The Maharaja shot a lighted arrow at the effigy of Ravana and his two brothers amidst loud cheering by the crowd that echoed all around.

After the wedding, my mother, however, had to go to our village, Hawal as Papa was still completing his education in Lucknow and had to return within a few days. Village life was tough on her and she would come back to Srinagar to her mother's house at the smallest pretext. She always felt that the village family didn't have much knowledge of current affairs, hygiene and common sense. One incident which put her off completely was when she injured her foot by hitting a sharp stone in the vegetable garden of ours and got a lacerated wound. She was asked by the family and the chief priest of the village to apply fresh cow dung on it. She had heard of tetanus as a killer with such applications. She cried and persuaded her husband's younger brother Som Nath to take her to Srinagar to her mother's place. She was allowed to go but this defiant act was not received well by the family. In short, she was never comfortable there.

While growing up, I had heard quite a few stories of village life from my mother regarding the way the Pandit community handled the Muslim workers. The Pandits considered themselves superior and pious. She narrated to me that the family didn't treat our Muslim servants well and would rebuke them at the slightest pretext. It was a patriarchal family. The men would eat first served by the women. After they were done with their meals, the women would feed themselves on the leftovers, eating usually in the kitchen. While mutton and vegetables would be served to the men, very little would be left for the womenfolk to eat. Often, they would just feed on the chutney made of chillies and *pudina* (mint)) and some Koshur *haakh*. *Haakh* is a staple Kashmiri dish made of collard greens. It is very crunchy and can be very delicious if prepared nicely.

Mutton was not available every day in Hawal as the butcher would only slaughter a goat if he was sure that customers would buy it. The closest place where it was always available was Rajpura, a larger village at a distance of a few miles from Hawal, after crossing a few streams on foot or on a horse. It was an important village and had a bigger market. Its main connecting road was from Pulwama but from a different direction. It had a Muslim majority and only a few Pandit families. This village was very important to our family because meat was readily available there. I remember my elder uncle Maheshwar

Nath going there on a horse whenever an important guest would reach our home and had to be served a meal. Presently, its importance has grown manifold because of the presence of a good community medical centre and a booming market.

My Birth

I was born in Srinagar on 14 June 1948. My mother didn't want to deliver at home with the village midwife. She spent the last few months of her pregnancy in Srinagar and went to Shri Maharaja Hari Singh Hospital where I was delivered by a British obstetrician named Dr D'Silva. She had to apply outlet forceps due to some abnormality in her womb. The right side of my forehead received a minor injury and I still have a small scar there. This is one of my two identification marks. However, my mother was very proud of the fact that her doctor was British. Although Papa had a job in Delhi, he was in Srinagar the day I was born. He, however, had to go back to Delhi after a few days.

I spent the first 18 months of my life in Srinagar and Hawal, flitting between both my grandparents' houses, although my mother was never at ease with her in-laws in Hawal. Papa was in Delhi during that time and was staying with *Tathya* at Gwyer Hall, a hostel of Delhi University. He was searching for a rented accommodation so that he could bring his family over.

While I grew up a happy kid, I started speaking late, which worried my parents. My cousin who was almost my age was speaking fluently by then while I was just mumbling some noises. When my parents consulted the family's head priest with some consternation, he advised that a tongue be made of silver, which had to be donated to the Devi at Kheer Bhawani temple, one of the most sacred places for Kashmiri Pandits in the valley. The temple is dedicated to Goddess Ragnya—

originally called Bhawani—and was constructed over a sacred spring. Devotees would bring kheer, or rice pudding, in the spring to worship the goddess, which became a part of the temple's name. My parents followed the head priest's advice diligently and a few weeks later I uttered my first sentence.

When I was 18 months old, my mother brought me to Delhi to join Papa. By this time, he had rented one room in Prem Nagar. There was a cloth mill nearby called Birla Mill. Most residents in that colony were shift workers who were employed at the mill, which used to run round the clock. The building had just one toilet without any sewerage and residents had to wait for their turns. The water supply was from a handpump bored into the ground and women had to wait in queues in the morning for their turn to fill as many buckets as they could possibly carry. Those were the days when electricity hadn't come to all areas and the kerosene lantern used to be the only source of light. There were other children in the neighbourhood, who had their parents working at the mill. I was forbidden to interact with them, probably because of social reasons. I remember they used to swear a lot and would even be abusive with their friends. Once, I heard one of the boys calling out to his friend in the choicest of Hindi abuses. I didn't know the meaning of the word then and when I went inside the house to ask my mother what it meant, I received a slap in response! Since that day, I wasn't even allowed to be near the window of our house while the boys played outside.

The only friend I was allowed was the landlord's son, Ashok. Ashok was a few years older than I was. He had a tricycle, which he used to occasionally share with me and his sister Usha. Ashok used to call his mother Amma. That intrigued me and I started calling my mother Amma too. She didn't seem to mind the change though!

Our landlord was a Gupta and the family was vegetarian. Kashmiris love their mutton but as per our agreement with the landlord, my parents couldn't cook meat at home. This increasingly became frustrating and my parents finally found a way. Papa started getting meat wrapped in layers of newspaper sheets from a place called Pulbangash, which was situated a few miles away from Prem Nagar. Amma used to cook it after bolting the door of our kitchen from the inside. Once the dinner of mutton and boiled rice was over, Papa would gather all the bones, pack these carefully and dispose them off near his office at Connaught Place, the following day. I remember Ashok once came to our place while my mother was cooking mutton. He was puzzled by the smell of the food and asked what we were cooking that smelt so delicious. Amma told him it was a special dal from Kashmir. He insisted that he would eat with us. My mother was mortified, not knowing how to extricate herself from this situation. She went to Papa and asked worriedly, 'Now what?'

Papa suggested, 'Give him some curry; that shouldn't be a problem.' Amma did what Papa told her. I remember Ashok actually licking the plate that day after he was done. Later, his mother had asked Amma for the recipe of that special dal her son had had. I am not sure how Amma handled it but it worked.

We stayed at Prem Nagar till I was five. Over the years, Papa had managed to improve our situation financially. We moved to a house in 3 UB, Jawahar Nagar, a colony near the University of Delhi. The area in its neighbourhood had sprawling bungalows with trees lining the pavement, which was an improvement from where we were staying at Prem Nagar. Though the new house only had one room, it had a small kitchen and a separate toilet as well as a bathroom. We also had the terrace, where we would sleep during the summer, drawing our mattresses outside. Our flat was on the backside of the building and the entry was through the service lane. There was a *halwai* (sweetmeat) shop right under our flat and whenever we would open the door to the balcony, the smell of the freshly fried *pakoras* and *samosas* (savouries) would waft through the house. We had no access to the front of the house, which was occupied by our Punjabi landlord, the Kapoors. Within a few years, we rented the room adjacent to us, which would be used when our relatives used to visit from Kashmir during the winters. Our next-door neighbour was Dr Govind Raj Sharma, who was a lecturer at the Hindu College. His daughter Neelu was of my age and we became great friends. She was the first girl who was my friend. When Dr Sharma and his family migrated to Canada a few years later, Neelu and I promised to write letters and maintain our friendship. Sadly, that promise wasn't kept by either of us.

3

My Schooling and Boyhood

My first school—Lahore Montessori School—where I joined at the age of six was close to where we lived at Jawahar Nagar. It was owned by Mr Bhatia, who had migrated from Lahore. He used to have a school in Lahore with the same name but had to leave it all after the Partition. Though the school was small with only five or six rooms, Mr Bhatia had a strict admission process and admitted only the best students. Naturally, my parents wanted me to study there but securing an admission was quite a task.

It was my *mami* (aunt) Shiela Dhar, who was an author as well as a Central government employee, who came to our rescue. She was a known name during that time as the author of the popular book *Children's History of India*. She happened to know the headmistress and wrote a letter to her about her dearest nephew who was a brilliant student and how the family would be so obliged if I could get admission. It worked and I was admitted to the kindergarten school.

I studied at Lahore Montessori School till the fourth grade. Those were unremarkable days as I was a shy child and barely could make friends. In the fifth grade, I joined Government Model School, Ludlow Castle. The school was housed in a colonial castle, which during the East India Company's rule in the first half of the 19th century served as the Residency of the British political agent to the Mughal Court. Later, it became the headquarters of the Commissioner of the Delhi Territory within the North-Western Provinces. At the beginning of the 20th century, it housed the Delhi Club where Nehru's *barat* had stayed in 1916. The admission was facilitated by Papa's friend Shamboo Nath Lahori, who came from Shopian town near our native village Hawal. As admissions to Delhi schools always required some string-pulling, my parents had no option but to seek assistance from others.

On the first day of school, I remember being awed by the colonial structure. Our class teacher, Dwarika Nath Ambardar, came to me and asked me if I could converse in Kashmiri. I just nodded and blushed. He patted me and took his English class. I remember Mr Garg, the mathematics teacher with no smile on his face, writing on the board with chalk explaining the equations. I never liked maths and would go to my dreamland. An exciting thing was that there was an Oberoi-owned hotel right next to the building, which often used to host cricketers during the Test season. Those were days when we would jump and hop near the boundary wall to catch a glimpse of the cricketers, often succeeding. I remember Wes Hall, who used to scare our batsmen by his tall stature, negroid looks and a fiery pace. He would occasionally wave at us, making our day.

I always looked forward to my summer vacations because that was the time we would visit Kashmir. Besides getting a respite from the scorching summer of Delhi, I revelled in the attention of my relatives, especially my mother's elder sister, Benigashee, and my cousins. Their house at Kanikadal was on the riverbank on a canal of River Jhelum.

We used to play on the wide stairs of the bank called the *chand* with the neighbouring children. Those were the days when the valley didn't start distinguishing between religions, and as children we never knew who was a Hindu or Muslim or belonged to which caste. We only saw who was nice or mean to us. During the summer, girls used to bathe in the river late in the evening. On moonlit nights, my cousins and I used to go to the top floor of our house and watch the beautiful women, risking the thrashing of our mothers if we were caught.

The visits to our ancestral village Hawal would also be delightful. In the evening, the children of the village used to go near the streams and play games using a wooden ball and a makeshift bat. At dusk, we used to pick up stones and go to the main Pulwama–Shopian Highway and pile the stones as a wall on the road. After six in the evening, no civilian vehicle would pass the road; there were only military vehicles that would use the road so late. During those days, Kashmiris, including children, had an anti-Army sentiment and we used to get a sadistic pleasure when the vehicles had to stop to clear the road. This, I guess, was the result of the historical fact that Kashmiris had always been exploited by invaders, Mughals, Afghans, Sikhs, Dogras and finally the dispute after the division of India in 1947. These feelings have multiplied several folds and the presence of forces has become a regular part of life there. Children and adults always felt that Kashmir was a country being exploited by outsiders. This feeling was expressed in many ways even by senior responsible officers of the government. I know whenever any officer of whatsoever seniority was going to Delhi or Bombay, they would say 'I am going to India', and this remained prevalent for several decades after the accession. This feeling has been there much more within the Muslim community. I also never liked to come back to Delhi and could well sense the feelings of people having to go out of the valley.

My brother Shankar was born in March 1961 when I was 13 years old. I was the proudest kid in my colony that day because I was finally an elder brother. Amma often used to tell me that I complained about not having a sibling. Sadly, I had another two-year-old younger brother whom we lost because of diarrhoea while travelling from Delhi to Srinagar. It was my father's youngest sister Jaykishiree's wedding and we had to go to Srinagar on a specific date. My mother told me that Pappu who was a year old was unwell and was feverish during the train journey to Pathankot, the last railway station on the way. Papa insisted that they must immediately take a bus to Srinagar. He was also carrying some important bridal wear for his sister. Meanwhile, Pappu became sicker, and started excessively vomiting and had diarrhoea. He passed away in my mother's lap with me on one side. I do not recall that incident at all being just three at that time.

Shankar's birth ushered good luck to our family. It was a difficult childbirth. Amma required a Caesarean section and she was admitted to a private nursing home near Papa's office on Asaf Ali Road. That year, we had to abandon our annual summer trip to Kashmir. Instead, we went to my mama Brij Lal's house in Pandara Road for two months. My youngest mama Makhan Lal was also staying with him. He was a huge fan of Hindi film songs and had a great collection. Both my mamas Makhan Lal and Brij Lal were bachelors and it was a lot of fun to be around with them. Their servant Gopal used to cook amazing meals and we used to spend the nights on the terrace, sleeping under a mosquito net. When we would wake up the next day, the bed used to be damp with dewdrops.

We bought a Philips radio that year. These were the days before television made its way in every Indian household. I was overjoyed when Papa brought that shiny contraption home. I was allowed to listen to the news broadcasts and *Bachchon ka Programme* (children's programme) on All India Radio. Till then, I would visit the local *paanwala*'s (betel nut seller) shop to listen to cricket commentary or sometimes the neighbours' houses for special events on the radio. *Binaca Geetmala* (a popular weekly programme of hit Hindi film songs) on Wednesday evenings used to be a big draw, and running commentary of popular sports was very sought after by us. Bapu Nadkarni, Rusi Surti, Budhi Kunderan and Pankaj Roy used to be my favourites. Cricketer Nadkarni used to be on the pitch for hours together and score just a few runs, testing the patience of the bowlers. Pankaj Roy was a very dependable opening batsman. Kunderan was a flashy wicketkeeper while Surti was a dazzling all-rounder.

Shankar's arrival made Amma and Papa very busy. I was fairly a good student and wouldn't require their supervision for my studies. My parents always insisted on education for a good future and I followed their words diligently. During this time, I became friends with a classmate named Sudhir Narang. Sudhir's father was the owner of a bustling chemist shop in Chandni Chowk. He used to help us procure baby milk for my brother as Amma couldn't feed the baby herself due to health reasons. Powdered milk often used to be in shortage those days and Amma did not trust any other milk powder apart from the one Sudhir's father provided. Sudhir was a boisterous fellow and loved watching Hindi movies. My parents had always considered that movies misled the youth and, naturally, I was prohibited from going to a theatre. But, one day, Sudhir gushed about the newly released Shammi Kapoor movie *Junglee* and said, 'Do you know that the film has been shot in Kashmir?'

'Really? I didn't know that,' I said, a little embarrassed at my lack of knowledge.

'Y-E-S!' Sudhir screamed, 'Come, let's go for the matinee show. Then you can see Kashmir from Delhi!'

I was tempted and we went, bunking school for the rest of the day. He had enough pocket money to buy my ticket too. When I watched the movie on the big screen, I was enthralled to see the valley so much that I watched it two more times after that day. Of course, my parents came to know nothing. The only movie I remember I was taken to was K. Asif's epic historical drama *Mughal-e-Azam* at a well-known theatre in Daryaganj called Golcha Cinema.

Sudhir introduced me to cricket, and we started playing it in the small compound of his house in Malka Ganj, which was just a kilometre away from my home. We started bunking school, resulting in abysmal neglect of our studies. The inevitable happened—we failed in the annual exam of the eighth standard. When I walked home with my report card, I trembled at the idea of what awaited home. My mother said nothing when I showed her the card, waiting for Papa to come back from his office. When Papa reached home to this shocking news, he thrashed me for the first time in his life. I was their star son, after all. How could I fail them so miserably? Amma kept her poise and counselled for reformation.

This was the month of May 1962 and the timing of this disaster couldn't have been worse. Every year, in May, we would visit Kashmir on our annual vacation for two months. While my school would be shut for the summer, Papa used to join us after a month. That year, Amma and Shankar, who was 15 months old by then, went. I was not allowed to go to Kashmir and was made to stay back in the heat of Delhi as punishment. This was the worst punishment ever as I loved Kashmir, and the annual trip was something I looked forward to eagerly. That night, when Amma and Shankar left, I resolved that to get over this humiliation, I would study seriously. I distanced myself from Sudhir and actually burnt the midnight oil. I used to carry a textbook and read while going to even buy milk from the depot every morning. I remember passers-by warning me to be careful so that I wasn't run over by a passing vehicle. When I finally appeared in the higher secondary examination, which was conducted by the Central Board of Secondary Education, I made my parents proud. As a reward for my performance, I was sent to Srinagar that summer.

My first recollection of a major public event of Kashmir was in December 1963, when news broke out of the theft of a holy relic from the Hazratbal shrine. Situated near the banks of the Dal Lake, the shrine hosted a strand of the beard of Hazrat-e-Muhammad. Historically, this relic was brought to the city of Bijapur (in Karnataka) in 1635 by Syed Abdullah, a descendant of the holy Prophet. His son passed it on to a Kashmiri businessman named Noorudeen. When Emperor Aurangzeb came to be aware of it, he arrested Noorudeen and kept it at the Ajmer Dargah. Aurangzeb, however, returned the relic in 1700 but, by then, Noorudeen was already dead. The relic was preserved by his descendants and later kept at the Hazratbal shrine. The theft of this sacred hair—an act of blasphemy against the Prophet—brought the valley to a standstill. More than 50,000 people protested with black flags, demanding the culprit be caught immediately. The situation was exacerbated with Pakistan's incessant coverage of the incident on their radio broadcasts, rousing the public outrage further. Nehru, who was the prime minister then, sent the Intelligence Bureau (IB) Chief B.N. Mullick to the valley to investigate the theft. The relic was finally restored on 4 January 1964. However, the government did not reveal the identity of the thieves that, to date, continues to remain a mystery. When Mullick informed Nehru about the recovery, he said, 'You have saved Kashmir for India.'

Meanwhile, Papa bought a plot of land in Greater Kailash I as the family was expanding. Papa had to go to the office during the day; so Amma supervised the construction and managed the labourers, keeping an eye out for any pilferage of building material. The family moved in within a year towards the end of 1964, while the work was still unfinished and only the front rooms were ready. We had a makeshift kitchen. There were only a few houses in the neighbourhood then and the colony was surrounded by green fields and tube wells. That was the time I had appeared for my higher secondary board exams. We had a three-month window of no studies between the exam and the announcement of results.

One fine morning, in July 1965, when we were still asleep on the veranda of our half-constructed house, we got a pleasant surprise. My *mama* B.L. Dhar, who used to live in neighbouring Hauz Khas those days and had an official jeep, came shouting jubilantly with a newspaper announcing that I had passed with a first division. The results along with marks used to be printed in the newspaper. Sweets were distributed to all the labourers. When the detailed marks were available from the school, I came to know that I had a distinction in Physics and good marks in all the five subjects.

Following the school-leaving exam, I got admission in premedical at Hans Raj College, University of Delhi. My mother wanted me to become a doctor. She always dreamt of becoming a nurse after she was forced to leave school. Unfortunately, nursing profession was not considered a good choice for the family's reputation, especially in Kashmiri Brahmin families. Medical was the right option for me as well because I never liked mathematics. Much like today, even then students who secured good percentages would opt for medicine or engineering. While the administrative services were coveted, it was a tough exam to crack. Subjects like biotechnology, commerce or business administration were just evolving. So, students had limited options for choosing their future career plans. In fact, we always thought we should accept whatever we get in good faith.

Hans Raj College, located in the north of the city, was far from Greater Kailash. I had to change at least two buses to reach college every day. After a few months, this became unviable and I shifted to my uncle *Tathya*'s house in the Institute of Economic Growth campus, from where I could walk to college. It was a good bungalow with Shiela *Mami*, her mother Bhuwajee and my two cousin brothers, Abhinav and

Madhav. They looked after me very well and gave me a room to stay. In my leisure time, I used to narrate stories to my young cousins and also make them cram some zoological terms like that of a cobra—*Naja naja*. I had realised that I must work very hard and take full advantage of the affection shown to me by the family. We had excellent teachers who inspired me to work hard. I distinctly remember Dr P.L. Soni, our chemistry teacher, who used to make us cram the periodic table, which I still can recite by heart after all these years.

At college, there were students from different cultural and socioeconomic backgrounds. I was from a government school whereas quite a few of my classmates were from the city's, and even the country's, most prestigious schools. There were boys from St Columba's, St Xavier's, Modern School and Doon School. Most of them would converse only in English. They would also never stand up in class while responding to questions from our teachers, which amazed me considerably considering we would be beaten up in our school for behaving like that. However, these were bright kids and everybody was competitive, with the sole aim of securing grades and cracking the medical college admission. Hindu College in the neighbourhood was another sought-after college. Hans Raj was a *brahmachari* (bachelor's) college whereas Hindu had co-education. The students of Hindu College used to look down upon us for reasons of their own. Since I had all along been studying in a boy's school, I never felt that I was missing out on anything. My focus was solely on my studies. The exam came and all of us put in the best of our efforts. It was a one-year course and we passed in the year 1966.

I left for Srinagar immediately after the exams, much to the annoyance of Papa. He wanted me to stay back and fill in application forms for the All India Institute of Medical Sciences (AIIMS), New Delhi, and colleges of Rajasthan and UP as soon as the results are declared. That was, I suppose, the practice that his colleagues in his office had briefed him. Kashmir, however, was more important to me. My cousins, the carefree atmosphere and the river with my childhood friends enticed me much more than the Delhi life, which for me was synonymous with studies. Moreover, having done well, I was confident of getting good marks to secure admission for an MBBS. These were days much before the entrance tests and Delhi had a quota for students who had studied in Delhi. Applying at AIIMS and other colleges would have meant entrance exams and staying back in Delhi.

4

Medical College Years

After I came back from the summer holidays in Kashmir, we awaited the declaration of the premedical results. When it was announced, my family was delighted to see that I had scored 63 per cent, which was considered very good those days. It was a huge relief for Papa too as he knew that 60 per cent and above meant one thing—an assured seat in a medical college. I returned from Srinagar, filled in the form and waited for the results of a medical seat, which would be displayed at Maulana Azad Medical College (MAMC), the only co-educational college in Delhi. Girls were luckier; they also had Lady Hardinge Medical College (LHMC) where they could apply, which was exclusively for women.

When the first list came out, my name was not on it, much to Papa's chagrin. It, however, used to be pure arithmetic because some toppers would go to AIIMS and few girls would prefer Lady Hardinge and some eligible students in other states would go to other state medical colleges. My name appeared in the second list displayed a few days later. Both Papa and I had gone to the college that day to check the results. When we reached the main corridor, where the list would be displayed, there was already a lot of hustle and bustle, with boys and their parents trying to check their names. When I pushed through the crowd and reviewed the list, I spotted my name immediately. Papa, however, seemed to have missed it and turned towards me with deep disappointment in his eyes. Before he could say anything, I calmly put my finger on my name on the list. When he saw his son's name in print, his face cracked into a smile of relief—I was all set now to start my medical career.

The admission formalities took a few weeks to be completed and the MBBS classes finally started in July 1966. Our roll numbers were determined by our first names. As I was almost at the end alphabetically, my roll number was 69, right along with Usha Sood, Usha Ahluwalia and Vimla Menon. We became lab partners while dissecting corpses as anatomy students. The only talk I used to have was about the subject of anatomy and nothing else. I was not interested in their gossips.

Vir Seth was the only other guy in this batch of dissection partners. He became a good friend later, and stayed in the college hostel. His father, Dr R.N. Seth, was a retired professor of Biochemistry in Patna, and his mother, Venetia, was a headmistress at a convent school. They had a house near ours in Greater Kailash I but used to live in Baghdad where his father got a job after retirement from Patna Medical College. Vir during his schooling used to live in a boarding school in Dehradun. His elder brothers—Aftab, Roshan and Kabir—were all in Doon School, Dehradun, and had guardians in Delhi. All the brothers excelled in their respective fields. Roshan became a screen actor who later played Nehru in Richard Attenborough's *Gandhi* (1982). Aftab, who joined the Foreign Service in 1968, served as ambassador to Japan, Vietnam and Greece.

There were two more Kauls in my class—Aditya Kaul and Manohar Narayan Kaul. Manohar was one of the toppers of the university.

However, they had little connection with Kashmir and had lived in Delhi all their lives. We were polite in our conversations, but while I loved reminiscing about Kashmir, they weren't familiar with the valley. There were also two nominees from the Kashmir government who had been chosen for the MBBS course—Shabbir Ahmad Andrabi and Iftikhar Ahmed Bukhari. Both became my best friends. Shabbir and Iftikhar couldn't be more unlike—while Shabbir was outgoing, a footballer and not at all hardworking, Iftikhar was very quiet, very religious and a regular student, who would attend all the classes and took fervent notes during lectures. The two would speak in Kashmiri with each other. I was not fluent in Kashmiri despite it being my mother tongue. As I was raised predominantly in Delhi, visiting the valley only for short periods, I did not have enough exposure to it. My friendship with Shabbir and Iftikhar was a godsend as I could finally practise my Kashmiri, which became perfect within a few months. My parents were surprised with this change. Now I could converse with my aunts and grandmother which was not possible till then. No longer was I called *Delhi ka babujee* (gentleman from Delhi) by my cousins in Kashmir. Although Amma was very happy seeing my improvement in Kashmiri vocabulary, Papa was not impressed. He always felt more at ease speaking in Hindi and would often respond to my mother's questions in Hindi. I found this strange. My mother would encourage my friendship with Shabbir and Iftikhar and would invite them home for meals off and on.

One of our class fellows, Anindya Kumar Sen, was the topper in premedical and a very bright student. He was the son of the then Law Minister A.K. Sen. As the son of a cabinet minister, he used to have an aura around him. He was from St Columba's and would come to college in a chauffeur-driven imported car and a servant accompanying him with a big box, containing his lunch and drinking water. He was a quiet fellow and a studious boy too. He didn't interact much with the rest of the class. His only friend was Rajeev Kumar also from St Columba's, a nephew of Ashwini Kumar, the former national hockey selector and an ace police officer. Anindya and Rajeev are now both in the USA and have excelled professionally.

After joining the MBBS, we studied anatomy and physiology for the first month. However, apart from studies, ragging was a huge rave and during lunch breaks or after college, seniors would haul us to the hostel for ragging. Ragging was a ritual in which the seniors, especially the *dada*s (big guys) of the senior classes, would harass, humiliate and sometimes abuse too. In our batch, they used to make us sit on the head of the femur bone of the skeleton. We were all supposed to buy a human skeleton in parts and carry the bone which was being taught in anatomy practical classes. This phase lasted for a few months and slowly fizzled out. I remember being taken to the lawns of the college and asked to undress by two seniors. One of them ordered me to go naked in front of the girl's hostel. I started crying and they took pity on me and just kicked me and went away, much to my comfort. Ragging used to be the worst for students staying in the hostel because there was enough time for seniors to catch hold of the newcomers. I was a day scholar so after 5 p.m., I would buzz off. The practice of ragging is similar to hazing in North America, *bizutage* in France, *praxe* in Portugal. These practices are prevalent in educational institutions across the world, especially for students joining medical schools and professional training institutes.

The one thing we didn't have during premedical was practical classes. Now in the first year, we were introduced to them and classes would take place in the dissection hall. The first few days were awful with the stink of formalin-doused dead bodies; their stiff, distorted appearances haunted me for days. Two students used to share one limb for dissection and our demonstrators would come and supervise us by rotation. Gradually, as the days passed, we started getting used to it.

The other tedious study was the classes on the human skeleton. We were supposed to remember the names of all the 206 bones which adults have. Incidentally, humans have 270 bones, many of which fuse by adulthood. There was a small book on mnemonics to guide students on how to memorise these difficult names. For example, for Carpal bones (wrist bones), it used to be the following:

Bone Names	Scaphoid, Lunate, Triquetrum, Pisiform, Trapezium, Trapezoid, Capitate and Hamate
Mnemonic	*Sohan Lata Tinday Paka Tere Tinday Cachai Hain*

While the names were important for bone specialists, it was not useful for a general doctor or a physician. On the other hand, the anatomy of abdominal organs, physiology and biochemistry were more interesting subjects, which made us feel that we are getting trained in becoming doctors. These were the three subjects that constituted the first year of MBBS, and we needed to appear in a university exam in 18 months before being allowed to enter the second year.

Classes, thankfully, used to be over by five in the evening and then we had the rest of the day to ourselves. As our college was located near the Delhi Gate, we were fortunate to have the Feroz Shah Kotla (one of India's historic stadiums and rechristened as Arun Jaitley Stadium in 2019) soccer and cricket stadiums just across the road. During the winter, the wildly popular Durand Soccer Cup was a tremendous attraction. We saw quite a few matches during those days. The popular teams then were Mohun Bagan, East Bengal and Mohammedan Sporting from Calcutta, now Kolkata; Dempo and Salgaonkar Club from Goa and JCT Mills Phagwara from Punjab. Shabbir and I used to watch these matches regularly.

Shabbir, Iftikhar and I always looked forward to our summer breaks when we would visit Kashmir. We used to travel to Srinagar together by road every year during summer vacations. We never planned our trips; it was always spontaneous. On the day of the journey, the three of us used to go to the train yard, well away from the platform, and get into the train that was being washed and being made ready for the journey to Pathankot (the last railway terminal on that route till 1971 when Jammu came on the train map). Occupying seats in an unreserved compartment was quite a task. There would be no electricity in the compartment till the engine was connected, which made us sweat profusely. But the fact that we were going to be in the cool and breezy climate the next day reassured us.

After reaching Pathankot, we would take a bus to Srinagar. The bus stand was right on the railway station campus. The bus used to stop at designated places. The first halt was at Lakhanpur, the border between Punjab and Jammu and Kashmir. In the initial years, after the accession of Kashmir to India, we had to get a permit to enter the state, which was scrapped later. A few small restaurants were overlooking River Ravi. Passengers used to take a break there. The next stop invariably used to be at Sambha, a town about 36 km from Jammu city. It was acclaimed for its *rajma chawal* (red kidney beans curry and rice) and we would make it a point to have it every time we visited. Before the Partition of India, the town was known for its colourful prints and fabrics. Once known as *Chittan da Shahar*, the artisans were mainly Muslims who later migrated to Pakistan.

The next halt was the tourist reception centre of Jammu city, located on the Residency Road. After a lunch break of about an hour, the bus used to leave for Srinagar, and then to our immense joy, the mountainous journey with winding roads used to begin. The next brief stop would come after crossing a small tunnel, which used to be famous for its milk products, especially paneer (cottage cheese). Many passengers used to shop there and buy bricks of paneer to be carried to Srinagar. The bus used to stop at regular intervals for passengers to have tea and snacks (mostly paneer *pakodas* with tamarind sauce). The journey ahead was hilly. Vendors sold anti-nausea tablets to passengers to avoid getting mountain sickness.

The bus used to halt for the night at Batote, where we would arrive after driving past the heights of Kud and Patni Top, the highest point in the Jammu area. It is a picturesque town in Ramban district, which serves as a summer resort. There were several small hotels where tourists would shack up for the night. Before signing off for the day, the driver of the bus would remind us to be ready in our seats before five in the morning so that we could cross Banihal tunnel on time and enter the valley, reaching Srinagar by noon. I remember on one of our trips, film star Shammi Kapoor was at Batote for a film shooting. We decided to throng his hotel as we were big fans of the flamboyant star. When we reached the hotel, there was already a crowd swelling to see him. After waiting for half an hour, he appeared on the balcony, wrapped in a towel, and waved at us. The crowd screamed and clapped in joy. That night, when I went to bed, I smiled to myself, remembering the days when I had bunked school with Sudhir to watch Shammi Kapoor on the big screen in *Junglee*!

The drive from Batote to Banihal, with the Chenab flowing alongside, was picturesque. However, the roads were very bumpy as there used to be several roadblocks and clearing operations by the Public Works Department. The bus would stop at Banihal for breakfast. The clean cool air and pines dotting the road with the Bichlari Nala flowing on one side was a balm to our battered city souls. Srinagar was now within our reach.

Once we crossed the Jawahar tunnel, the view of the spectacular lush green valley used to thrill me. While going down, the conductor used to give the passengers an option to take a diversion and take us to Verinag for an extra ten bucks. Most of the passengers used to be tourists and they would enthusiastically agree to a trip to Verinag.

Verinag (or Vernag as that's the correct name) is a spring located about 78 km from Srinagar in Anantnag district. It is 28 km from Anantnag town. This spring is also mentioned in the famous book by Kalhana that chronicled the history of the kings of Kashmir and Northern India—*Rajatarangini*. It is the pre-Islamic history of the region. Vernag was brought to its current form by the Mughal Emperor Jahangir in AD 1620 by building an octagonal tank of sculptured stones around it. The purpose was to store water within it. The architects were brought from Iran. A garden was built by Jahangir, which demonstrates how pre-Islamic historical places changed with the spread of Islam in Kashmir. The temples around it lost their importance. There is still an ancient Shiva temple there but not of any touristic significance. This ancient temple is supposed to be of the times of Kashyap Rishi, who, according to legend, made an outlet to drain out the water so that the valley could emerge out of water. It is believed that the valley was submerged under a mammoth lake. For this reason, Kashmir is also still called *Kashir* in Kashmiri language after the name of Kashyap Rishi. Emperor Shah Jahan further improved the surroundings of this spring by constructing aqueducts and cascades in straight lines through the garden. The water in the spring is crystal clear, with many fish in it. However, fishing is strictly prohibited.

Vitastatra, another spring a few kilometres from Vernag, is the source of Jhelum. However, all the seven springs in the neighbourhood—called Sapta Rishi—merge at Sangam and form the source of Jhelum which is also joined by many large water bodies, including Liddar from the mountains of Pahalgam, to become a mighty river on the banks of which the city of Srinagar is situated.

After spending an hour or so at Vernag, we would then board the bus for the last leg of our journey to Qazigund, the first township of the valley after passing through the tunnel at Banihal. Then comes Khanabal. This is followed by Awantipora with its ruins of the Martand Temple built by King Avanti Varman during his reign from AD 855 to 883. These were destroyed by Sikandar Butshikan of the Shah Mir dynasty during his rule between 1389 and 1413. The ruins of this massive temple still stand there. The description of this Shiva temple is found in *Rajatarangini*. According to the description, the temple was situated in a courtyard made of a huge beautifully decorated stone wall. The broken down gateway is in the middle of this wall which is divided into two chambers and its remains are still there. There is a nice park made around it which is well maintained even today. Some visitors still visit the place but this could have been developed as a much better place of historic interest with guided tours to attract tourists. Unfortunately, most of the tourists are not even aware of this historic temple.

This temple is situated on the bank of River Jhelum which winds like a serpent with boats plying it. After Awantipora the road to Srinagar continues with poplar trees on both sides and lush green paddy fields which are a treat to watch during the summers. One can also see the snow-clad Pir Panjal Range and the mountains around Gulmarg, including the Apharwat Peak. The road then passes through Pampore, the saffron belt of the valley which is in bloom in autumn during the months of September and October, before reaching Srinagar. Many equate the valley of Kashmir with Switzerland, some even consider Kashmir to be more stunning. Frankly, I couldn't agree more even after all these years and having visited several European countries.

Once we would reach the bus terminal of Srinagar, Shabbir and Iftikhar would bid goodbye, promising to meet up after a few days of rest at home. My first stop would always be at my *masi*'s (maternal aunt) home in Kanikadal. I would take a *tonga* (a single horse carriage) from the tourist centre during my college days. Now, the *tongas* have been replaced by tempos, three-wheelers and minibuses. The *tonga* drivers were given loans by the government to purchase tempos and three-wheelers when the new vehicles were introduced. Once in Kanikadal, I would have a jolly time with my cousins and the neighbourhood children. The neighbourhood was a mixed one. One of our next-door neighbours were the Tikoos. My aunt's house shared a wall with the Khans on the other side. They were two cousins, Gulam Hussain Khan (popularly known as Hassa Khan) and Qadir Khan, who lived together with their families. Their children were my friends. One of their sons, Aurangzeb, was an adopted child. He had been abandoned while a baby and was sighted by Hassa Khan one morning floating in the river at Kanikadal in a basket made of grass. While people gathered by the riverside to see the wailing baby, Hassa Khan jumped into the river and brought him to the shore. Despite having six children, he and his wife Taja raised Aurangzeb as their own. Aurangzeb grew up to become a tailor. He is still a good friend of mine and we meet often even now whenever I visit that part of the city.

The children in Kanikadal used to play either in the narrow lanes or in people's courtyards. Boys used to assemble in their ground and play cricket. The rubber ball often used to be hit hard and would drop in the river. My cousin Durga used to jump and get it after swimming. These were the acts I used to miss in Delhi, and would make me always look forward to going to Kashmir. One noteworthy thing was the perfect harmony between the Pandits and Muslims with each group respecting their beliefs on religious matters.

Kashmiris are very conscious of national and world matters. Most would listen to Radio Kashmir for news, current affairs and special popular programmes and dramas like 'Zoona Dub'. Farooq Nazki was one of the most popular Urdu newsreaders during the period between 1965 and 1970, and Prem Nath Harmain in Kashmiri. Farooq Nazki was also a very popular Urdu poet. For international news, Kashmiris would trust BBC; additionally, the Pandits would listen to All India Radio news where Melville de Mellow was the most well-known broadcaster. The Muslims would tune in to the news bulletin from Radio Pakistan. Interestingly, the timings of the main news bulletins from India and Pakistan would never overlap.

Kashmiri surnames are often very peculiar, like *Gaggar* (rat), *Haakh* (an edible leaf), *Mujhu* (radish), *Kachru* or *Kachur* (blonde), *Malla* (boatman), *Kral* (potter) and *Wugra* (rice mixed with excessive water to feed more people; this later became Ogra). The genesis of these names is quite intriguing and often linked to the neighbourhoods these people lived in or their likes and dislikes. For instance, there is this story about a poor Pandit whose name was Vasadev. He had a mulberry tree in his courtyard; people, therefore, called him Vasadev Tul, *tul* being the Kashmiri word for mulberry. Vasadev was infuriated with the nickname and cut down the mulberry tree one day. But a *mond* (trunk) remained and now people started calling him Vasadev Mond. Irritated, the Pandit immediately removed the trunk. This, however, led to a *khuda* (depression) and now he became Vasadev Khuda. This incessant trend of peculiar nicknames kept nagging him and he got the depression filled up but the ground became a bit *teng* (elevated). Thus, he was re-nicknamed as Vasadev Teng. Exhausted, he finally gave in and accepted Teng as his surname, which passed on to his progeny.

Just like a beautiful dream, the two months of summer vacation used to be over and it would be time to return to Delhi, which always was an alien land to me. The politics in the valley was also interesting with the party of Sheikh Abdullah being referred to as *sher* (lion) and the party of Mirwaiz, the religious head, who had a lot of influence in the downtown, was called *bakra* (goat, nicknamed because of their flowing beards). Children also used to take sides with these two groups and used to have mock fights.

It was soon time again for college and MBBS classes, with a lot of studying and cramming. By the time of the final exam, we had completed anatomy, physiology and biochemistry, which was a part of physiology. A few days before the theory exams, we would always meet Professor I.D. Bajaj, Head of the Department of Anatomy, and seek his blessings. Our seniors had told us that meeting Prof. Bajaj would give us a hint about the exam questions. While we were absolutely clueless about how this would happen, a bunch of us went to meet him one afternoon. Prof. Bajaj was in his office and was gracious to meet us. He wished us well and said, 'Keep your head on your shoulders and keep smiling.' We came out puzzled. Was he hinting at something specific about the body parts? We started analyzing and brainstorming, and finally deduced what could come in the paper—the bones of the skull, shoulder joints and face muscles. We studied this fervently for the next few days. Well, we did get some short notes on some of these but I think it was just a coincidence.

Physiology was an easy subject and some of it was a repetition of what we had already studied in premedical and higher secondary in Zoology classes. One funny incident I remember involved Dr U.C. Rai, the head of the Department of Physiology. He often used to say, 'You see (U.C.) my name is U.C. Rai', which used to bring some cheer, otherwise it was a drab subject. One of the demonstrators in Anatomy, Dr Triloki Nath, who was a bachelor, would give special attention towards the girls. We used to feel ignored. He had a long nose, and was nicknamed *Trikoni Nak* (triangular nose). He would retaliate by saying that all of us would fail in Anatomy. We also had a witty demonstrator in Physiology named Mrs Pandey. She would crack jokes and would often say that the HOD (head of department) should be sent to Bihar for a few months and then she would be able to exhibit her teaching capabilities.

We had only a few weeks' breather between our exam and the results. Most of us passed except a few. However, there used to be another exam within six weeks of the main one and the students who had flunked the first one could clear the second and join the batch in the second part of MBBS. I found it to be more interesting. What we studied was closer to treating patients. Also, we could hang a stethoscope around our neck and attend clinical classes in the medicine and surgery wards, which we did with a lot of enthusiasm. In the second part, we studied pathology, pharmacology and forensic medicine.

The head of the Department of Pathology was Dr Gauri Bazaz Malik. I was elated to know that she was a Kashmiri-speaking Kashmiri like my friends Shabbir and Iftikhar. She was an exceptional teacher and an acclaimed professional with several international publications to her credit. She was the daughter of Prem Nath Bazaz, a veteran Kashmiri politician and scholar, who had raised the slogan—'Kashmir for Kashmiris'. He was a close comrade of Sheikh Abdullah and opposed the Maharaja's rule. Bazaz, however, had a difference with Sheikh Abdullah on the accession issue with India. As a liberal Kashmiri, he was outspoken about the accession for which he was hated by most Kashmiri Pandits and even a few Muslim groups. Pandit women even ridiculed his wife by concocting a hymn in Kashmiri: '*Batnee batnee Dodyay Mas. Ye Kehai Korthum Prem Nathas?* (Hey Pandit lady, your hair should be ablaze. What have you done to Prem Nath?) The desire to have a unique identity as a result of centuries of oppression by Afghans and Mughals had been forming for quite some time. This sentiment is not favoured by a majority of the Pandits, but the Muslims, who are the dominating group, continue to share this feeling. This difference of opinion between the two groups has continued to increase over the years. Bazaz, however, left Kashmir and spent his last years in Delhi after the accession of Kashmir with India in 1948. A well-acclaimed author, all his books are critical of the deliberations on the history of Jammu and Kashmir acceding to India in 1948.

Coming back to our classes, Pathology and Pharmacology were interesting. Pathology involved reading about physiology gone wrong with all the diseases and how the organs get affected. Besides theory, we would also be shown specimens of diseased organs and their histology. This would help derive a good clinicopathological correlation (CPC). Demonstrators who were PG students would also participate in giving us practical training.

Pharmacology was interesting as we were introduced to medicines—antibiotics, painkillers, antidiarrheals and the lot. We started gathering some confidence about treating our families and friends for simple ailments and felt that we were closer to our goal of becoming healers. During our Pharmacy practical classes, we were asked to make liquid mixtures and powders by using pestle and mortar. This process was called trituration, which is a method of grinding the material into very fine powder. Our Pharmacology professor, Dr Sinha, was a very meticulous man. He used to start his lecture sharp on time and used to dictate notes from cards that he always carried with him. Interestingly, he used to carry an alarm clock, which he would place on the table near the blackboard. The first day he did that, we were puzzled, whispering to each other what could the clock mean. However, after an hour, when the clock buzzed, indicating that an hour was up, he immediately walked out of the class. The college bell rang too and then it dawned on us—the alarm was so that he could begin and end his class dot on time. There had been numerous instances when the alarm clock would go off and Dr Sinha would walk out from the class, even when he was in the middle of explaining something or writing on the board! But we loved his classes nevertheless.

Once Dr Sinha was discussing the formation of faeces and its importance in terms of appearance, smell and colour before one can prescribe appropriate medicines. Some students at the back of the class started giggling. Dr Sinha stopped his lecture in the middle, and taking his glasses off, sternly said, 'You are laughing now. But remember, a few years from now when you will be in your clinic, a patient would walk in with his stool sample and you would be the happiest person then since it would be your bread and butter.'

I was a day scholar during my MBBS days, except during the weeks preceding our final exams when I would stay at the hostel, sharing the room with Shabbir or Iftikhar. This gave me a glimpse of hostel life. It was nice and being so close to the college was a great advantage. Despite this, many hostellers would always be late and were called *late-lateefs*. Gossiping was a pastime for some students. Going for late-night movies was easy with a few cinema halls like Delite and Golcha at walking distances. For a delicious meal, once in a while, we would go to Peshawari or the well-known, stylish Moti Mahal restaurant in Daryaganj, very famous for its tandoori chicken. I recall once we took out a friend of Shabbir to Moti Mahal. After lunch, they brought warm water with a lemon slice in a silver-plated bowl meant for cleaning fingers. Not knowing about this, he quietly squeezed the lemon in the water and gulped it down. We later corrected him on this. I also remember a few guests from Srinagar staying with Shabbir. Most of them were very pleasant persons. One was Mohd. Ashraf Batkoo, who stayed for more than a year. He was an engineering student in Srinagar but because of his political views on independence for Kashmiris, he was expelled from the college. During this one year, he learnt professional photography and French. Back from French classes, he would teach us a few French words like *bonjour* (hello) and *merci beaucoup* (thank you very much). Eventually, Ashraf became an adventure tour guide and later was taken by the tourism department of Jammu and Kashmir. He finally rose to the post of Director of Tourism. He became a good friend and we were very pally till we lost him in 2020 due to a complication of Covid-19.

One of the interesting hostel characters, who was also a fellow in my class, Surinder Sachdeva, used to pose as a drunkard, which he actually wasn't. He would say that a tablet of APC (aspirin, phenacetin and codeine), a popular painkiller those days, would give him a kick. He always used to keep a quarter bottle of whiskey in his hostel room cupboard and used to take a teaspoon of that every evening and roam in the corridors of the hostel staggering and singing like a drunkard. It was an interesting sight and sound. He was very fond of Moti Lal, a film actor who used to act as a drunkard in Bollywood films, and I suppose he used to imitate him. One evening, I went to his room with Shabbir and found his cupboard open. I took the bottle out and finished it which did not have more than 100cc of the drink left. Surinder had gone out on his singing spree. The next day, he realised that the bottle was empty. He was very upset and was going from room to room complaining about the theft. When he saw me, I asked him to show me the bottle and accompanied him. The bottle had no cap on it; I immediately told him that the whiskey must have evaporated in the summer heat. Poor fellow accepted it and was reconciled.

As there were very few buses from Delhi Gate to Kalkaji, commuting home from college was always inconvenient. There were times, especially on days when there were football matches at the Kotla stadium and the buses would spill over with people coming for the match, the quickest way was to walk back home. Even if I did shortcuts, the distance was 12 to 13 km. While it would take an inordinate amount of time, I would console myself thinking that it was good for health, after all!

The second year of the MBBS exam was not difficult, and mostly the college witnessed a good percentage. Besides, even if one failed to get to the final year, supplementary exams were held twice in the year for students who had failed. The final year of the MBBS had five subjects:

Medicine, Surgery, Obstetrics and Gynaecology, Ear, Nose and Throat (ENT) and Ophthalmology. Medicine and Surgery were the real subjects unless one wanted to go in for Obstetrics and Gynaecology, which was mainly dominated by women. In North India, there are very few male gynaecologists, unlike in the eastern and southern parts of the country where males are preferred. Medicine and Surgery bedside classes used to be very important. We were allotted cases and two students would work on them—one would present the case history and the other would provide the clinical examination. Typically, an admitted patient would be allotted. Two students would take the patient's history and examine the person as per the methods written in our books, which were fairly detailed. The allotted patient sometimes used to get irritated by this examination, would not cooperate and act difficult. This would invite criticism by the teacher who would scold us and advise us to learn the art of winning the confidence of the patient. This would make us successful clinicians. The students would, however, not agree because it was not their fault. The patient knew that we were trainees and not full doctors.

The prescribed textbooks mostly were by British authors and not the American ones. This was obviously because of our British heritage of more than a century. By the time we started our postgraduation, American books had become popular.

When I see the new generation of doctors these days, my impression is that the art of bedside clinical sense and reaching a diagnosis has remarkably come down. The reason for this is the availability of prompt diagnosis by modern imaging techniques, such as ultrasound, echocardiography and Doppler evaluation along with computed tomograms (CT scans) and Magnetic Resonance Imaging (MRI), all of which give a ready accurate diagnosis. However, while these are positive developments, clinical examination and examining patient history should not lose significance. This will avoid many redundant investigations as well as unnecessary radiation exposure and prevent wastage of money for those who find it difficult to afford medical expenses. It is not uncommon for a physician to order a CT scan of the head in a stable patient and then follow it up soon by ordering an MRI brain. This is a drain on the pocket of the patient.

The final-year MBBS examination constituted five subjects: General Medicine; General Surgery, including Orthopaedics, Obstetrics and Gynaecology; Ear, Nose and Throat (ENT); Ophthalmology; and Preventive and Social Medicine. It was an exhaustive preparation. During the last few months, I used to study till very late and try to remember as much as possible. There was a scientific method of doing that. A drug by the name of Dexedrine (dextro-amphetamine), a potent central nervous system stimulant which is used for several indications and is now a drug which you can get only by a special prescription, was very popular with the students in our times. It helped us in aborting sleep. I also used to take it during my preparation days. These late hours of work used to give us a feeling that we have done our best. My mother would plead with me to go to sleep and not ruin my health, but it was easier said than done when five theory exams were conducted within 10 to 12 days with barely a day's reprieve in between.

The theory exams got over with much sweat and strain. It was now time for the practical examinations, which were scheduled in the wards of Irwin Hospital (now known as Lok Nayak Hospital). For the Medicine exam, one of the external examiners was Professor Syed Naseer Ahmad Shah from Srinagar Medical College, whom we knew about from the newspapers. Once, while travelling from Srinagar to Delhi, the Indian Airlines aircraft in which Dr Naseer was travelling was hijacked to Lahore (on 30 January 1971) and burnt at the behest of Pakistanis by the hijackers. The plane was a Fokker Friendship aircraft captained by a Kashmiri pilot, Captain Kachroo. The hijackers were the Qureshi brothers, Hashim and Ashraf. India retaliated to the hijacking and the subsequent burning by closing the Indian airspace for Pakistani aircraft. The ban, occurring in the run-up to the December 1971 war between the two countries, had a significant impact on troop movement into erstwhile East Pakistan, now Bangladesh.

Dr Naseer was a kind examiner and when it was my turn, he asked me my name. As I mentioned my surname, he looked up and asked, 'Can you speak Kashmiri?' I said, '*Ahnaz* (yes sir).' He smiled at me, which boosted my confidence and I had an excellent exam.

We had another examiner, Dr Chander Prakash, who was from Rohtak. Both Dr Prakash and Dr Naseer were smokers. Dr Prakash preferred Charminar, a strongly flavoured cigarette brand from Hyderabad, whereas Dr Naseer, who was an FRCP (Fellow of the Royal College of Physicians) and a sophisticated man, smoked only Gold Flake, an international brand which was much coveted. Shabbir told me an interesting story about Dr Naseer's smoking habit. He had his clinic in Dalgate, Srinagar, which was close to Shabbir's residence. Shabbir once told me how Dr Naseer would never smoke more than one-third of his cigarette and would throw the rest of it. As his clinic was near the tonga stand, the boys manning the stand or the carriages would pick these discarded butts and have a nice time puffing high-quality cigarettes. Dr Naseer was quite popular among them!

Passing the MBBS final year exam at one go is a Herculean task; so I was pleasantly surprised when I got to know that not only had I passed but I had been awarded a gold medal in Surgery. This was quite unexpected as I always considered myself an average student. When the award function was held, my parents were thrilled to be celebrating me; Amma even cried when I went up on the stage to receive my medal from M.C. Chagla, who was the education and external affairs minister then. He was also a former Indian Ambassador to the USA. Delighted that her son was now an awarded doctor, Amma, in her simplicity, told all our neighbours that I had received a 'golden medal', which, ironically, was correct as it was indeed a gold-plated medal with no selling value—unlike the real gold medal, which her father had received for crossing the Wular, the largest freshwater lake of Asia, which is 16 km long and 10 km wide. Its area varies according to the seasons and rainfall. According to Amma, my grandfather crossed it at a stretch. As this was an extensive swim, his coach, nicknamed Nanak Batuk (Nanak, the duck), followed him in a boat, throwing bread over the water which would sustain him. That coveted medal, which brought enormous pride to the family, was finally melted by the goldsmith to make jewellery when his eldest daughter, Bengashi, got married. My gold medals, which came much later and are of no use to any goldsmith, are lying securely in Papa's locker!

5

Life as a Junior Resident Doctor

After passing the MBBS exam in 1969, the 12-month rotatory internship was mandatory before qualifying to practice independently as a doctor. We used to have two months posting as an intern in each of the major subjects—Medicine, Surgery, Obstetrics, Gynaecology, and Preventive and Social Medicine. The remaining four months were spent in minor subjects, such as Paediatrics, Orthopaedics, ENT, Ophthalmology, Skin and Venereal Diseases and so on. We were paid a stipend of Rs 200 per month.

In most of these postings, we were made to work like clerks to fill in forms and do dirty jobs of dressing the wounds of patients with burns or colostomies, etc. and nothing was exciting. Patients also considered us as trainees and wouldn't take us very seriously. However, the Preventive and Social Medicine posting turned out to be quite interesting. I was posted in Barwala village in Delhi NCR for two months during this time. I was accompanied by other interns—Gurpreet Singh Brar,

Shabnam Kapoor and Kanwaljeet Pahwa. It was a residential posting and we were allowed leaves only on Sundays and public holidays. The village had limited facilities; there was just a health centre where we used to conduct our OPDs. Medicines were scarce too. However, the OPD used to be very busy. We had been allotted a small house with a compound inside the village. The place had a cook, but I often used to cook and I was a better one. Brar had an Army background; his father was a brigadier from Ferozepur, Punjab. He loved whiskey and preferred his liquor to be served in shining, clean glasses. Every evening, after the day's work, he would sit with a glass on the lawn of our small house. I didn't deprive him of my good company too! The girls, however, poor souls, deeply censured this and would lock themselves in their rooms, refusing to even eat dinner with us.

This was the year 1971, with the Bangladesh Liberation War raging across the country's borders. Brar and I used to enjoy talking about it and thrashing Pakistan. Somehow, the Pakistan phobia of Indians was always there since the Partition in 1947.

During the war, Pakistan also postured to attack from its western front of Punjab and bomb Delhi—their national radio used to bombastically declare how Pakistan would bomb Delhi and capture the Red Fort under them. I remember mock drills and sirens going on at night with people running here and there trying to go to safer places, just like they do during an earthquake. During this period, I was an intern working in Irwin Hospital. One evening, I remember, the blazing noise of sirens started when I along with my friend Vir Seth and a Lebanese friend, Dayab Zeelani, were sitting on a small hillock in our block in Greater Kailash I. Dayab had a torch which he started flashing towards the sky. This attracted the attention of some other people watching the sky. They came and threatened to report us to the police. Vir and I became very nervous and apologised on behalf of Dayab. Dayab, the son of a senior diplomat of the Lebanese embassy, was Vir's friend. Vir was having an affair with his sister May and, therefore, used to entertain him. Eventually, Vir got married to May and left for England and became a geriatric consultant. Dayab also went back to Beirut after his father's tenure in India was over.

Regarding the start of a war on the western front, I was sure this would not happen and used to listen often to Radio Pakistan and then All India Radio sequentially. Interestingly, the news used to be diametrically opposite. According to Radio Pakistan, their jets were hovering over the Punjab region in India and going to hit vital installations of Ambala and Delhi. According to our radio, Lahore was being evacuated and Ichogil Canal on way to Lahore had been struck by brave Indian soldiers. In the absence of TV coverage, it was not possible to verify anything. The version from the eastern front was more interesting, where the Mukti Bahini (Bangladesh freedom fighters) and the Indian forces had an upper hand with regard to the airspace. Since India was not allowing Pakistan to use its airspace, Pakistan was cornered and eventually had to give up. It was the huge public support of the Bangla masses for an independent country which was supported by the Indian armed forces by helping the Mukti Bahini, which cost Pakistan its eastern sector. A new country Bangladesh thus emerged on 26 March 1971.

The internship was followed by junior residency for 12 months, which was a necessity before applying for postgraduation. The postings were allotted based on the MBBS results. I secured both Medicine and Surgery—the most sought-after subjects—for six months each. It was in January 1972 that I started with medicine at Irwin Hospital. The posting was with Professor Chuttani as the chief and Dr Subhash Naik as his registrar. Subhash was a bright doctor and was actively interested in engaging with our batch. Often, he would take us out for coffee. However, as it got revealed a few weeks later, this special interest in us was because he was interested in one of our batchmates, Sita

Ramanathan, a charming girl who would always sport a black bindi on her forehead that never got wiped out even after a hectic day's work. Sita was a diligent student too and would quietly listen to Subhash when he would teach us. Subhash and Sita eventually got married. This relationship ensured that our batch received special attention. We learnt the treatment of medical emergencies besides doing procedures, such as lumbar puncture, liver biopsy and bone marrow aspiration.

Irwin Hospital was constructed during the British era. It has walls made of red sandstone, like the ones seen at the Rashtrapati Bhawan. There was another hospital attached to ours—G.B. Pant Hospital. As Prof. Chuttani was the head of Gastroenterology, he had a ward there as well. The head of the Department of Medicine was Prof. Hari Vaishnava. It was a very peculiar trait of these two professors that in all difficult-to-diagnose cases, Prof. Vaishnava would make a diagnosis of tuberculosis and Prof. Chuttani of amoebiasis. Prof. Vaishnava, a tall fair man from Garhwal (earlier in Uttar Pradesh and now part of Uttarakhand), invariably used to make the diagnosis of tuberculosis for most intricate problems during his rounds. Once his favourite registrar dared him and asked him, 'Sir, but where is the evidence?' The Professor immediately retorted, 'Rizvi *Sahib*, you should understand that TB is a *bahrupiya* (mimicker).' Everybody became silent. On the other hand, Prof. Chuttani was a short, stalky, bald doctor with thick spectacles. He had a special interest in gastroenterology. He had a habit of asking the residents, 'Doctor, stool?' A stool was pulled for him and he used to sit on that. His next demand used to be 'Doctor, stool?' This demand would require for the person to pull out the bedpan in which the patient had passed the faeces. He would carefully look at it and would remark, 'I bet it is amoebiasis'. He often jokingly used to remark, 'Amoebiasis can cause all the conditions in the body except a pregnancy'. Both diseases were common and also reflected their line of thinking.

All the wards in the hospital were big rectangular halls with beds on both sides in a row. There were a few rooms outside the ward along with the doctors' and nurses' duty room and storeroom. No sick patient was refused admission those days, a thing that has become a trend these days. There were very few private hospitals in Delhi then and the big hospitals were mostly the government's, such as AIIMS, Hindu Rao, Kalawati Saran and Safdarjung. Missionary hospitals, such as St Stephen's and Holy Family, were quite popular too.

The Surgery posting was more rewarding personally. My unit head was Professor S.K. Nair, a gentleman with a good reputation and an excellent team; his registrar Dr Vinay Sehgal was very friendly. He used to allow us to operate in the operating room. Hence, by the end of the posting, I could successfully do laparotomy and appendectomy and assist efficiently in gall bladder surgeries. One of the specialised surgeries our unit used to do was called portacaval shunt. This was meant to decompress the portal vein in portal hypertension. Extensive preparations were made and the surgery used to last for a whole day. There were two teams of surgeons and we, as house surgeons, were only allowed to watch it from a distance.

Our ward sister in charge, Mrs D'Souza, was a very pleasant elderly lady who used to often feed us Goan dishes. As we mostly hung around the wards all day without food and drink most of the time, perhaps she felt sorry for us. She also introduced me to Feni, Goa's own alcoholic drink made out of cashews. Mrs D'Souza lived alone but she was a strong disciplinarian. In my long career, I still consider her the best sister in charge I have come across so far.

Ms Fernandez, one of the staff nurses, was a young charming lady in the same ward who became very friendly with me. She also belonged to Goa. We used to chat for hours in the ward on night duties and on phone during off duties. The topics of our talks used to be varied, discussing the beautiful Goa and Kashmir. She liked my fair colour and I liked her hairstyle and the capturing smile. There were no mobile telephones in those days so we really needed strong motivation to carry on. We went to watch a few movies together; I was always a very shy person and could never propose to her despite making plans. The other issue was that she was a nurse, which would not have been appreciated by my family. The friendship went on for more than six months happily. I used to get her small but pretty gifts like perfumes and once a dress. One evening, she gave me a shocker on the phone call. She told me that she was going to Canada and getting married to a white Canadian gentleman! I was so upset that I put the phone down and did not ask for any other details. Obviously, I did not like it and lost my cool. We never contacted each other after that. My only feeling was that she ditched me and I became a fool.

The Surgery posting got over in December 1971. It was time to apply for postgraduation, which would commence in July. As there was still time, I started working as an Assistant Casualty Medical Officer (ACMO) at Irwin Hospital. The shifts would last for eight hours during which all patients coming to Casualty were our responsibility. We used to report to Senior Casualty Medical Officers. Patients, for whom we felt admission was necessary, were referred to the unit of Medicine of Surgery on call. The emergency ward was adjacent to the Casualty.

The hospital was adjacent to Turkman Gate, Daryaganj and Jama Masjid, which are some of the most populated localities in Delhi. Hence, the Casualty department used to be exceptionally busy. We had a police post in a room next to the department, which was necessary as there would be numerous patients arriving after suffering traffic accidents, stabbings and poisonings—these had to be reported to the police. They had a readymade register to record all information. During these days, I observed closely how the police functions. There was a small room in the Casualty premises, where a police constable used to be always available. The purpose was to keep a watch on the medico-legal cases (MLC). The hospital used to get a number of cases of stab injuries and injuries during scuffles. One of the constables, usually on night duty, was Niranjan. He was specialised in reaching out to both the parties involved in these incidents. He would offer a settlement instead of making it an MLC. These cases, if registered, would drag them into court and lawyers would make a fortune from the involved persons. Many cases were immediately settled by the police personnel, of course, with money exchange. There never seemed to be any misunderstanding about this as all the parties were content after such settlements. Niranjan was a man in his forties then. He handled quite a few cases and we quickly became good friends. MLC cases most often used to reach the hospital during night hours. This provided a good opportunity for the constables to make easy money. Niranjan was paid so low by the government that it wouldn't have been possible to care for his family without some additional income. He was a man stuck in the system and I understood his compulsions.

Niranjan was fond of his whiskey and always had a bottle of Blue Bull (a cheap and strong brand) with him in the police post. Whenever I had a bit of spare time, I would join him in his duty room. After a few drinks, we used to walk across the road and visit the *dhabas* (small eating shops) near Delite Cinema. The *dhabas* wouldn't charge Niranjan and his friends anything, a prevalent custom of sellers when it comes to policemen. During the winter nights of Delhi, nothing would be more delicious than a smoking plate of *aloo* paratha, with dollops of butter melting on it, and an omelette.

One night, I got an emergency call and rushed out to the department to see a group of men coming through the door with lacerated wounds. It turned out that they were a team of pop singers who were employed at the Oberoi Maidens Hotel in the posh Civil Lines area. After their shift, they were returning home when their cab met with an accident.

A few doctors and nurses took them to the minor operating room to suture their CLWs (clean lacerated wounds). Niranjan and company came to fill in the medico-legal details. We prevailed on them to leave them since they are professional guys. They agreed. The rock group head gave me his phone number which I preserved.

After a few days, I met my friend and class fellow Vir who was from Doon school and was himself a guitarist. He was thrilled and said we must call them and meet the group at the Maidens Hotel which was not far from our college. We contacted them and got an invitation to visit them on a Saturday afternoon. On the appointed day, I accompanied Vir on his two-wheeler Vespa. The group welcomed us in the lobby of the hotel. After a light lunch, we went to the jazz club. They played music and Vir also sang. Once the performance was over, we sat down in a circle. From one end of the circle, one of the guys lit a cigarette, took a puff and handed it to the guy next to him. This guy again took a drag and passed it on. I looked at Vir quizzically who winked at me. That didn't clear matters and when the cigarette finally reached me, I obliged the others and took a few puffs. The young chap sitting next to me elbowed me for his turn and I handed the cigarette over. A few minutes later, I started feeling a bit weightless, and, intrigued, I took a few more puffs. I was starting to feel giddy now. The warm glow of the sunset was enveloping Delhi and Vir, who was very punctual, indicated that it was time to go home.

When we left, I asked Vir, 'What was there in that cigarette? Was that charas?' Vir laughed and said, 'My friend, is this your first time? The way you took the puffs, I thought you knew what you were having!' I slapped him on the back and as we rode through the city on his scooter, I felt as if I was flying through clouds of air. Vir, however, was a sensible driver and we reached home unscathed. I was living with my parents at the time.

My first experience with charas fascinated me. I decided to probe this further and enquired around discreetly; a friend turned out to be a regular and I accompanied him one afternoon to the Jama Masjid. We arrived at the *tonga* stand and walked back and forth for a few minutes. Soon, a man appeared. He was wearing a pair of white trousers and a pale shirt, which used to be white but now looked yellow. He sauntered towards us and coming uncomfortably close, whispered in my ear, '*Maal chahiye?* (Do you need the stuff)?' I nodded nervously. He flashed a grin and in a crisp, business-like manner explained that the minimum quantity available was priced at Rs 10. My friend and I hastily agreed to the bargain. The man wrapped the charas in a silver foil and took the 10-rupee note that we forwarded him. Our expedition was successful, we caught the next bus and came back home.

The next step was to learn how to make a cigarette roll with the charas. This was a lesson that required tremendous patience and deft fingers. It involved emptying the contents of a Charminar cigarette (a cigarette brand without a filter and with very strong tobacco) without damaging the paper. The next step was mixing the tobacco with the charas very well and then refilling it into the same cigarette. I always had a stack ready but would only take one after dinner. The safest place in our Greater Kailash house was the roof, where my parents wouldn't come. I used to watch the sky, puffing away, almost feeling I could touch the celestial stars. Fortunately, I wasn't ever caught and this never became a habit. It remained just an experiment and after a few months, I gave it up.

Our emoluments during house job in 1972, now termed as junior residency, were Rs 250 only, which we realised was very little. Even the senior residents with postgraduate degrees would get Rs 650 only. There was a resident union of Delhi doctors which included all the government hospitals. Our leaders put in a representation to the health ministry which was not taken seriously at all. We, therefore, went on a strike, and paralysed the work in all the hospitals. The union came to know that my uncle Prithvi (P.N. Dhar) was the Principal Secretary to Mrs Indira Gandhi, the then prime minister, so I was also roped in as a member. The usual tricks of bureaucracy were tried, that included dividing the unity, followed by threats of evacuation of the residents from the hostels. The hospital services were restricted only to emergency services and indoor patients discharged. All this did not work, and our leaders would make passionate speeches to keep the flock together. We also went on a *dharna* (sit-in) outside the Health Minister Dr Karan Singh's residence at Nyaya Marg (Nyaya in Hindi means justice). Our slogan was '*Nyay marg ke Karan Singh nyay karo*'. (The resident of Nyay Marg, Karan Singh do justice.) We also met the Principal Secretary, my mama, officially in his office. Apparently, Mrs Gandhi wanted an end to this nuisance, with newspapers giving it a lot of coverage. Finally, after a few weeks, the ministry formed a committee to look into the demands with a time-bound commitment. This led to an increase in our stipends.

This was the time to get admission into postgraduation. After completing MBBS and the compulsory internship, there was a chance to go abroad, either to the UK, the USA or Australia. For the USA, there was an exam called ECFMG (entrance test for foreign medical graduates) which was conducted in major metros of India. Australia was also encouraging applications from young Indian doctors for its General Practice (GP) in cities which had a shortage of personnel. Many of my classmates went abroad, including Gurpreet Brar, who was so close to me. He went to the USA. Another friend, Virendra Berera, went to Melbourne, Australia. This was very tempting and I too thought of applying to get a foreign degree. I, however, had no desire to settle down abroad like many of my colleagues. I brought forms for both the destinations, and as I was filling these lengthy documents, Amma asked me what I was doing so seriously. I told her the truth. She remained silent for a while, then with moist eyes she told me that after all their hard work in making me a doctor, I too had some responsibility towards them. I got the point and immediately tore away those forms, which brought a smile to her face.

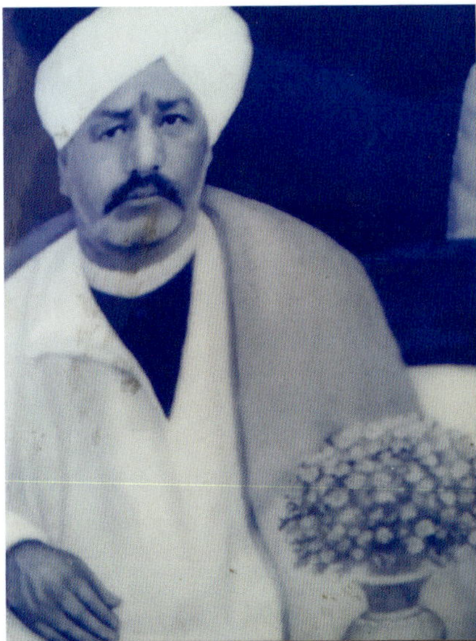

The author's late grandfather Prasad Joo Khan, a well-known Pandit of Hawal village, Pulwama district, Jammu and Kashmir

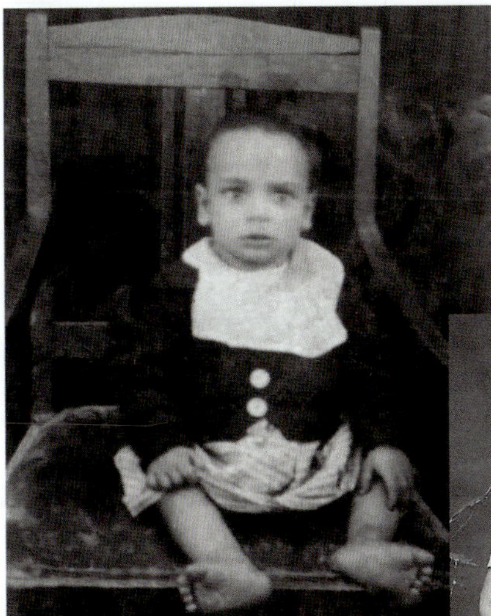

The author as an infant

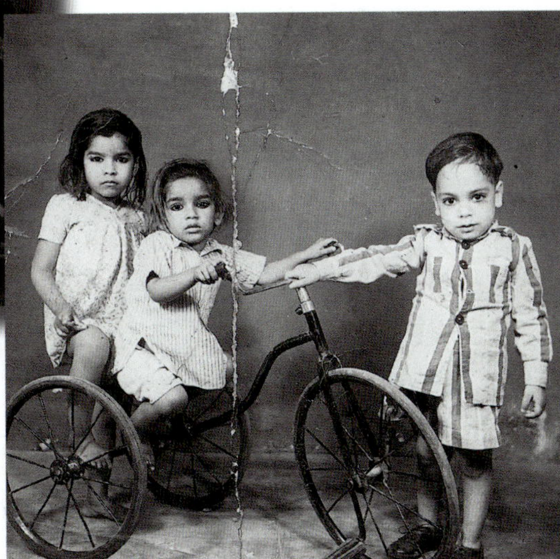

The author (right) with his landlord's children who had a tricycle

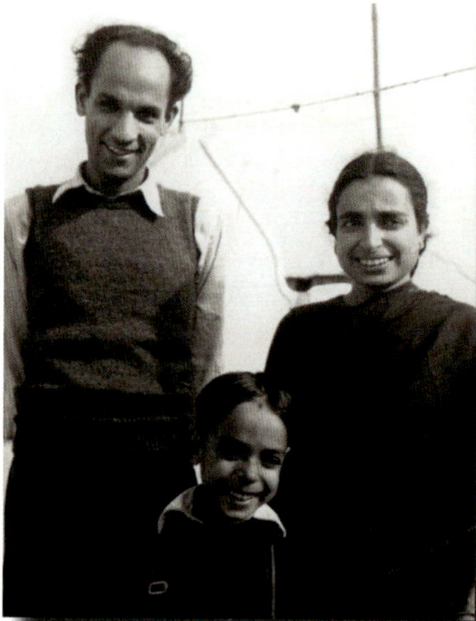

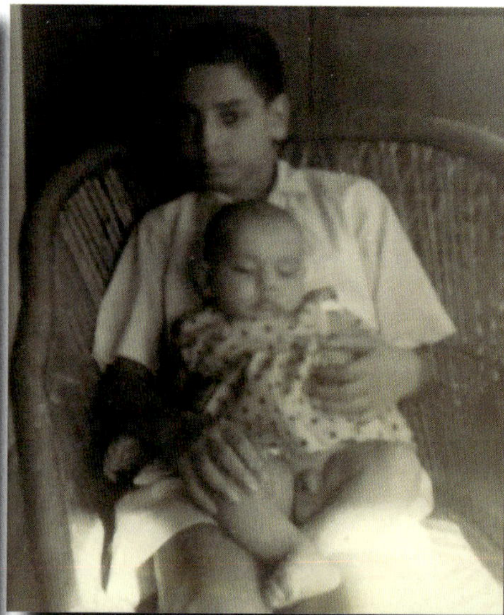

(Clockwise) The author with his father and mother, 6-month-old brother Shankar, *mama* (uncle) and childhood friend Neelu

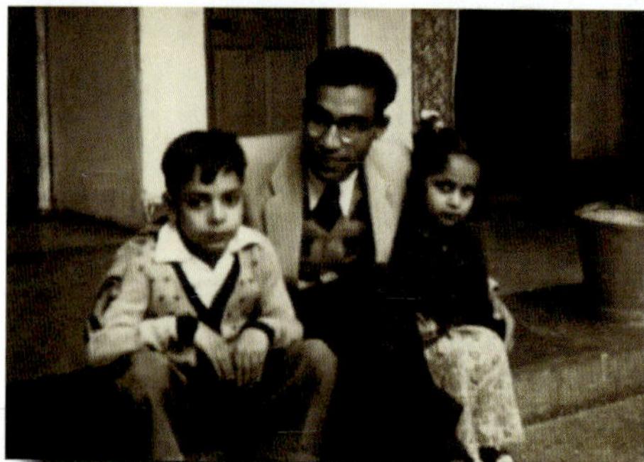

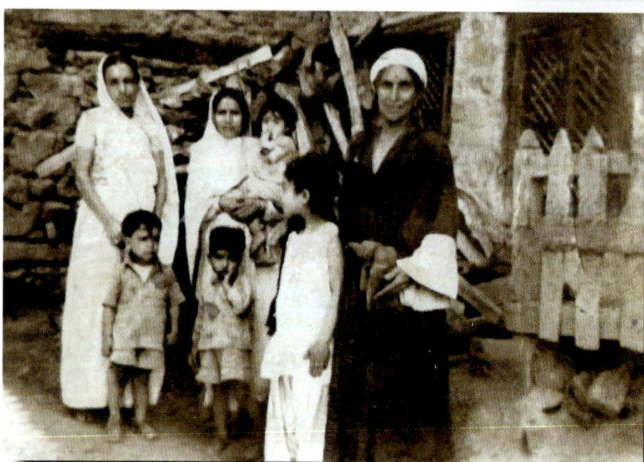

The author with his mother's family—grandmother Radha, mother, *Benigashee* (aunt) and cousins

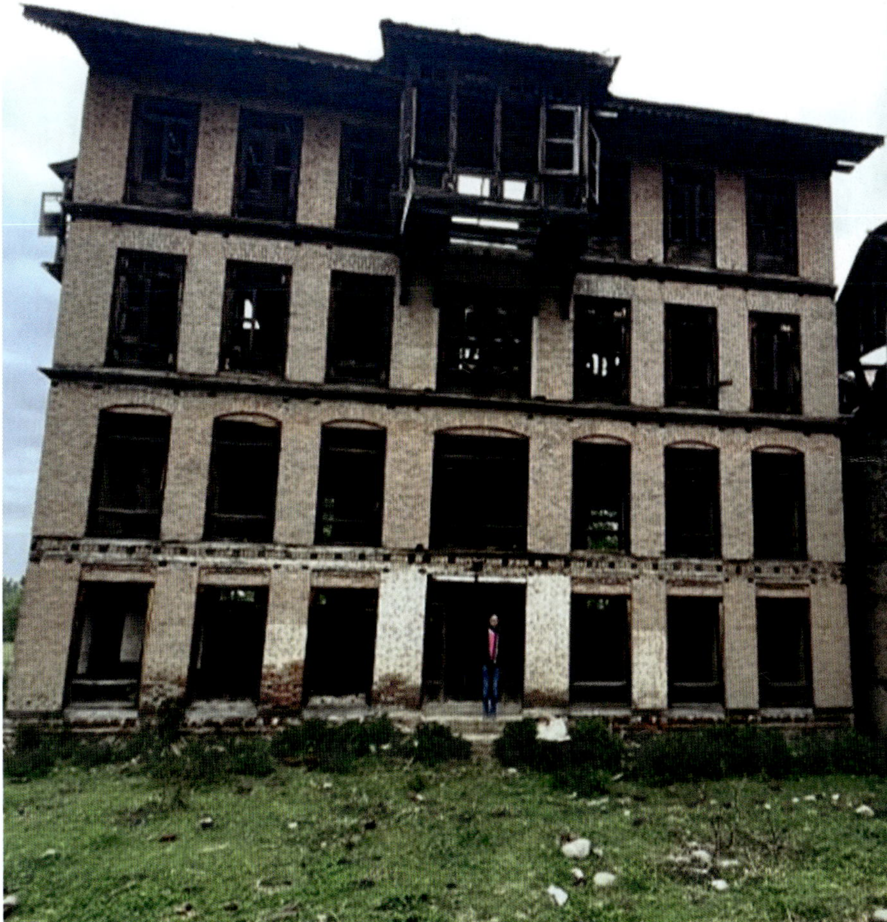

A recent picture of the author's ancestral house in Hawal, Pulwama

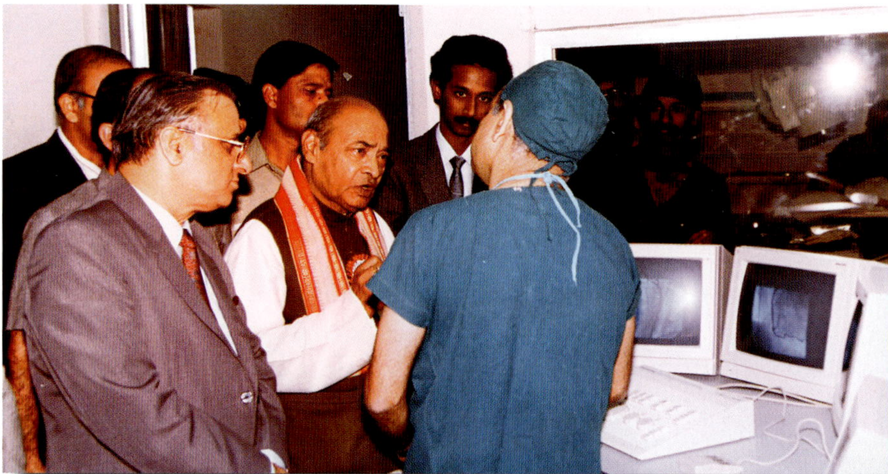

The author interacting with Prime Minister P.V. Narasimha Rao and Sathya Sai Super Speciality Hospital Director at the inauguration of the Cardiology Department in Puttaparthi on 21 November 1991

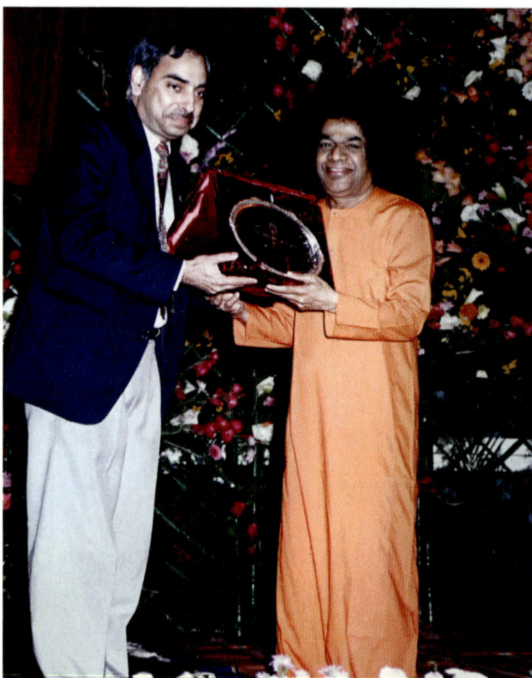

With Sathya Sai Baba during a scientific meeting organized by SSIHMS, Puttaparthi, Andhra Pradesh in 1995

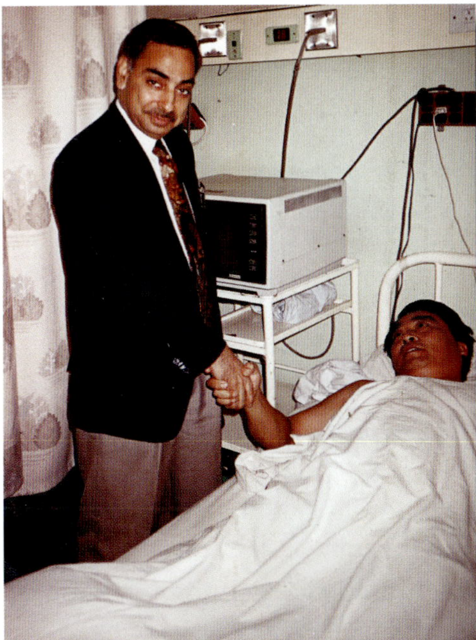

With Beijing's first angioplasty patient after he was operated on by the author in 1995

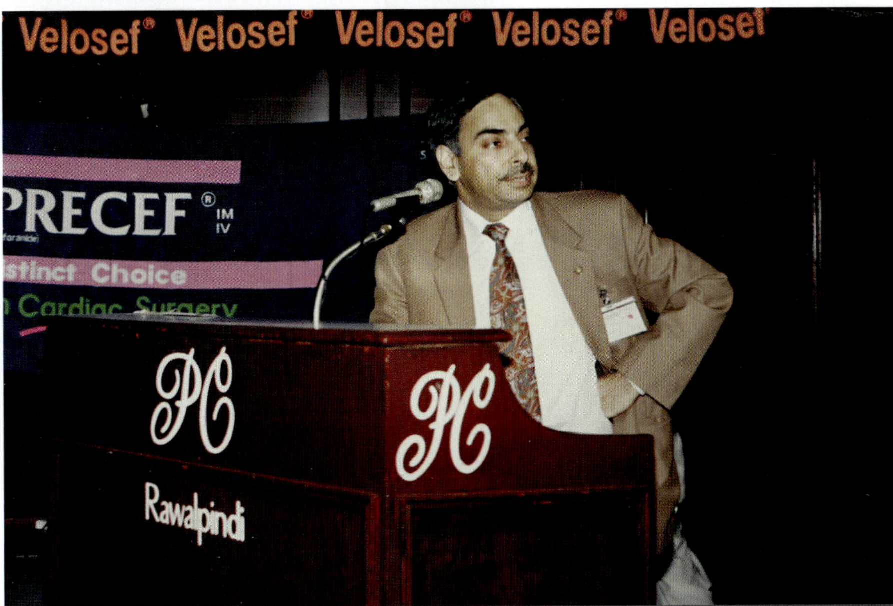

During a cardiology summit in Pakistan in 1996

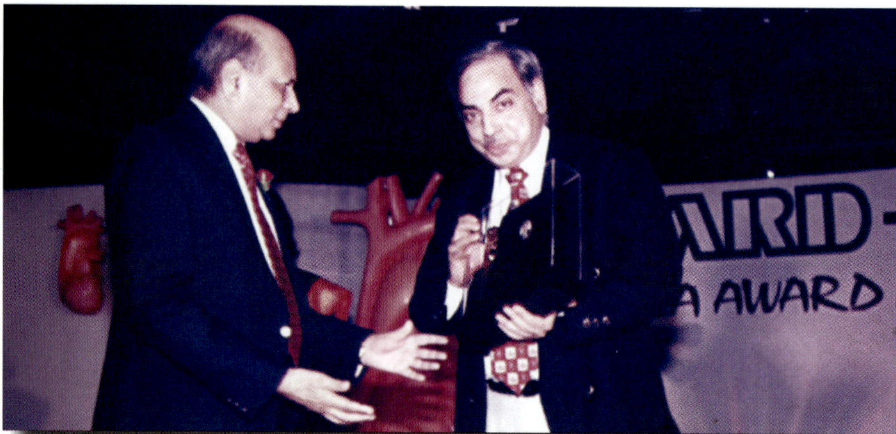

Dr N.S. Dixit, Chairman of Batra Heart Centre, welcoming the author after he received the Andreas Grüntzig Award on 15 August 1998 from the Cardiological Society of India for promoting Coronary Angioplasty in India. Andreas Grüntzig, considered the father of interventional cardiology, performed the first balloon angioplasty in the late 1970s—a technique that revolutionised cardiology

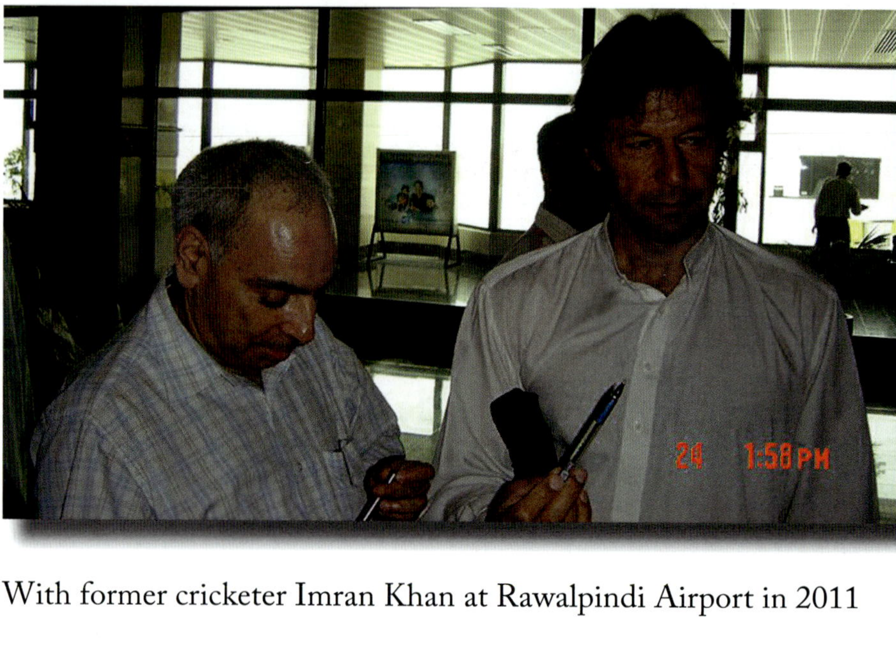

With former cricketer Imran Khan at Rawalpindi Airport in 2011

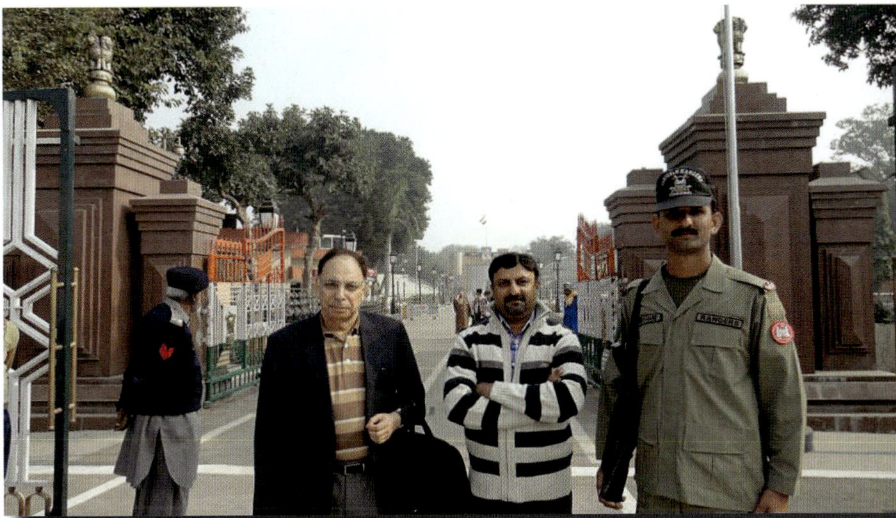

With Pakistani Rangers at Wagah while returning from Lahore after a teaching assignment in 2012

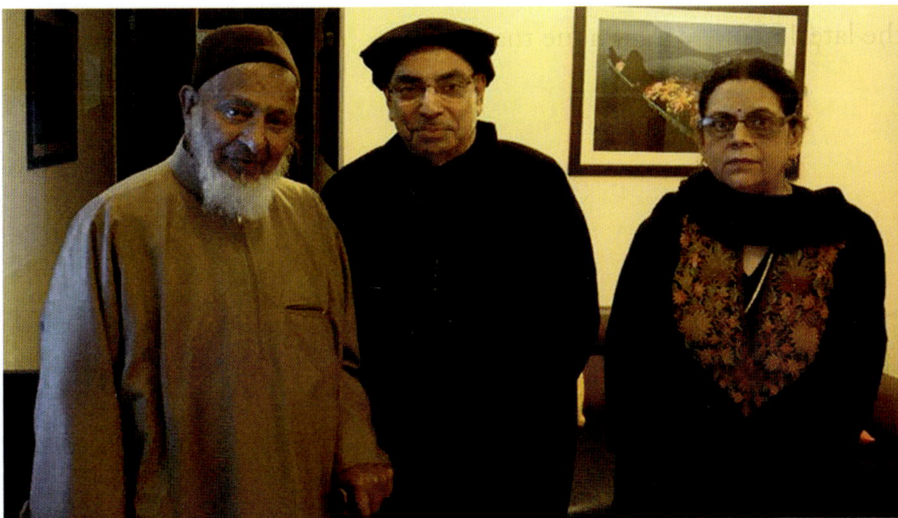

J&K's Sufi saint, Gujjar leader and social reformer Mian Bashir Ahmed Larvi with the author and his wife when he visited the author's house in New Delhi in February 2016

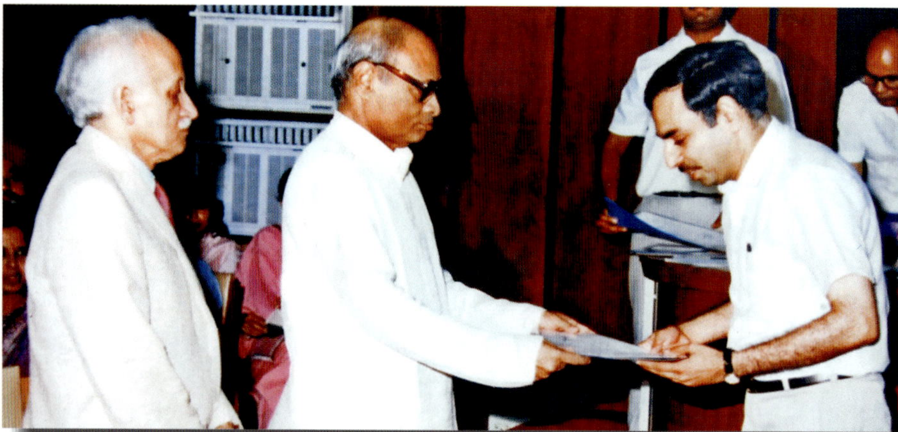

Congress MP P.V. Narasimha Rao presenting the Shakuntala Amir Chand Prize for young scientists, instituted by the Indian Council of Medical Research, to the author in 1987 for his research work in the field of Cardiac Pacing and Electrophysiology. ICMR Director-General Prof. A.S. Paintal is also seen

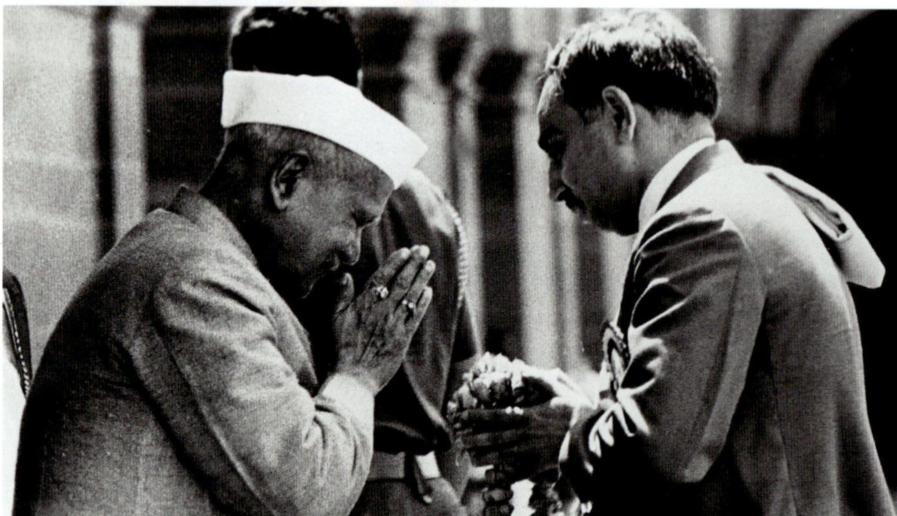

Receiving the Press India Award for achieving excellence in the medical field from President Shankar Dayal Sharma in 1992

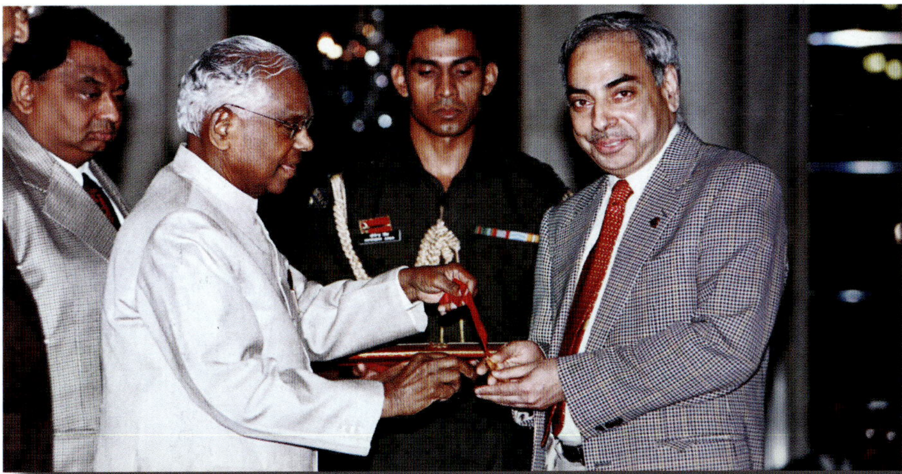

Receiving the Dr B.C. Roy Award—the highest Indian award in medical category—from President K.R. Narayanan in 1999

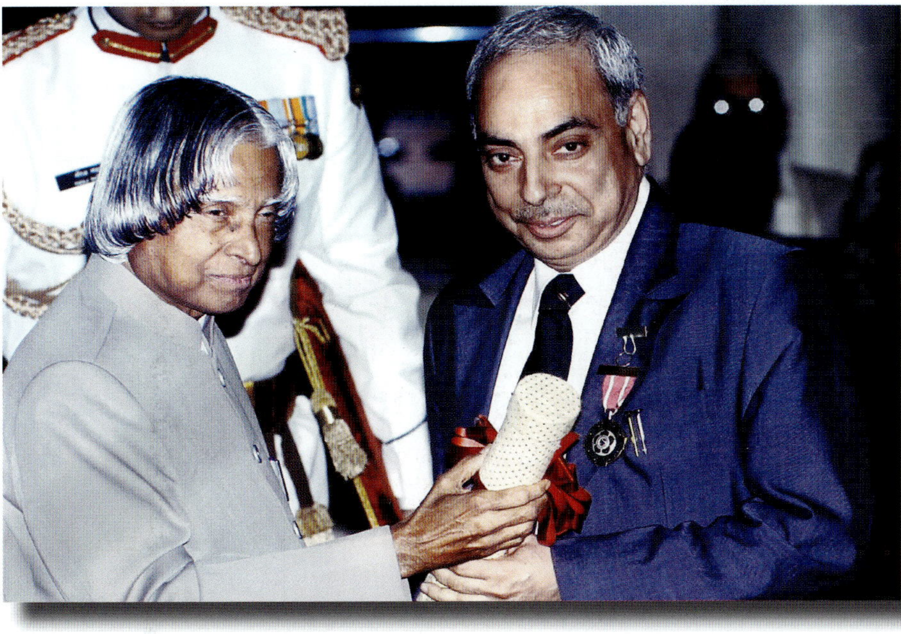

President A.P.J. Abdul Kalam awarding the Padma Shri to the author in 2006, for his contributions to Indian medicine

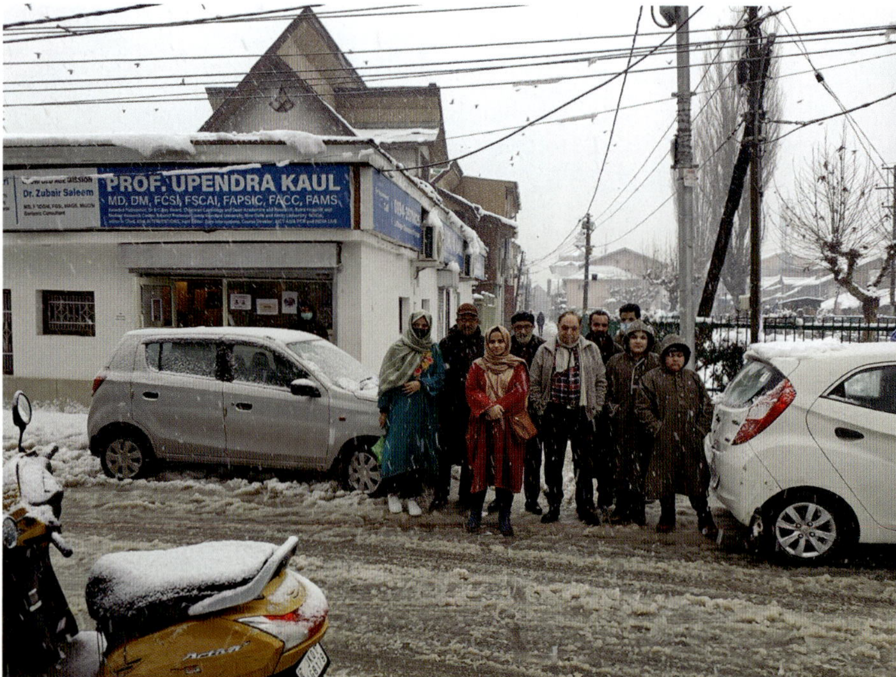

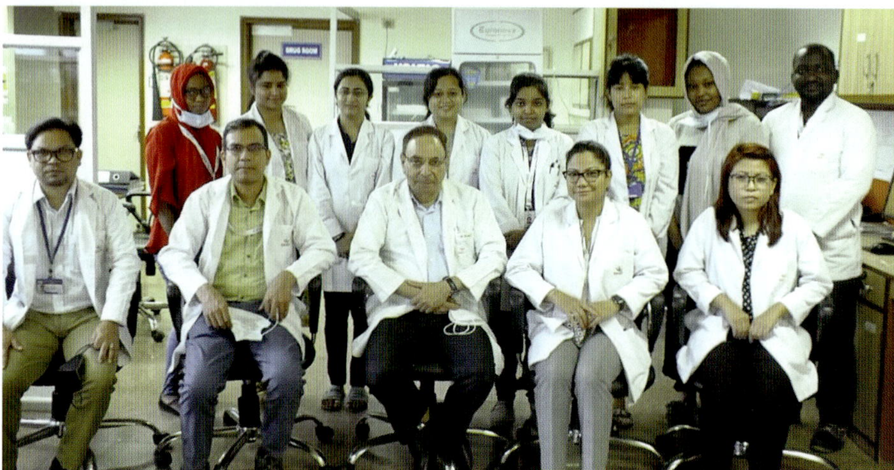

With colleagues of Gauri Heart Centre, Srinagar (above) and the Academics and Research Department, Batra Hospital and Medical Research Centre, New Delhi

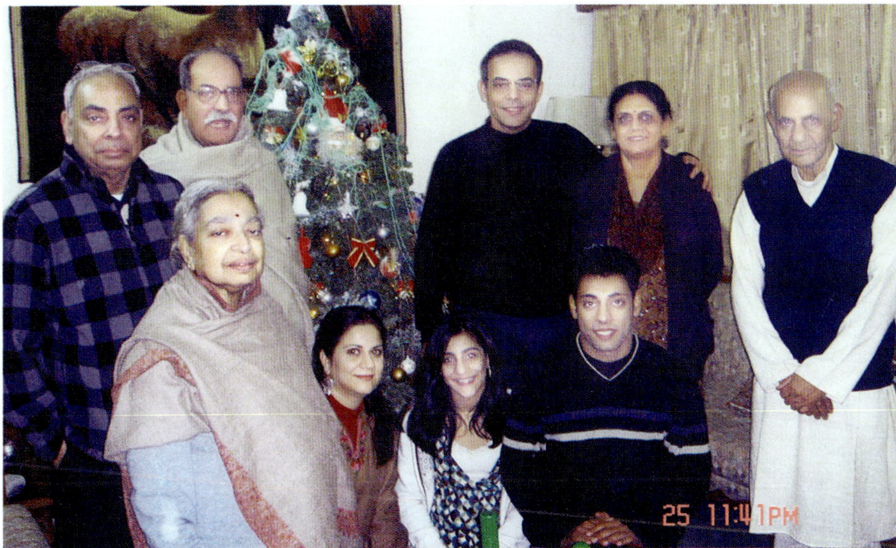

The author with his parents, wife, son, brother, his wife, niece and *mama* (uncle) B.L. Dhar

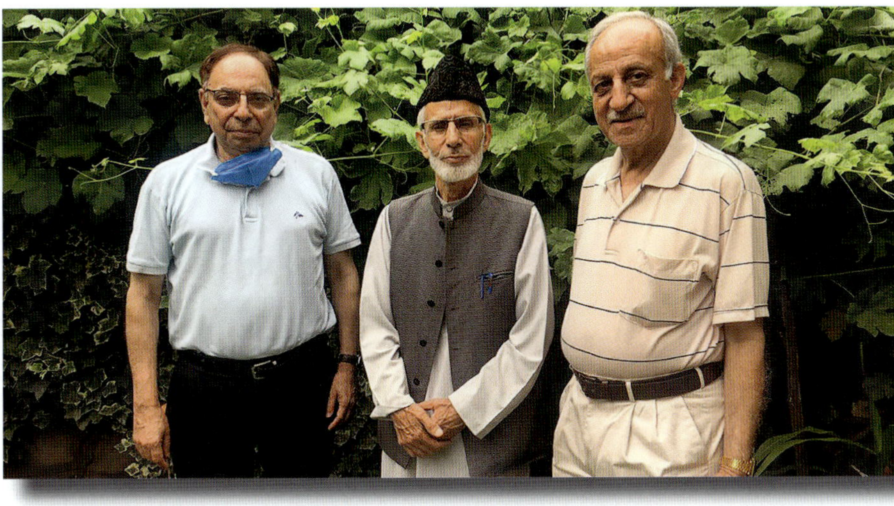

The author with Kashmiri poet, historian and environmentalist Zareef Ahmad Zareef (centre) and the late Mohammad Ashraf, a doyen of travel and tourism in Jammu and Kashmir, in Srinagar in 2020

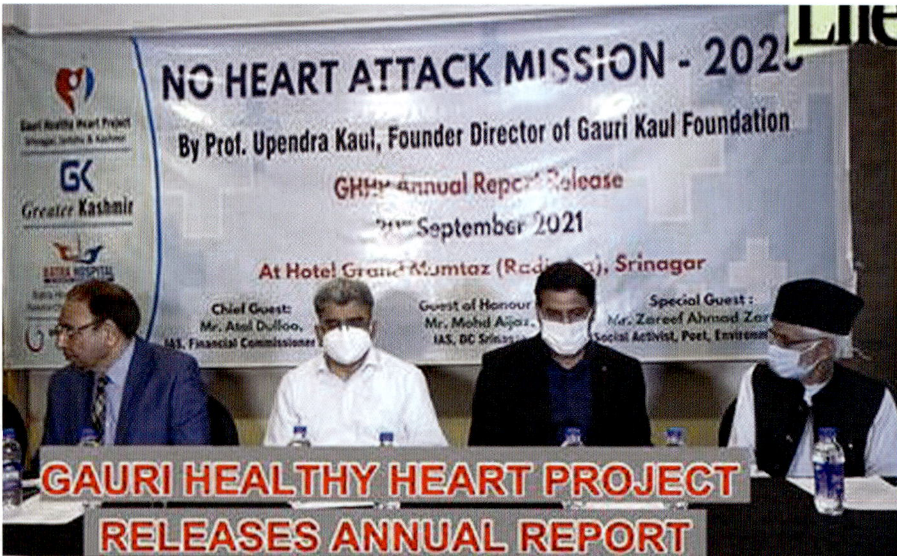
NO HEART ATTACK MISSION - 202
By Prof. Upendra Kaul, Founder Director of Gauri Kaul Foundation
September 2021
Srinagar
Greater Kashmir
Chief Guest:
Mr. Atul Dulloo,
Special Guest :
GAURI HEALTHY HEART PROJECT
RELEASES ANNUAL REPORT

The author at an event commemorating World Heart Day 2021, during which the Gauri Healthy Heart Project ('No Heart Attack Mission-2025') also released its annual report

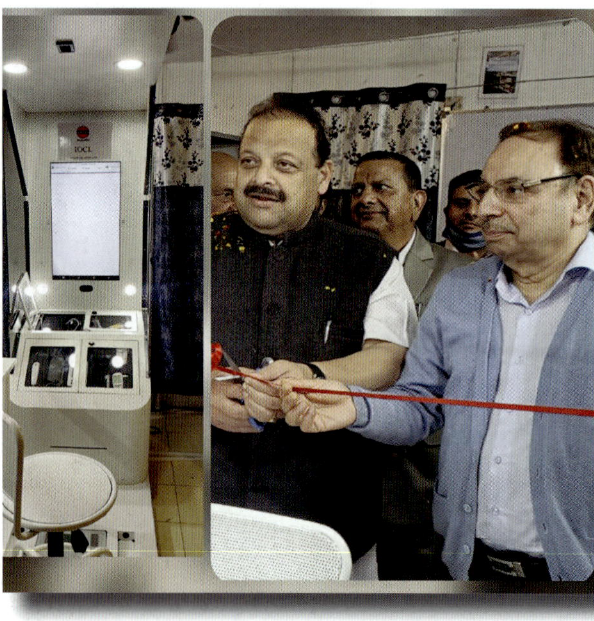

With chief guest Mr D. S. Rana during the launch of the telemedicine facility, organised by the Gauri Heart Foundation, at Jagati Camp, Jammu in early 2022

6

Postgraduation and Becoming a Cardiologist

In our times, to go in for postgraduation didn't entail having to sit for a separate examination, unlike these days. The MBBS marks decided the specialisation. I got admission in both Medicine and Surgery. I opted for Medicine and got it at Maulana Azad Medical College. After the admission, we waited for the guides to be allocated. Most students wanted to work under the heads of departments but it wasn't possible to accommodate all such requests. No criteria were established for who got whom as guide. *Chamchagiri* (flattery) often worked; flattery, after all, is a potent weapon. Being connected with senior bureaucrats or politicians too helped one in getting the coveted role. I fitted no such category—neither could I flatter someone nor did I have any connection that could be put to use. Papa and Amma believed one should deserve their achievement based on merit, and absolutely nothing else. So, I landed up with the junior-most faculty member who was getting a student for the first time. He was interested in lung diseases. I wanted to make the best of the situation and met him one morning. He received me politely and asked me to select a topic in Pulmonology after visiting the pulmonary lab. I went to the lab and to my utter surprise found only a spirometer and an empty tin of Dalda Vanaspati (a popular cooking oil brand) there. When I looked at him puzzled, he said, 'Well, this is all we have. You will have to set up the laboratory before you can start working.' This was not acceptable and I left upset.

I discussed the matter with a few of my colleagues, who told me that there was a vacancy in Cardiology under Dr M.P. Gupta at G.B. Pant Hospital—a part of the same institution with super specialities. Usually, very few students would opt to go to G.B. Pant Hospital as we had to spend time mostly in the main Irwin Hospital for most of our classes and postings. There were very few students posted at G.B. Pant Hospital and it had a lonely atmosphere. Another important reason is that the internal examiners during the finals would be from Irwin Hospital. I had done my two-week elective posting during my internship in Cardiology in G.B. Pant Hospital and knew that hospital very well. It had a better building and was less crowded, no emergency and Casualty department of its own. This would deprive us of seeing serious patients. In addition, it had private wards, where the patients and their families were usually snobbish. They would not be happy being examined by students and would not cooperate. Moreover, most of our training would be in Irwin Hospital and only thesis work would be from G.B. Pant Hospital.

There were some positives too. The hospital had a modern coronary care unit (CCU) to manage patients with heart attacks. The CCU is an area where sick patients with acute heart problems are treated. It was equipped with electrocardiography (ECG), blood pressure (BP) monitors, defibrillators and other types of equipment for prompt resuscitation. Besides this, it had trained personnel, including nurses and doctors, under one roof. This was possibly the first CCU in India. The history of CCUs dates back to 1964 when Dr Desmond Julian from the Royal Infirmary at Edinburgh set up the first organised CCU. When Professor Julian visited India in 1982, I had the opportunity to meet him. He told me that before he went to England, he was toying with this idea when he was in Sydney. He used Coca-Cola bottle caps as contact points to transmit the ECG to the monitor. That is how the CCU concept came in the year 1961, and was followed by a similar unit in Kansas City, USA. The landscape of the CCU today, however, has changed vastly from that of the 1960s. No longer is it simply an observation unit for patients with acute MI (myocardial infarction/ heart attack), but rather it has become a dynamic and diverse arena of patient care. Dedicated CCUs that were developed in the 1960s have been transformed into combined units such as CCU and high dependency units. When I look back, I am proud to be associated with CCU care in its early days in India.

I decided to opt for G.B. Pant Hospital and went to meet Professor M.P. Gupta, with whom we had a few classes during MBBS. He had been trained at AIIMS and qualified as one of the first trained DMs (Doctorate of Medicine), a post-MD degree. He promptly accepted me as his postgraduate student and his words were very encouraging. He said he remembered me as a hard-working intern and would gladly accept me. He also invited me to his bungalow, which was on campus and introduced me to his wife, Dr Mala, who was working as a general duty doctor in a New Delhi Municipal Council (NDMC) dispensary. My senior in the department, a second-year postgraduate student, was Dr Prem Pais from Bangalore, now Bengaluru. He had already completed his Doctor of Medicine (MD) thesis on 'Systolic time intervals', which focused on calculating intervals during the pumping phase of the heart. He was a very soft-spoken man but extremely intelligent. Dr Gupta allotted me a thesis subject which was sort of a continuation of Dr Prem Pais' thesis subject. The topic involved the study of the 'Effects of Contrast Media on Systolic Time Intervals'. Dr Pais, though a very innocent-looking man, was actually quite romantic. He had an affair with one of our class fellows Nalini Verma, who subsequently became Nalini Pais. One day, I saw them hanging around in the lawns of our hostel. They saw me and Prem really blushed. Nalini just smiled. Later in life, they moved to Bangalore and excelled in academics and research. He became HOD Medicine and Clinical Research at St John's Hospital and is currently working for the Manipal Group of Hospitals in Bengaluru. We meet whenever he comes to Delhi and talk about the good old days. The thesis work in G.B. Pant Hospital kept me very busy because I had to go to the catheterisation laboratory whenever a case was being done. It was, however, rather easy because Prem had already reviewed the entire literature on the subject and I just had to fill in the blanks on contrast media used in angiography procedures.

I used to sit with Dr M.P. Gupta in the OPD and work up his patients. He usually used to agree with my analysis of the case. In cases where I missed important findings, he would call me and make me listen to the sounds and murmurs using his stethoscope. In one of the cases with a birth defect who also had high blood pressure, I got so busy working up that gentleman for high BP that I totally missed examining his heart, which had peculiar murmurs. Dr M.P. Gupta pointed out my mistake and called me to his room and admonished me regarding missing this vital finding. I remember that mistake to date and always do a thorough examination and have realised that one patient can have multiple problems.

G.B. Pant Hospital had a separate hostel for postgraduate residents. It had eight floors with small single-occupancy rooms and common washrooms. The ground floor had a dining hall and a few rooms with attached baths for registrars (senior residents). As junior residents, it was a lot of slogging as we worked as a physician and then as a student, burning the midnight oil working on our thesis. We used to have a lot of fun interacting with a few students who had failed several times in succession. One such doctor was Kasturi Lal, who was a chain smoker and always sitting on a parked motorcycle outside the hostel, passing remarks on junior students along with his other friend Dr Bhagwan Das who also had a similar experience of repeated failure. They used to abuse the external examiners with the choicest words and also guide us to the shortcuts to success and some tips and tricks. I used to wonder why they did not use these tricks and pass.

My visits to home used to be once a month on a post-duty off day, usually very tired. Mother used to feed me and feel very satisfied that her son was becoming an MD doctor. Usually, our evenings on post-duty off days were something to look forward to. After an exhausting 36-hour continuous duty, often a bottle of beer would be very welcome. The mess staff would procure it for a small tip. This was followed by dinner outside at one of the *dhabas* after which we would crash on our beds till the next morning's arduous schedule began.

During these months, I received excellent training from my mentors; the variety of clinical cases was exceptional too. As G.B. Pant was a general hospital, there was no problem in taking a detailed history of the patients; sometimes, students would examine and elicit signs in the same patient repeatedly as that was a part of our study. Patients, to their credit, were especially cooperative and understanding. The same cannot be said of colleges attached to private hospitals and nursing homes. The patients there would be very reluctant to allow examination more than once to confirm clinical findings, which restricted the training of medical students. This problem is seen in most private colleges also. In addition, the teaching staff in such institutions is not so dedicated as they also are busy practicing in their chambers.

Besides regular bedside discussion classes, there were very few formal lectures, unlike what we experienced during the MBBS. Every evening, after the day's work, a few of us would go and see cases with good clinical findings and discuss amongst ourselves. This sadly is a habit which is not practised much by the present generation of students. The art of clinical medicine and approaching the problem systematically—like Sherlock Holmes used to investigate—has its own charm. The final evidence of your success comes when you see the diagnostic test reports, such as an echocardiogram or a CT scan in a cardiology patient. Ordering appropriate tests for a patient is an important part of the training, and as a doctor one must approach it step by step. Every patient doesn't require a battery of tests for the right diagnosis to be identified. This distinguishes a good doctor who is well trained from an average one who is not sure of his findings and is unable to justify the tests.

With the MD training completed, finally it was exam time. Theory exams had very little value. It was the practical and bedside examination that mattered more. Practicals were scheduled at Dr Ram Manohar Lohia Hospital, formerly known as Willingdon Hospital. This hospital was founded by the British Raj in 1932 for its government staff. Since then, it has grown enormously and today is one of the biggest hospitals for both the general public and government staff. This was the first time I visited this hospital and was quite impressed with the sprawling premises.

I did well in the final MD (Medicine) practical exam held in 1975 on two successive days. I hadn't met any of the four examiners who took the practicals. The practicals preceded three theory papers, which most students do well. These theory papers are sent to external examiners, who are hardly interested in reading them. It is the practical exam which decides your result. Had it been in Irwin Hospital, at least the internal examiners would be our own teachers and that always was a source of comfort. The practical exam at Ram Manohar Lohia

Hospital consisted of examining two patients, and for each evaluation, we got around 90 minutes. These cases are tougher than the cases kept in MBBS and the cross-examination is fairly detailed. It is very difficult to get to know these patients usually brought from different hospitals. I remember having got a case with a hole in the heart. The patient in addition had a rudimentary finger deformity. I picked up the finding because the patient who had been kept as one of the cases for other students had told me that I should not miss this finding. Case examination is followed by a viva on recent literature and showing some graphs of ECG, etc. to identify. I passed the exam, as did most students in our group who used to study together. Although the university declares the result after a few weeks, most often the examiners at the end of compiling the result call the students and congratulate those who have passed. For those who did not, they usually point out their shortcomings. It was such a piece of great news when they told me that I was through. I remember I was so relieved that I could not sleep the whole night out of excitement.

The big question now was what after MD. This was a critical question that I took some days to mull over; after all, it was the turning point in my career. My choices were to either become a registrar and look for a job or be a consultant internist either at a teaching hospital or a nursing home. There weren't too many good private hospitals those days and a few handful ones were already saturated. Post-doctoral courses (DM) from the University of Delhi were limited to Cardiology, Neurology and Gastroenterology. Professor Padmavati, an eminent cardiologist, had recently taken over as the director of Maulana Azad Medical College. She was a well-known figure in Delhi's medical circles. Incidentally, her younger sister, Professor S. Janaki, was the chief of Neurology at G.B. Pant Hospital.

Professor Padmavati was credited with starting the DM Cardiology programme at the university. The other two DM Cardiology programmes running in the country were at AIIMS, by Professor Sujoy B. Roy, and Christian Medical College (CMC), Vellore, Tamil Nadu, by Professor Vytilingam. Interestingly, both Professor Padmavati and Professor Roy received their initial medical training in Yangon and were contemporaries.

Most postgraduates in the 1970s weren't keen on joining post-doctoral courses as these didn't bring much value. Special jobs were unavailable; nor did the hospitals have special facilities to utilise that training. Hence, it just meant losing two years of seniority in a teaching or a non-teaching hospital. But Professor Padmavati had kept an eye out for me; she knew me as I had done my MD thesis at G.B. Pant Hospital on a subject related to Cardiology. She called me to her director's office and treated me very well. She had an affectionate charm and convinced me how a Cardiology career would help me. She told me rather than joining the bandwagon of physicians, it would be much better to choose a subject which has a great future. She pointed to some of her students who were doing very well and were respected doctors of the city. Five doctors had done their DM Cardiology ahead of me. The most senior of them was Dr Suresh Gupta, who later started a cardiology set-up at Defence Colony. He was followed by Dr (Mrs) Ramesh Arora, who had joined G.B. Pant Hospital and continued working there till her retirement. Then there were Dr K.G. Balakrishnan, who joined Sree Chitra Tirunal Institute in Thiruvananthapuram and finally migrated to the Middle East, and Dr N.K. Mahapatra, who worked at a government medical college in Cuttack. The fifth one was Dr C.G. Venkitachalam, fondly called Venky, who left for Kerala for a few years before settling down in Abu Dhabi. In fact, Dr Mahapatra and Venky were still students when I joined DM Cardiology at G.B. Pant Hospital.

Venky, a bachelor, was a happy-go-lucky guy, a pleasant, short-statured person with a dark complexion with pimples on his face.

He was fond of keeping his hair oily and shining. He used to spend long hours in OPD and wards examining patients. He also was very popular with the nurses and lady doctors of the hospital and would take them to the coffee house and dress up in glistening white clothes. On the other hand, Mahapatra was a very mature man with a family of three daughters and a charming wife Anju. He was staying in a flat with the family. Both of them became very good friends of mine and were staying in the hospital quarters on campus. I was junior to both of them but they treated me as an equal.

As senior residents, we had to spend long hours at the hospital, caring for patients both in OPD and wards. The department had a cardiac catheterisation laboratory where angiographies and haemodynamic studies were regularly done. The only other such facility in Delhi during that time was in AIIMS. We also were doing electrophysiology studies to diagnose problems related to the heart rhythm and the conduction system of the heart. Dr M.P. Gupta and Dr Khalilullah were the faculty doing procedures in the lab. All graphic tracings of these investigations were reviewed and calculations were done by the DM students till late in the night. Computerisation and digitisation were in their infancy and everything had to be done manually. Hence, this taught us to work the harder way. It, however, was an excellent learning experience, which the present-day students and consultants are not required to do because the values now come digitally on the monitor and in the records. I firmly believe that learning from studying the curves, tracings and graphs makes you perfect in learning the principles of cardiac pressures and electrical activity. Sadly, this training has vanished from most of the training programmes in Cardiology these days.

In July 1975, during my first year of DM training, I got married to Upkar, whom I had met at G.B. Pant Hospital. She was a registrar, who had done her Cardiology training from Beth Israel Hospital,

New York. She seemed to be a loner and was older to me by four years. Somehow, I became friendly to her. Her parents were Sikhs from Peshawar who had migrated to Meerut. She had her schooling there and later MBBS in Lady Hardinge Hospital, Delhi. From there she went to the USA and returned in 1974. After returning, she got a registrar Cardiology job in G.B. Pant Hospital where I was a post-MD cardiology student. She used to stay in the girl's hostel. I used to see patients with her and she was my boss. Her training in Cardiology did not have a fellowship degree and hence she was not eligible to get a faculty post. Our friendship became more intimate and I used to take her to Lodhi Gardens and occasionally to a five-star hotel on Mathura Road near Faridabad. I told my mama B.L. Dhar about this relationship. He strangely encouraged it. He asked me to invite her to his place in Greater Kailash close to my home. Finally, the day of reckoning came and I had to nervously tell my mother who was looking for a Kashmiri match for me. I was a very eligible bachelor but never used to show interest in her choices. When she came to know about this relationship, she was not at all happy. She raised the topic of Upkar being a Sikh and being older to me. But love has no logic and I did not budge. It was a court marriage solemnised at the residence of my mama P.N. Dhar. We have two children. Amita, a well-known paediatrician in Pune, is married to a bright engineer and entrepreneur Ashish Kulkarni. My son, Samir who is younger to Amita, is a management trained person from Perth, Australia, and is at present a senior executive in Citibank in Mumbai. Both have one child each.

One of the shortcomings of the G.B. Pant Hospital was that the cardiac surgery department was not very active and the hospital was famous for its Cardiology and not the surgical speciality in those times. As part of our postgraduate training in Cardiology, we had to spend a month in Vellore. As a result, I along with my colleague Dr Umesh

Gupta had to go to CMC. In 1977, CMC was a private, minority-run educational and research institute founded in 1900 by an American missionary, Dr Ida S. Scudder. CMC has brought many significant medical achievements to India.

Umesh and I started our journey to Madras, now Chennai, on a superfast train, called the Tamil Nadu Express, which used to have limited stoppages. This was my first trip to South India and I was excited to travel. We boarded the train in the evening, expecting to reach 36 hours later. I could see the transition from the north of India to the south around Nagpur. While Nagpur is in the central part of India, the passengers who boarded the train now spoke a different language. The vendors were selling *vadas* and *dosas*, instead of *samosas* and *poori choley* (popular North Indian snacks). The *chutney* became coconut-based and it was *rasam* and *sambar* instead of *daal* (lentil soup). The countryside landscape too was transforming—the huts had different roofs; people were mostly in *lungis* (a white sarong-like garment worn by men) instead of *pajamas* that one would see in the North. Even the cattle looked different with cows and bulls sporting vertically pointed horns. Temples had a different architecture and were painted in riotous colours; the temple tops carried intricate details which fascinated me. With people from southern India settling across the country for work, these temple structures are now seen even in North India, but during the 1970s it was a wholly different experience in cultural diversity for me. I realized the greatness of our country with different languages, food and lifestyle. Travelling provides a learning experience like no other.

Finally, we reached Madras on time, partly worn out by the journey, in September 1976. Venky's friend Dr Bala, whom I knew, took us to his nursing home in Anna Nagar so that we could freshen up. Once we had washed away the grime of a two-day journey, we went to a local restaurant for a vegetarian thali. When the waiter brought the plate, it turned out to be this round, brass plate with steaming rice in the middle, surrounded with *rasam*, *dahi*, seasonal veggies and *papad*. A totally delectable gastronomical experience—more so as we were on train food for the last two days—we finished our lunch quickly. When we paid the bill, I was surprised to see how economical it was. Gradually, I realised that the cost of living in Madras was quite low—people appeared simple without any need for show-off and pretensions.

We took the evening Nilgiri Express to Katpadi junction, the nearest railway station to Vellore. This was a shorter trip and lasted only a few hours. After reaching Katpadi, we got on an eight-seater tempo that took us to the CMC gate. We managed to find accommodation at a nearby hotel in front of the hospital complex. Umesh and I took one room with double beds. The next morning, we went to meet Professor Stanley John, the head of the Department of Cardiac Surgery, who was taking a round of post-operative patients, mainly valve replacement cases, and grown-up kids with corrected Tetralogy of Fallot, a condition with multiple heart defects making them blue babies. Our aim, however, was to follow the rounds of Professor George Cherian (who was fondly called GC) and gather pearls of wisdom so that we could answer him well both in Vellore and in our final exam in Delhi. He had been one of our external examiners for the last few years. We found him to be a soft-spoken man and would diligently listen to us whenever we ventured to propose an opinion.

The other well-known cardiology personalities at CMC were I.P. Sukumar, who specialised in Paediatric Cardiology, Shankar Krishnaswamy, who was an expert in Coronary Angiography, and Krishnaswamy's protégé, K.A. Abraham. Paediatric Cardiology procedures and coronary angiographies were not performed at G.B. Pant Hospital those days. It was thus a good learning experience. We also met a young, pleasant physician, Satyavan Sharma, from Jaipur posted in an area where ECG during and after exercise is recorded. It is called the Exercise ECG Lab. He was a friendly man and was also visiting and making an effort to join the DM Cardiology course there. He eventually managed to get into KEM Hospital, Mumbai. Satyavan became a great friend later and is an academic cardiologist practising in Mumbai today.

After spending long hours at the hospital, I would take a stroll through the local markets in the evening. I observed that the shopkeepers conversed only in Tamil among themselves and would feign ignorance if we asked for any local information. However, the moment we wanted to buy something, they would start talking in broken Hindi or English, whatever they could muster, to push in a sale. But it was quite clear that they resisted Hindi. The anti-Hindi movement that raged across Madras leading to riots and deaths was still a fresh memory. The movement, which sprung as a response to make Hindi the national language of India, was a contentious issue for decades. The first agitation was launched by E.V. Ramasamy (Periyar) in 1937 when he opposed the compulsory introduction of Hindi in school education in the Madras Presidency as mandated by the first Indian National Congress government under C. Rajagopalachari. This later saw the beginning of the Dravidian movement and the emergence of C.N. Annadurai (popularly known as *Anna,* the big brother in Madras) and the birth of Dravida Munnetra Kazhagam (DMK) as a leading political party. The most virulent agitation took place on 25 January 1965, when a scuffle broke out between protesting students and members of the Congress Party in Madurai. The protest spread across Tamil Nadu and continued unabated for two months, resulting in weeks of violence, arson and looting. Trains and buses were set on fire. Tragic cases of self-immolations happened on the streets. It was only when the then Prime Minister, Lal Bahadur Shastri, assured that English would continue to be the official language as long as the non-Hindi-speaking states wished that the agitation was called off.

After 1967, no North Indian party could ever come into power in this southern state.

One day, I wished to eat a simple chicken meal and looked around in the local market. The signboards usually hanging in front of restaurants would say 'Meals Ready' or 'Breakfast Ready', depending upon the time of the day. The typical boards were Udupi restaurants, Woodland and Brahmin hotels, which were chiefly vegetarian. But try as I did, I couldn't find a single restaurant with a non-vegetarian signboard, which was odd considering there were many Muslims and Christians in the city. Exhausted, I took a vegetarian *thali* for lunch that day and went back to the hospital disgruntled. When a fellow doctor saw me sweating and irritated that afternoon, he asked what had happened and I shared my plight with him. He laughed and said, 'You poor man! You just had to look around carefully. All you had to do was look around for signboards saying "Military Hotels". They have all the good stuff!' He guffawed and left. It turned out that all these military hotels were the places the armed forces officers would go and they served the best non-vegetarian stuff. This came as a big relief as a Kashmiri can only survive on dal and veggies for just a few meals!

Tamil Nadu was a dry state those days and we were told bootlegging was widely prevalent. One Saturday evening, we craved for a drink and were advised by our hotelkeeper that the safest way to get an alcoholic beverage would be to take a bus and go to the nearest town of Andhra Pradesh, which was 30 minutes away. We acted on his advice and went to a bordering town and got four bottles of Golden Eagle beer in a bag, which was camouflaged well. Our mission of smuggling alcohol was successful and we celebrated over a few drinks and a fantastic assortment of chicken and mutton appetisers from our local military restaurant. Prohibition can never succeed because whether we approve or not, alcohol is a part of human civilisation. Prohibition is usually a political gimmick and costs many lives due to illicit drinks, which are easily available, and takes a toll on the poor and uneducated population. It also affects the revenue of these states because alcohol taxes are a good source of income, and nobody, except the manufacturers, can object to this. Prohibition also leads to police corruption as this is a good opportunity for bribery after they raid these *theka*s (joints). The only state which has been able to sustain prohibition is Gujarat, the birthplace of Mahatma Gandhi, as people have deep respect for the man who practised abstinence on several levels. Bihar has been practising prohibition too for a while to secure women's votes.

It was finally our turn to say farewell to Vellore and go back to Delhi in October 1976. The feelings were mixed; going home was a great thought but it appeared that we had a good educative dose of the southern part of our country. The people there are simple, not flashy, very hard working and have over the years learnt to have good relations with people from North India. We retraced our journey from Katpadi to Madras and then Delhi in Tamil Nadu Express. Dr Bala who had received us came to see us off and had also brought some snacks for us for our journey. We knew what to expect on the train and had also carried some pickles and snacks to supplement the food distributed on train, along with a few magazines. We reached Delhi and went to our homes. My parents and wife were waiting for me and showered their affection by feeding me my favourite mutton dish, the Kashmiri *rogan josh*.

The experience at Vellore allowed us broader exposure to the subject. A year later, before our final examination, one of my abstracts got selected for an oral presentation at the Annual Conference of the Cardiological Society of India, which was held in Bangalore in September 1977. The paper was on our experience of aortic stenosis at G.B. Pant Hospital. Umesh, who was a co-author, and I were allowed to attend the meeting. The hospital took care of the registration fee but travel and accommodation were our responsibility. When we reached Bangalore, we found it to be pleasant and cool, which was such a departure from the sweaty, hot weather of Delhi. This was my first visit to this southern city. Umesh had arranged our stay at the State Bank of India's guest house, which was located in a lovely, green neighbourhood. Umesh's father-in-law was a high-ranking officer at the bank, which made the arrangement easy.

The next morning, we left for the presentation, which was being held at Hotel Ashok. This was my first presentation in front of such a large audience of cardiologists and that made me nervous. I must have rehearsed the 10-minute presentation at least 50 times and had hardly slept the previous night. Umesh watched me getting nervous and knew that he is going to face the same music one of these days. I gave the presentation, which turned out superb. I could answer all the audience questions and received warm applause when it was over.

That evening, we had a plan to visit our senior colleague Venky's home who lived in Calicut and was already there for a vacation. Umesh and I left Hotel Ashok and reached the bus stand from where we took a state government bus to Calicut. It was a night bus which took us through the Western Ghats and the hills and forests of Wayanad. The weather was quite chilly and the route was dark. While we couldn't see much of the forests in the night, we, however, did see a few elephants crossing our way. After a few hours, the bus stopped at Sulthan Bathery—a town in the mountainous Wayanad region of Kerala. It takes its name from the ancient Bathery Jain Temple on the edge of the town, which was used as a place to camouflage an ammunition depot called battery by Tipu Sultan's army in the 1700s. In the Ambukuthi Hills to the southwest, Neolithic carvings are preserved on the walls of Edakkal Caves. Close by, the Wayanad Heritage Museum displays archaeological and tribal artefacts.

We, however, just had the bus stand to roam about as it was too dark. Umesh picked up snacks and then half a bottle of rum to keep us warm.

Although at first we hesitated drinking in public, our co-passenger, a man in his fifties, gave us courage since he also was drinking the local *arak*. The rest of the journey was comfortable and Umesh and I had good fun over the rum. Finally, we reached Calicut where Venky and his brother Ramji, who had a good business of paper, were waiting for us. Venky, our friend from G.B. Pant Hospital days, was smiling and hugged us on our arrival. Ramji, his younger brother, a short fellow sporting a lungi, also greeted us. They took us straight to their home. It was a typical Kerala house with a large compound lined with coconut and palm trees and was absolutely lush green. Venky's parents greeted us at the doorway. After having a sumptuous breakfast consisting of *dosas,* coconut *chutney* and *sambar*, we rested for a few hours.

The following day, Venky took us to see the historical city of Calicut. It is a coastal city and was a significant spice trade centre. After decades of sailors trying to reach India, Portuguese explorer Vasco da Gama eventually landed at Kappad Beach, Calicut on 20 May 1498. Unopposed access to the Indian spice routes by the Portuguese boosted the economy of that region. The main spices at first obtained from Southeast Asia were pepper and cinnamon, but soon included other products, all new to Europe.

The central Calicut beach, which had a lighthouse overlooking it, had a crowd of people that evening watching the sunset. The tree-lined Mananchira Square, with its musical fountain, surrounded the massive Mananchira Tank, an artificial pond, which was quite fascinating. While the trip was short, it was a memorable one and Umesh and I reached Delhi feeling fresh after a vacation.

The pressure of the final DM Cardiology exam was building up. The Cardiology exam besides theoretical parts had a lot of clinical case discussions with viva on catheterisation laboratory procedures. This was the time when a lot of innovations were happening, including the beginning of balloon angioplasty to open blocked arteries of the heart by Andreas Gruentzig in Zurich, Switzerland, in 1977.

Our final exam for DM was conducted in G.B. Pant Hospital in April 1978. Dr George Cherian from Vellore and Dr K.K. Datey from Bombay were our external examiners. I remember Dr Datey, a short and lean person, was carrying a very impressive stethoscope made of gold. The examination was taken very seriously. The theory part was already over. The two external examiners came in with Dr Padmavati and Professor Vishwanathan, our internal examiners. The allotted cases were examined by me one by one. Dr Datey looked very impatient but Dr Cherian was very understanding and was in no rush. He seemed to remember my Vellore posting, addressed me by my first name and allowed me enough time to overcome my initial nervousness. I answered most questions while he kept on nodding affirmatively. After the first case having gone well and for more than an hour, they decided to shorten the presentation of my second case. The viva based upon recent advances, including the new and evolving procedures, went smoothly in spite of the questions being tricky. The examiners at the end of compiling the result called us one by one and told us that we had passed and our life as a cardiologist starts now. Professor Cherian went ahead and advised that we need to select and develop a subspecialty in which we were interested the most. It was a matter of great satisfaction that I along with Dr Umesh Gupta and Dr N.K. Shreshtha, another candidate from Nepal, who had done his initial training from Patel Chest Institute, passed in our first attempt.

Thus, we became cardiologists finally. Incidentally, I was the first qualified cardiologist of Kashmiri origin—a fact which made my parents very proud.

7

Early Years after Becoming a Cardiologist

I had now successfully become a cardiologist. But what now? I had to plan my next step.

Dr Shreshta was from Nepal. He eventually returned to Kathmandu from where he went to the Philippines for a few years before again returning to Kathmandu. Dr Umesh Gupta intended to start a small hospital in Greater Kailash I, which would have simple diagnostic facilities. His hard work and polite manners paid off, and within a few years, the hospital started doing well. Umesh started admission facilities for patients and slowly expanded his business by opening a bigger hospital in Gurgaon, which he named Umkal Hospital—'Um' after Umesh and 'Kal' after his wife Kalpana.

I had no such extensive plans and wanted to practise cardiology at a place with good facilities. In 1978, such facilities existed only at AIIMS and G.B. Pant Hospital in Delhi. Unfortunately, there were no vacancies there. I had finished my three years of Senior Residency in

Cardiology and had no job. In the interim, I got a tenure attachment of a Pool Officer under a scheme of the Council of Scientific and Industrial Research (CSIR) and continued at G.B. Pant Hospital. This scheme was meant to give opportunity up to one year with a meagre stipend to work in a hospital of one's choice till one got a job. While I tried my luck at places, a lot of the opportunities were outside Delhi. But now I had my little Amita, who was born in April 1978, so we couldn't leave Delhi now.

This was a period of uncertainty and taught me many lessons. One could not depend on friends and guides, who though wished me well, didn't do much beyond their words. A few of them counselled me to join anything which came my way—like being a physician at the New Delhi Municipal Council (NDMC). But I was more inclined to do something close to my heart, something that would inspire me. As I was emotionally very attached to Kashmir, I sought an appointment with the then chief minister of Jammu and Kashmir, Sheikh Mohammed Abdullah, to offer my services to the state. Sheikh Abdullah was the patron of the Sher-i-Kashmir Institute of Medical Sciences (SKIMS), which had come into existence a year earlier. He did meet me briefly in a corridor at his office after his secretary Om Jee Gupta had arranged the meeting. I told him that I would like to serve my people and join SKIMS. However, he didn't look interested and barely exchanged a few words. In the end, he said that it was God's will and I would be directed by Him regarding my *aab a daana* (bread and butter). I knew I was dismissed and was rather disappointed having travelled all the way from Delhi to Jammu. I had thought he would at least ask me to meet the director of SKIMS or ask for my resume.

Finally, in response to an advertisement for two positions from the Postgraduate Institute of Medical Education and Research (PGIMER), Chandigarh, I got the position of assistant professor. The vacancies arose because two assistant professors, Dr R.P. Sapru and

Dr Khattri, got jobs as HOD at the Sree Chitra Tirunal Institute, Thiruvananthapuram, and Mahatma Gandhi Institute of Medical Sciences, Wardha, Maharashtra, respectively. My family, even though I had to move out, welcomed this development and assured me that it was much better than going to South India since Chandigarh was much closer to Delhi and the position has prestige associated with it. The other position was given to Dr Inder Singh Anand. Professor P.L. Wahi was the cardiology chief and the other colleague was Dr P.S. Bidwai, a cardiologist interested in paediatrics. I immediately accepted the position and joined PGIMER on 15 May 1979.

Chandigarh is one of the earliest planned cities in post-Independent India, and is acclaimed for its architecture and urban design. The master plan of the city was prepared by Swiss-French architect Le Corbusier. Most of the government buildings and housings in the city were designed by Chandigarh Capital Project Team headed by Le Corbusier, Jane Drew and Maxwell Fry. In 2015, the *British Broadcasting Corporation (BBC)* named Chandigarh as one of the perfect cities of the world in terms of architecture, cultural growth and modernisation. Founded in 1962, in the erstwhile state of Punjab, PGIMER aimed to encourage medical research and impart medical and paramedical training. It was declared an Institute of National Importance by an Act of Parliament in April 1967.

This was my first academic assignment as a cardiologist and while I was excited about the prospects, I was nervous too. I took my Fiat car from Delhi and stayed for a few days with a family friend, Dr M.K. Bhan, who was based in Chandigarh. The next morning, I went to meet Prof. Wahi at the appointed time before he started his ward rounds. A warm, pleasant man, Prof. Wahi told me that since summer vacations have begun and Dr Bidwai was off, I should, along with Inder, take care of the cardiac catheterisation laboratory besides the routine work. I welcomed the idea of independently working in the laboratory. The day coincided with the final day of the DM Cardiology examination of the department. I was asked to sit with the examiners. The candidates were Dr V.K. Chopra and Dr Ram Gopal Singh Shahi. Both passed and it was a joyous day at the department.

Prof. Wahi helped me in getting a rented apartment in Sector 8C. It was a two-room apartment with a huge, open terrace. The house belonged to Mr Sachdeva, an officer retired from the Punjab government and originally from Jammu. The green hills of Kasauli could be seen from the terrace and at night it was quite a sight with twinkling lights. I used to cook dinner myself and became a good cook in the process. Since I had a car, commuting to and from PGIMER was easy. For several months, Prof. Wahi used to bring lunch for me since he knew I was living on my own and Upkar was in Delhi in a teaching job at G.B. Pant Hospital.

Independent work in the cardiac laboratory was very educative and I found that senior technicians were a great help. They had all the troubleshooting methods in case of machine failure. In fact, the chief technician one day confided in me that since Prof. Wahi was not trained in doing invasive procedures, he never made serious efforts to get modern equipment. He compensated for this lacuna by keeping his theoretical knowledge up to date and encouraging bedside discussions.

Since this was my first teaching assignment as an assistant professor, it gave me a lot of satisfaction. However, I did feel a bit embarrassed because many of the post-doctoral students were older than me and were already in jobs in their states for several years. I put up a good show and used to prepare for my classes and at the same time was very friendly with them. Since my family was in Delhi and I hardly knew anyone in Chandigarh, my relationship with Col. B.N. Shahi and Bashir Ahmad, who was also an associate professor in a medical college in Srinagar, became very friendly. I used to invite them home for a Kashmiri dinner. I used to travel to Delhi frequently in state transport buses while going and used to return to Chandigarh in the overnight Kalka Mail train. This would give me at least two full days at home with my family. My second child, a son, was born in April 1980 while I was in Chandigarh. He is two years younger than Amita. These were the days of no mobile phones. I used to call from public telephone booths although my landlord had a telephone. On 25 April 1980 morning, my mother had called me on Mr Sachdeva's number to give me the good news and congratulated me on becoming the father to a son, whom we named Samir alias Manu.

Things moved very smoothly despite living alone. In August 1979, I was informed by the administration that Dr Sapru and Dr Khattri were returning to their posts because of personal reasons. I had to move out and start looking for alternate opportunities. Fortunately, there was a vacancy for an ad hoc lecturer at G.B. Pant Hospital in September 1980. I met Professor M.P. Gupta who was kind enough to take me on. I moved back to Delhi to my family's delight. However, having worked in an institute of national importance as an assistant professor with so many distinguished faculty members was a huge learning experience. The atmosphere at G.B. Pant Hospital after seeing the work culture of PGIMER was not at all to my liking. Most people tended to leave the hospital at 5 p.m. with a poor sense of commitment. I was sharing time in the catheterisation laboratory with Professor Khalilullah. He would not allow much work and would like to do the procedures himself when he was around. I found a way out. He used to come to the lab at around 10 a.m. but the working hours were from 9 a.m. The best thing I realised was to reach early and put the first patient before his arrival and start the procedure. My desire of leaving this place, however, was very strong because I felt being a faculty in the same place where you were a student is not the best way to grow in your career. I was, therefore, looking out for an opening outside G.B. Pant Hospital.

8

Joining AIIMS and the Australian Fellowship

Faculty vacancies were advertised at AIIMS for an assistant professor's post in October 1980. I applied, but did not get selected in the first selection interview. I was told that Professor M.L. Bhatia had a poor opinion of people who were not trained at AIIMS. He hardly asked any questions during the interview and only looked at my application perfunctorily.

My luck improved in the next interview held in March 1981. By this time, the rules for entry-point consultants had changed and the heads of the departments were not allowed to be on the board. This change ensured my selection. I got selected for assistant professor and Dr K. Srinath Reddy got the post of lecturer. There were several other candidates for these posts.

Established in 1956, AIIMS is a premier medical college in India. It operates autonomously under the Ministry of Health and Family Welfare. It was the vision of Rajkumari Amrit Kaur, the first health minister of India, and Prime Minister Nehru—both wanted to establish an institute of medicinal excellence after Independence. One of the most coveted medical colleges in the country, AIIMS boasts of some stellar faculty members. When I cracked the interview, my family was elated at this prestigious appointment. I joined the department as soon as the letter of the appointment came, lest somebody challenged the interview results. I joined and met Professor Bhatia. His reception was not very warm and he asked Mr Khurana, his PA, to show me around. I got a chair and a shelf to sit in the teaching block opposite his office. Mr Khurana, of course, had a much bigger office.

My initial few days were spent just familiarising myself with the Cardiology ward, CCU and OPD. I was also given a slot in the catheterisation laboratory.

During the first month of joining, while performing a cardiac catheterisation procedure, a wire inadvertently slipped into the heart. It was the fault of a DM cardiology student Dr Seshagiri Rao, and we were in a terrible soup. There was a commotion in the lab and obviously Dr Bhatia was informed. Cardiac surgeon Dr Sampath Kumar was informed of this mishap and he came to the lab to consider removing it surgically. He was fuming with anger and looked at me as if I had committed a crime.

I did not accept surgical intervention so easily and thought out of the box. I asked Seshagiri to go to the urology department and get a Dormia basket catheter, which is used to pull out stones from urinary passages. He got a sterile device. I inserted it into the vein from where the wire had slipped in while looking at the X-Ray image to guide it. Eventually, I got hold of the wire and snared it out. These procedures which are well described now were novelties in 1981. I published it as a case report in an indexed cardiology journal with the names of Seshagiri Rao, myself and Professor Bhatia. When I got the hard copies, I gave Professor Bhatia one with his name as the last author.

He was very pleased and said 'Well done'. This incident proved to him my sincerity at work and he became fond of me thereafter. He gave me a few projects on new drugs, which were very exciting, and I not only completed these satisfactorily but also had the results published.

Another confrontation with Professor Bhatia is again worth mentioning. The one-thousandth case in the catheterisation laboratory was approaching in 1982. Prof. Bhatia wanted this event to be done by Dr Savitri Shrivastava, my senior colleague and a paediatric cardiologist. She was the blue-eyed lady of Prof. Bhatia. However, I had a desire to be the person doing this celebrity-numbered case. Lo and behold, the 999th case was performed by me and that was the last case of the day. I asked the nurses and technicians if I somehow got another case for angiography, would they cooperate and allow me to do it. My friendliness with the non-medico staff worked in my favour. I got a patient who was waiting for a surgical procedure pending an angiography and I did the procedure making it the coveted 1000th case in the catheterisation laboratory of AIIMS. Thus, it was me rather than Dr Shrivastava who performed the desired case and upset her plan. The moment Prof. Bhatia came to know about this, he became angry. I was summoned and reprimanded by him. He called me a 'runaway pacemaker', an allusion to a faulty pacemaker that instead of 70 beats per minute, suddenly goes berserk and starts beating at a dangerously fast rate. I told him that I thought a sick patient in need of surgery should have been a priority rather than who does the 1000th case. He smiled with sarcasm and let me go, but Dr Shrivastava did not like this move of mine.

Professor Bhatia was a teetotaller but he was gracious enough to keep a good brand of Scotch whenever he invited the department for parties, usually at the time of the final examination with the examiners. Dr (Mrs) Bhatia was an excellent host and we were always treated to a delicious dinner. Prof. Bhatia retired from AIIMS service in 1985 and after a brief stint at Escorts Heart Institute, he joined the Sitaram Bhartia Institute in South Delhi.

He was succeeded by Professor R. Tandon as the head of the department at AIIMS. Professor Tandon was the most well-known paediatric cardiologist in the country. Before coming to India, he had worked in the USA with many celebrities. He was a teacher par excellence and his book on the approach to congenital heart disease is a treat to read. In spite of being a paediatric cardiologist, he never refused to treat adults and would refer many of them to me for procedures like angioplasty.

Fellowship in Australia

In 1983, I got an opportunity to go for a short three-month fellowship at Epworth and Royal Melbourne Hospital, Australia. This was funded by the offices of Dr Grahm Sloman, an Australian cardiologist who had visited Delhi on behalf of the World Health Organization (WHO) several times between 1981 and 1982. He made a report on priorities in Cardiology for India and its neighbouring countries. I remember him walking in AIIMS in shorts with a tie and shirt—an Australian style of dressing. We became friends and our friendship eventually got me an invitation to visit Melbourne. Going abroad for higher studies has always been a very sought-after assignment. I had to secure the necessary permission from AIIMS and the Health Ministry before I could accept the offer. This incidentally was my first visit outside India. As I took the Singapore Airlines flight from Bombay to Singapore in December 1983, I felt a thrill of excitement washing over me. My mama B.L. Dhar accompanied me to Bombay to see me off.

The Singapore–Melbourne sector was long in its duration and it took seven hours to reach Australia. As it was December, it was summer in the Southern Hemisphere, with bright sunshine and very long days. I reached on a weekend. My stay was arranged with my class fellow Virender Berera and his family in a suburb of Melbourne. The second most populous city of Australia after Sydney, Melbourne is situated on the banks of river Yarra and had a buzzing social life with plazas, bars and restaurants. The dazzling night lights and the spotless, broad roads of Melbourne were mesmerising. Virender had a beautiful house and his family entertained me very well. On weekends, we watched Hindi movies.

The next day, Virender dropped me at the Nurses Hostel of Epworth Hospital, located in Richmond, which was walking distance from the Melbourne Cricket Ground and the majestic Flinders Street Central Railway Station. The hospital was in a neighbourhood where Vietnamese refugees had been rehabilitated following the communist Northern Vietnam's takeover of southern Vietnam. This locality had many Vietnamese and Asian food restaurants, which I found preferable to the Australian diet of meat, corn and potatoes.

Epworth Hospital was a private establishment—the cardiology and IVF departments were strong units. Nurses were the main force managing coronary care patients; they would call doctors only for emergencies and were proficient in their jobs. Likewise, in the cath lab, they used to prepare and assist the operator without any resident doctor's assistance. This was starkly different from the Indian hospitals, where a nurse's main job was to administer drugs, keep stock of disposables and carry out the doctor's orders. The hospital, wards and intensive care units were shining and the administrative staff used to routinely clean the corridors. There were small, wall-mounted trails that carried drugs being sent from the pharmacy. No visitors were sitting with the patients, who looked well taken care of. The state-run Royal Melbourne Hospital, which I visited a few days later, also had a similar interior, though it had a lot more patients in the outdoors. It was very clear to me in the first few days how our country's medical service was far behind compared to Australia. The hospitalisation periods were very short and nurse educators would explain treatment protocols to patients and their attendants. All these protocols would improve the outcomes of their patients. Even doctors and paramedics appeared relaxed and never looked overworked, which amazed me because as Indian doctors, we were so used to the stressful working conditions that we never could imagine it otherwise. This taxing environment was aggravated due to the doctor-to-patient ratio in India, which was and continues to be skewed with significantly lower proportion of doctors in India. In addition, the government expenditure on health has remained significantly low and insurance schemes are largely not available to the public, all of which have stalled the advancement of the public health system in India. One of the nurses of the CCU became very friendly with me. She was living in the hostel but had a home in the city. She wanted me to come with her for a weekend to her place but I made an excuse and did not go. Later I thought that I was too shy a person not to accept an invitation.

I chose Dr Peter Valentine, a senior consultant known for doing percutaneous coronary angioplasty (PTCA) procedures, as my mentor. He had started this technique in the state of Victoria. He gave me the privilege to wash up during the procedures. This was how I got inducted into the field of coronary interventions. Peter and I soon became friends. He later introduced me to his friend Fren. He used to invite me often for weekends and I would prepare Kashmiri meals, which left them very impressed with my culinary skills.

They took me to Canberra, the capital city of Australia, housed in the Australian Capital Territory (ACT), in a flight and showed me the city. The city exhibits impressive government offices and Royal mint buildings beside the Parliament house. I remember we went for dinner to a Chinese restaurant where I heard of the dessert fried ice cream for the first time. It turned out to be a sizzling hot egg-shaped dish, steaming from the outside but filled with ice-cold vanilla ice cream. The city had a lot of tourists, enjoying the balmy summer weather.

I found it to be a city without a soul and aptly so because it was made as a compromise capital city since both Melbourne and Sydney were claiming to be the ideal contenders based upon the history of Australia following the British occupation in 1778.

We went around the city and had a wonderful weekend before flying back to Melbourne. The three months of fellowship were like a dream come true. It not only taught me coronary angioplasty and associated patient care but also how the practice of medicine can be enjoyable and gratifying. Besides, the exposure to a liberal society increased my self-confidence and improved my spoken English. I met a Kashmiri family while in Melbourne—Sohan and Vijay Kaul, whose daughter, Jasmine, was an adorable little girl. Sohan was a physicist trained in Norway and belonged to a village close to my ancestral place of Hawal. Vijay was a botanist trained in Srinagar, working now in Melbourne University as a research officer. Sohan had done his PhD in biophysics following which he got a job in Melbourne. He got married to Vijay, a girl from a rich Pandit family from Srinagar. In spite of Sohan being trained in Europe, his roots were from a village in Kashmir and getting a girl from Srinagar city was considered a big achievement.

Sohan had got a job as a physicist where he used to analyze stones and rocks from various sources, including a bit of a rock brought from the moon. He had bought a house in Wantirna South, a suburb of Melbourne. He was making a passage for this house, which needed cutting of bricks to conform to the shape. He took a stack of bricks to his office on a Sunday and took me along. There he used a sophisticated laser cutter to shape the bricks. I thought it was a misuse of office equipment and spoke my mind. He just smiled. My weekends used to be at his place. I used to go there on a suburban train. One weekend, his friend from Singapore, Romesh Koul, had come on a business trip. He took me out in a rented car to a flea market of the neighbourhood. I found a lot of Greeks there selling goods from Greece including woollens. These were quite affordable for me and I did a bit of shopping for gifts for the family back home. It was a happy coincidence that I met Romesh Koul at Sohan's place, and we became friends. Romesh was originally from Srinagar but now settled in Singapore. This allowed me to stay for a few days in Singapore with him.

Before returning to New Delhi, I visited Adelaide to meet my colleague from AIIMS' cardiac surgery department, Dr Balram Airan. He was there for a one-year fellowship at the Royal Adelaide Hospital; he had taken his family along too. He was gracious enough to send me an air ticket for my travel and I spent a few lovely days there. Adelaide is South Australia's capital city, situated on the banks of River Torrens. The city had a distinctly cosmopolitan flavour and was well known for sprawling art galleries, collections of indigenous art and South Australian museums devoted to natural history.

We hired a car and went around the countryside, which was dotted with wineries. We stayed at low-cost motels that had clean kitchenettes for making simple meals. Most of the wineries were owned by German settlers; a lot of these had freshwater streams full of trout fish. The predominantly green and blue landscape, with the smell of fresh fruits wafting in, reminded me of my homeland Kashmir. Dr Balram and family were vegetarians and would eat only potatoes, salad and yogurt besides fruit. It was Christmas time and the markets were very nicely decorated. I found him always looking forward to returning to Delhi after completing his assignment and training in advanced cardiac surgery. The few days spent with him were very enjoyable besides seeing another part of Australia.

Before returning, I had to visit Sydney as well, as, without that, the trip wouldn't have been complete. It was a 10-hour journey on a bus with a stop at Canberra. I could not afford an air ticket. My stay was arranged. I stayed with Anil Bakaya, who was a family friend; we had known each other for years. Sydney, the capital of New South Wales and one of Australia's largest cities, is synonymous with the Sydney Opera House. It's one of the most recognised landmarks of the city. The Massive Darling Harbour and the smaller Circular Quay port are the hubs of waterside life, with the arched Harbour Bridge and the Royal Botanic Garden adjacent to these. I used to walk around all these places, which are next to each other. I feel people born in such countries are indeed very lucky as they get better opportunities for career advancement. I was amused to see so many Indians selling cheap models of the Opera House and doing a good business. I used to leave Anil's house in the morning and return late in the evening.

Anil and his family were living in a spacious apartment, which was situated on a very busy road near Bondi junction. The road outside would have traffic throughout the day and even had cars honking late in the night. The clamour outside gave me sleepless nights, and before leaving I told Anil that it would perhaps be best if he could relocate to avoid suffering early deafness! Anil agreed with me wholeheartedly, and a few months later even called me to say that he had taken my advice and was moving to Papua New Guinea. Later, he moved to the USA where his elder brother got him a job.

Returning Home

Soon, time to return home had come after getting a brief but useful professional and social experience in a developed country. I was feeling good at the thought of getting back home and also adding something to my department at AIIMS. My return journey had to be through Singapore. After meeting Romesh Koul in Melbourne, I had made my stay arrangements with his family in Singapore.

I left Melbourne carrying a certificate from the Australian Postgraduate Federation of Medicine. My feelings were mixed. I wished I had migrated to this wonderful country after MBBS when I had ample opportunity like my friend Virendra, but at the same time felt the decision was good since I became a specialist. Romesh picked me up from the Singapore airport and took me to his home, where his charming wife Malu welcomed me. They lived in a quaint apartment at a place called Truro Road. My mission was to do shopping and I had a list with me. I had been told to buy electronics from a place called Mustafa's supermarket. The list sent by my wife included a radio-cum-tape recorder, saris and anything which would be better than what we get in Delhi. Mustafa's famous shopping mall was on Serangoon Road. This area is also called Little India because there are several shops owned by Indians and restaurants catering to the Indian palate.

The Mustafa Shamsuddin brothers had a roaring business and were very well known for electronic goods, watches, cosmetics, garments and condiments. Malu took me there to buy the Sony 2-in-1. For the saris, we went to a silk store, owned by a Sindhi gentleman. Malu managed to get receipts from both the shops, understating the actual price of the items to help me with the customs on my arrival in India.

My return journey was again via Bombay. Customs clearance those days was a big hassle, unlike today. Had I returned to Delhi directly it would have been easier being a doctor at AIIMS. As luck would have it, the inspector at customs was a shrewd man who knew all the tricks that passengers from Singapore would resort to. He had the actual costs of electronic items with him; so there was a duty on the 2-in-1 that I had to pay despite the bill I produced. For the saris, he had a yardstick and I couldn't escape that either. However, when he asked me what I did and I told him that I was a cardiologist from AIIMS, he was nice enough to reduce the amount I had to pay.

9

Beginning of Coronary Angioplasty in India

After my return from Australia, bubbling with enthusiasm to show my newly-learnt skills, I had a meeting with my colleagues and motivated them to start balloon angioplasty programmes at AIIMS. The technique had just started almost around the same time in Chennai, Hyderabad and Mumbai. Each operator was going to press claiming to be the first to do it in India.

We took a different route altogether. Having got the equipment from major European companies, we did a series of cases beginning in 1984 and published them in *The Indian Heart Journal* rather than a newspaper. Professor Venugopal, the chief of cardiac surgery at AIIMS, provided back-up support which was essential in those early days. We also followed up with our patients and reported our long-term results. The recurrence of blocks was a major problem in those days. We started research in that direction and used many agents given as tablets to see whether any relief comes.

All the studies came negative. Fish oil capsule administration seemed to hold some promise in a few published studies. We did a meticulous study to look into this hypothesis. The study again showed that it did not work. The results of our findings got published in a reputed international journal. A few days after this publication, I was pleasantly surprised when I received an invitation from a Japanese group, working on edible oils, to present this data in Tokyo. My travel, accommodation, food and conference registration were paid for by the group and I had no reason to decline this offer. I promptly accepted the invitation and reached Tokyo within a month to deliver the lecture in March 1993.

My audience mostly comprised non-doctors—people dealing in oils—and might not have understood a word of what I said but as per the Japanese tradition, they made me feel great and gave a standing ovation once I was finished. I was even more flattered when they handed me a beautiful memento and thanked me repeatedly for gracing their event.

My host had budgeted a few leisurely days in my trip and once the presentation was finished, I had the whole of Tokyo to myself. This was my second international trip and the bug of adventure was taking its roots inside me. I walked around the streets of Tokyo aimlessly, absorbing the local culture. The next stop was the famous Mount Fuji—the highest mountain in Japan and a dormant volcano that had last erupted in 1707–1708. Mount Fuji lies about 100 km south-west of Tokyo and can be seen from there on a clear day. The mountain has an exceptionally symmetrical cone, which is snow-capped for about five months a year. A well-known symbol of Japan, it is frequently depicted in art and photographs as well as visited by tourists and climbers. I was taken in by the spectacle of its majestic view.

My last evening in Tokyo was another walk on the busy and colourful streets of Tokyo. I took a ride in the metro, which was yet to debut in

India then. It was thrilling to imagine a ride under the city in tunnels. While I worried a bit about whether it would be dark and drab, I was pleasantly surprised to see the Japanese metro swanky and running efficiently. As it was evening, there were a lot of commuters. When the automatic door opened, passengers got down and those who were waiting to get on board stood aside to give them space and boarded only when the last of the passengers had alighted. The compartment was packed like sardines. Tokyo is the most populous metro city in the world and people clearly preferred the underground for their commute.

The next morning, when I got up in my hotel room and drew the curtain aside, I was amazed to see Mount Fuji, with its snow peak shining in the blue sky. It looked like a painting, serene and almost ethereal. The view was breathtaking and I continued staring at it for a long time. When I narrated this experience to an English-speaking Japanese gentleman sitting next to me at the breakfast table, he said, 'This means that you are coming again to Tokyo very soon!' It turns out that the Japanese believe that if the mountain is seen by travellers to Tokyo unexpectedly, then they would visit again. While I laughed hearing this and dismissed the idea from my head, a month later, I was stunned to receive an invitation from the Japanese Pacing Society, requesting me to give a talk on the cardiac pacing situation in India. I don't know whether this was the victory of belief or a coincidence, but I was delighted to go back to Japan.

The second time when I was travelling to Tokyo, I had the country chief of a cardiac imaging company sitting beside me on the flight. When I introduced myself, he recognised me as a member of the panel of the board which had to decide on the new cath lab for AIIMS. The gentleman became very friendly and engaged me on various subjects, even my hobbies—he even probed my interest in classical music. I didn't want to expose my ignorance and said I loved it. He pressed for more and enquired whom I liked. Confused, I could come up with only one name and blurted out, 'Beethoven!' He smiled in appreciation and said, 'You really are fond of the best.'

A few days before I was returning to Delhi, the gentleman called on me at my hotel and gifted me a portable bass CD player and a box of CDs of Beethoven. I was embarrassed because I had no idea of Beethoven and his classical music but graciously accepted the gift as he had remembered what I had said. I could not refuse him and brought the small box containing the music system to Delhi. Reading about Beethoven, I came to know that he was a celebrity followed even now.

This was the beginning of my international presentations. It gave me the impetus to start more studies in the department at AIIMS. We started a project on various drugs to reduce restenosis (when a section of the blocked artery that was opened up with angioplasty or a stent has become narrowed again) after balloon angioplasty, none of which worked, unfortunately. By this time, non-balloon techniques had started emerging in the field. New techniques like removal of the blockages produced by fat deposits in the arteries by shaving them off or by drilling them using a device called rotablator came into vogue. I introduced these techniques at AIIMS. Unfortunately, these techniques remained sidelined in the practice of angioplasty. When I used to mention these to my non-medical friends, they used to laugh and compare me with a plumber or a carpenter. All these efforts meant long hours in the hospital for me. I was invariably the first consultant to reach and the last one to leave the campus. Our OPDs also used to be in the evenings. All this meant very little contact with the family. Home for me meant bed and breakfast.

Being on the cutting edge of new technology, I used to travel a lot for meetings, sponsored by various companies, to European countries and also to some exotic places in the USA like Hawaii. I attended one course in Kauai, an island in Hawaii. It was an exotic and remarkable experience. More than learning angioplasty, it was fun. The course used to be held in the forenoon between 8 a.m. and noon followed by lunch after which we used to have free time. It was a three-day programme. Kauai is Hawaii's fourth largest island and is also called the 'Garden Island'. It seemed to be draped in emerald. I saw the beautiful Wailua River, spotless beaches and hiking trails. The entire course was sponsored by a company based out of Hong Kong. I must say the companies are really helping in disseminating the new techniques and making us better and more skilled professionals. These were also occasions to meet senior persons and real pioneers and legends. They were friendly and always ready to communicate.

I along with a few like-minded colleagues started angioplasty training courses, since those days there were no didactic books available to teach the intricacies of the techniques used. These became very popular and young enthusiastic cardiologists sought permission for attending. The industry did sponsor these activities. We created a registry called the National Angioplasty Registry of India which grew steadily and later became the National Interventional Council of India, a body still continuing under the Cardiological Society of India. The programme of coronary angioplasty that started with us in 1981 with simple procedures went on to become highly technical. We learnt it from courses conducted by experienced persons in Europe and the USA which were very sought after by the younger cardiologists who wanted to get into this area. The industry used to sponsor the talented doctors to these courses taking care of their travel, stay, etc. I along with my colleagues also went to some of these courses in France and the USA. One of the courses I recall was in Toulouse in southern France—a small city that we had heard of as the manufacturing hub of the Airbus. This historic city had a lot of terracotta tiles lining the walls of houses and the streets giving the city a red colour. The course was very educative because the number of attendees used to be small. Besides learning angioplasty it gave me the opportunity to make friends with top French cardiologists like Jean Marco and Jean Fajadet. They visited Delhi on my invitation and we conducted small teaching courses with them. They were fascinated by seeing our cities like Jaipur and Udaipur with their palaces.

Attending these international courses also allowed me to visit exotic places like Hawai and the surrounding islands. In fact, I can say that angioplasty not only gave me my expertise in cardiology but also made me a globetrotter.

Meeting Dr Shawl

I heard of Dr Fayaz Ahmad Shawl, a cardiologist originally from Kashmir, through professional colleagues in India. He was apparently doing very well at Washington Adventist Hospital (WAH) in Maryland, USA. In March 1990, I was supposed to travel to the USA for the annual meeting of the American College of Cardiology (ACC), being held in New Orleans, Louisiana. I sent a request to Fayaz to allow me to visit his centre for a week before the meeting. He promptly agreed and offered to arrange my stay at a hotel near the hospital. I went to Maryland on my way to New Orleans. In fact, I was also invited by the ACC to give a talk on the scene of 'Interventional Cardiology in India'. This opportunity was wonderful but it also made me work hard to prepare for an international talk especially as I had to represent my country.

I had been once before to Washington for a meeting called by the World Congress of Cardiology a few years before this. That meeting was a congregation of more than 15,000 delegates and I hardly understood what was going on. It was my first visit and I had a terrible jet lag, and that possibly was the reason for the confusion. I was taken aback at the number of attendees—our meetings of the Cardiac Society in India those days had a maximum of 800 to 1,000 people visiting, though, over the years, these have become considerably bigger.

I reached Dulles Airport in the afternoon and took a taxi to my hotel, Holiday Inn, in Maryland. The taxi driver looked South Asian, possibly even Indian. It was a long ride and I struck up a conversation with the driver, something uncommon in India but quite prevalent outside. When I asked him where he was from, the driver smiled cheerily and said, 'Lahore, Sir. Lahore in Pakistan.' I was delighted to meet someone from my side of the world and we started chatting in Hindi. It turned out he was in the US for more than two decades. He had a diploma in mechanical engineering but this was the most lucrative job he got. His children were studying in college and had the best education that he could possibly give. A God-fearing family man, he told me, 'Sir, I know we are supposed to hate each other but I really want India and Pakistan to be friends. We have the same history, the same culture. Why are we fighting all the time?' I wondered whether it takes people to get out of the subcontinent to realise this.

When we reached the hotel, he offered me assistance of any kind if needed during my stay in DC. He gave me his card and when I tried to pay him, he folded his hands and refused, saying, 'You are my guest. How can I take money from you?' Of course, I wouldn't hear any of that and even insisted on paying the customary tip. During my travels in the US, I learnt how tipping is customary in this country. Once, I had a Caucasian taxi driver, who was very well dressed and had an imposing personality. He didn't look like he needed the money and I was hesitating to tip him—suppose he got offended? And then I recalled how in Japan once a taxi driver had returned me the tip. So, I asked this Caucasian driver very politely whether he would accept a tip. The man cracked a smile, took the money that I was holding out and said, 'Sir, we Americans live and die for tips.'

It was a Sunday when I checked into the hotel. I had to stay till Friday before leaving for Emory. As the day passed, I realised it was very difficult to spend time alone in the room. The only relation I knew in that area of the world was a distant cousin of mine Dr Lokesh Bazaz, a nephrologist who lived in Virginia. I felt hesitant in calling him lest he should feel disturbed. In the evening, I went out for a stroll. There were very few people on the roads—only cars zoomed around—which, I later found, is typical of any suburb and residential area in the US. I decided to walk and explore the area. After half an hour, I saw a shopping mall, which was yet to debut in India then. As it was a weekend, it was quite busy with people thronging the stores. Stores such as the chain KMart seemed very reasonable in their prices. A few shops down, I spotted a McDonald's. As I had heard my foreign-returned friends go on and on about this place, I decided to try a few items and zeroed in on two different kinds of burgers. I packed these for my dinner at night and got a few cans of beer on my way out. I reached my room, put on the television, watched a few news channels and devoured the burgers.

Finally, ennui overcame me and I rang up Dr Shawl to tell him that I was in Maryland. Dr Shawl was surprised but pleased to hear my voice. He told me that he would pick me up on his way to the hospital and I should be ready by seven in the morning. He added, 'I will call you three minutes before reaching so that you have time to come to the driveway with your luggage.' I was impressed by this precision of timing. The next morning I was ready well before time. I was anyway up from three in the morning due to jet lag. We went together in his beautiful Mercedes car fitted with many gadgets that I had yet to see in Indian cars. Once we reached the hospital, he took me to his office and introduced me to the staff.

Dr Shawl was always dressed in his greens and would talk animatedly for hours about his cases that had been rejected for angioplasty because of being very complex. The cases he took up were really difficult and at times very risky, often turned down by surgeons. During that week, Dr Shawl had three cases where he did the procedure after putting the patient on percutaneous cardiopulmonary support (PCPS). The procedure was done without opening the chest, which is usually the way surgeons do it. He put the large bore cannulas through the groin by puncturing the femoral artery and the vein under local anaesthesia. This tubing comes in a kit named after him—Shawl Kit—which he helped design and was manufactured by BARD-USCI. Patients sustained the procedure admirably and were discharged within a few days. After returning to Delhi, I persuaded our centre chief, Professor Venugopal, to procure the PCPS, which he could also use in his department in emergencies. He was always very positive and would bulldoze the finance and purchase departments and get things done. We got the system within a month. However, it cost a bomb—a whopping sum of Rs 25 lakh those days—and I had to show results to justify the purchase. We started doing very high-risk cases, usually referred by the cardiac surgery department. Eventually, we gathered data of 25 patients, the first-of-its-kind from the Asia-Pacific region. This prompted us to embark on a randomised study comparing two forms of hemodynamic support, which we published in an international journal. My takeaway from the whole experience was that international cooperation in modern techniques is the best way to start new procedures.

One day, while we were in Dr Shawl's office, a gastroenterologist came in and introduced himself as Dr Farooq. When I introduced myself, he immediately started talking in Kashmiri and hugged me. Meanwhile, Shawl came in and was surprised to see me conversing in my mother tongue. 'Why didn't you tell me that you were from Kashmir?' he asked. That evening he took me to his palatial home in the Potomac area—one of the costliest places around DC and

Maryland and adjacent to the River Potomac around which the city of Washington is built. The house was built by a designer, decorated with the choicest Kashmiri and Persian carpets. The living room was huge and reminded me of Bollywood films. We had a nice dinner of fish, rice and green vegetables washed down with some delicious white wine. I met both his sons who were studying. Shawl and I talked late into the night and I stayed over at his place. The next morning we were back in the hospital by 7.30 a.m. During his conversation, I came to know that he came to England from Srinagar after his MBBS. He was an average student as later narrated by his class fellows. In England, he got a residency and trained in cardiology and did his MRCP before coming to the USA where he got a job, completed his fellowship in cardiology and got a position in the WAH, his current place of work.

My observations at the WAH were very educative. I had to leave for New Orleans, Louisiana, for the ACC meeting. A friend had put me in a motel not very far from the venue. The next few days, I kept working on my slides for the invited lecture so that I didn't fumble for words, had the perfect pronunciation and didn't exceed the time. It was finally showtime and I was introduced as a young cardiologist from AIIMS, India. When I finished the lecture, I sighed in relief as I thought it had gone off pretty well. There were a few comments and questions from the audience. I felt that their impression of our work in this area had improved significantly after my talk.

While I was interacting with the audience, I suddenly saw that some of my distinguished colleagues—we had worked together to reach this stage—were walking out of the hall. For a few seconds, I was perplexed but pushed it out of my mind. I got to know later that Wali Kasim from the device company had been asked by the organisers of the meeting to name a few eminent persons from India for this lecture. He had suggested a few names but the organisers in their wisdom chose me. These colleagues got very upset about why I was chosen for the lecture.

While I was unhappy to learn this, I consoled myself thinking that the lecture was a success and I had done my bit in sharing my knowledge.

After the lecture, we socialised with the guests and I met several Indian-origin cardiologists who congratulated me for my talk and invited me out to dinner. Delighted to have a free meal, I happily obliged them. We went to an Indian restaurant in New Orleans. The city is the capital city of Louisiana state and has an interesting colonial history. It was a French-administered area from the 17th century, followed by a Spanish rule of four decades before again coming under the French. Finally, in 1803, it became part of America, when Napoleon sold it to them. Today, Louisiana is one of the 50 states in the USA.

From New Orleans, I flew back to New Delhi by KLM, a Dutch Airlines. KLM eventually became my favourite airline. One delightful experience on the airline was that every business class passenger was gifted a Delft Blue miniature traditional Dutch house, filled with Dutch gin, also known as Genever. I have several of these beautiful items kept in different parts of my house. With my penchant for travelling with them while flying abroad, they awarded me a lifetime Platinum Membership of Flying Blue, which is one of the few things I cherish dearly!

10

Coronary Stents, Pacemakers and a Horrid London Experience

One of the limitations of balloon angioplasty was the unpredictability of the procedure and frequent recurrences of the block within a short period of time. The problem got circumvented by the use of metal meshes called stents, which were left in the artery to support it and prevent a recoil. These came in 1986 but became acceptable for use around 1990. We at AIIMS started using them in 1992 after being proctored by the French cardiologist Jean Marco. Following this, we started using these products made in the USA and published our experience, around the same time in 1994 as the Europeans and Americans. We also started using them in treating patients with heart attacks. Ours was one of the first reports for their use in patients with fresh heart attacks. It came one year before the US cardiologists published it.

We also encouraged Indian companies to make these devices and published the safety and efficacy of Indian products. The concept of 'publish or perish' was well understood by me and it gave me a lot of satisfaction. I worked with a Surat-based company and did studies on their stents. These brought credibility to the company at a time when stents were a monopoly of European and American companies.

During the same period, I became interested in treating diseases of the heart rhythm—either very slow or very fast heartbeats. I promoted the idea to my colleague, Dr Balbir Singh, and convinced him to get involved. The set-up was primitive but we started radiofrequency ablations, a non-surgical procedure of using heat to break the unwanted connections of nerves in the heart. This would cure some varieties of serious palpitations. This we started in our CCU procedure room. Balbir, a product of my alma mater Maulana Azad Medical College, joined AIIMS after 10 years of my entry. He was a very bright and meritorious student and I could see his talent. Today, he is a very well-known cardiologist of the country practising in Delhi. He worked very hard under my supervision and in 2004 decided to join Escorts Hospital as a Principal Consultant. However, I found in him a man in a hurry and would at times be not very respectful to seniors. I gave this feedback to him through his wife Urvashi since I always wished him well. He has taken over as the Chief of Cardiology of MAX group of hospitals in NCR. I am proud of this fact. However, his reciprocity towards me has been lukewarm. I had asked him if he could take me to MAX as the Chief of Research since this is an area for which MAX is not so well known. He never showed any interest in my proposal. I found it disappointing.

In 1993, I attended a meeting in London on pacemakers and related advances. It was a usual industry-sponsored meeting with a low budget for travel. For this reason, I chose to travel by Gulf Air which had the lowest fares. It took off from New Delhi very early in the morning and had four stopovers till London—Dubai, Doha, Qatar and Bahrain—which is their base. We reached London late at night despite the time difference of just four and a half hours. Despite hopping around in all these places and changing planes, I had a pleasant trip and enjoyed several meals and the hospitality of European air hostesses.

The meeting did not involve much teaching and mainly was for socialising. It, however, gave me ample opportunity, two days to be exact, to roam about the streets of London, something about which I had only heard of from my parents and relatives, and had watched in movies. It was sad to see Indians working as cleaners at the airport that I witnessed upon my arrival. They seemed to be unhappy. I decided that there was no point brooding on their fate. Instead, I should focus on the good things. The weather was cool and pleasant. The gardens were lush green. River Thames and Buckingham Palace were imposing. I really enjoyed having beer and fish and chips during my tour of the city. The London Tube was again a good experience and a good way of commuting and seeing the city. There were very few Indian cardiologists at the meeting so it was mostly a brief trip without friends. My stay was arranged at a five-star hotel with complimentary breakfast. Lunches and dinners were expensive in the hotel. I found it better to go to a McDonald's for an affordable meal.

The return trip to Heathrow airport from my hotel was an experience that I would never forget in my life. The flight back to New Delhi was early in the morning and I hired a cab to go up to the Tube station closest to my hotel. Now, during my stay in London, I had saved a good number of coins while shopping and commuting. When I reached the station, I gave the cab driver the exact fare in coins. I had thought he would appreciate the coins as back home taxis prefer the exact change. My boy, I was so wrong! The driver, a white guy who looked in his early fifties, almost threw the coins on my face and started abusing me. He called me a black ass. It was very derogatory and humiliating. He was probably expecting crisp notes, including a good tip, and there I was, his customer, a poor junior medical faculty from India, drawing a salary of only Rs 18,000.

A bit shaken after this unpleasant encounter, I started getting down the stairs of the Tube with my suitcase. Suddenly, I found a bunch of white-skinned boys almost pouncing on me and calling me a 'blackie'. I was under the impression till then that I am a fair-skinned Kashmiri and not a 'blackie'. It was good learning to realise that only Caucasians are considered non-blacks. I literally ran with my heavy bag, not daring to look back till I boarded the train to Heathrow.

11

A Dark Era in Kashmir Valley

During this time of my medical career, something else was brewing in my motherland that would have devastating repercussions—the unfortunate Kashmiri Pandit exodus from the valley in the 1990s. Trouble in the Kashmir Valley, with the radicalisation of the peace-loving people, reared its head first in 1975 when Sheikh Abdullah signed an accord with the Government of India to have complete integration of the state with the Union. Things went on smoothly till the late 1980s when Jamaat-e-Islami Kashmir, Jammu Kashmir Peoples League (JKPL) and Jammu Kashmir Liberation Front (JKLF), based out of Pakistan Occupied Kashmir (POK), along with their sympathisers in the valley, started joining hands. Pakistan's Inter-Services Intelligence (ISI) had been persistently trying to Islamise Kashmir and replace Sufi Islam with the more rigorous Wahhabism. The aim was clear—to create an atmosphere of religious unity in Kashmir which would be following Pakistan.

In the late 1980s, a series of international events—the Islamic revolution in Iran in the late 1970s, the Afghan jihad against Soviets for a whole decade after that, and the armed struggle of Sikhs in Punjab in the 1980s—inspired Kashmiri youth. Both the pro-independence JKLF and pro-Pakistan Jamaat-e-Islami mobilised the fast-growing anti-India sentiments in the Kashmiri population. The execution of Maqbool Bhat, the JKLF leader and a designated militant by the government, on 11 February 1984, led to more unrest with widespread protests that were handled with heavy reprisals by the state forces. The situation kept on simmering towards lawlessness, with the security forces taking over intermittently. After the death of Sheikh Abdullah in 1982, his son Farooq Abdullah took over. In 1983 despite his party winning the elections Farooq was replaced by his brother-in-law, G.M. Shah, with the support of the Centre. Mufti Mohammad Sayeed was the elected representative from Anantnag at that time. The law and order situation in the valley remained very fragile with many curfews imposed to maintain peace. G.M. Shah was also nicknamed 'Gulla curfew'.

In 1986, G.M. Shah got a mosque constructed inside the premises of a Hindu temple in the civil secretariat complex in Jammu. This prompted widespread protests in Jammu. He went to Srinagar and proclaimed that '*Islam khatre main hai*' (Islam is in danger). The same year the Babri Masjid in Ayodhya, UP, was opened for Hindus to go in and worship. This led to a violent reaction in several areas of Kashmir with temples being burnt, particularly in Anantnag district. The Hindu properties and shops were looted and burnt in Anantnag. The Islamists organized under the banner of the Muslim United Front (MUF) became very active in these acts of spreading hate and arson. The result was many Pandit families from Anantnag district fled to Udhampur and Jammu. This was the first exodus of Kashmiri Pandits from the Kashmir Valley in 1986. The worst, however, came in 1987 when the MUF declared their determination to usher in Islamic unity and stand against political interference from the Centre. The MUF, which was becoming popular because of its anti-India posture, decided to contest the 1987 state elections. It is widely believed that these elections were rigged and the MUF was made to lose. Many reliable sources vouch that Syed Salahuddin, the extremist leader (presently chief of the Hizbul Mujahideen), now in POK, was made to lose by manipulating the counting of votes to bring the secular parties (National Conference and the Indian National Congress) in Kashmir at the forefront. This coincided with the beginning of insurgency in Kashmir. Militants killed anyone who openly expressed pro-India policies. Kashmiri Pandits were targeted specifically because they were seen as representing the Indian presence in Kashmir due to their faith. The insurgency had been launched by JKLF but the Islamist groups rose over the next few months, advocating for the establishment of *Nizam-e-Mustafa* (Rule of Allah). These groups desired the Islamisation of the socio-political and economic set-up, merger with Pakistan, unification of the *ummah* (community) and establishment of an Islamic caliphate. The extermination of Central government officials, Pandits, liberal and nationalist intellectuals, and social and cultural activists was declared as a necessity to rid the valley of 'un-Islamic elements'. Although the relations between the semi-secular and Islamist groups were generally poor and often hostile, their common agenda was to establish an Islamic state, and they were showing this intent with slogans of *Ya Raliv ya Galiv* (either convert to Islam or die).

In July 1988, the JKLF began a separatist insurgency for the independence of Kashmir from India. The group targeted a Kashmiri Hindu for the first time on 14 September 1989, when they killed Tika Lal Taploo, an advocate and a prominent leader of the Bharatiya Janata Party (BJP) in Jammu and Kashmir, in front of several eyewitnesses.

This instilled fear in the Kashmiri Pandit community, especially as Taploo's killers were never caught, which further emboldened the terrorists. The Pandits felt that they weren't safe in the valley and could be targeted at any time, especially after a prominent politician was killed without any repercussion. The killing of Kashmiri Hindus, including of many prominent people, continued. On 4 January 1990, a local Urdu newspaper, *Aftab*, published a press release issued by the Hizbul Mujahideen, asking all Pandits to leave the valley immediately. Another local paper, *Al Safa*, repeated this expulsion order. Explosive and inflammatory speeches were broadcast from public address systems of the mosques frequently. This sense of vulnerability and insecurity was exacerbated by attacks on prominent Hindu politicians, the putting up of 'hit lists' with the names of specific Hindu individuals and various violent episodes in Srinagar and other places.

Farooq Abdullah, son of Sheikh Abdullah, was the chief minister of the state during this time while his political opponent, Mufti Mohammad Sayeed, who was founder of the People's Democratic Party (PDP), was the union home minister. Mufti convinced the then Prime Minister V.P. Singh to send tough man Jagmohan as the governor to the strife-torn state against Abdullah's wishes. The day Jagmohan took over, Abdullah resigned. Jagmohan dissolved the assembly and President's Rule ensued. On 21 January 1990, two days after Jagmohan took over as governor, Indian paramilitary troops opened fire on Kashmiri protesters at Gawkadal. While the official casualty figure was 50, many more were believed to have died. The Gawkadal massacre led to a huge public uproar. Lawlessness took over the valley and crowds shouting slogans and toting guns started roaming the streets. Rumours abounded and news kept coming of violent attacks on Hindu minorities and brutal murders and attempted rapes of their women. Those who survived the night saved their lives by travelling out of the valley. Within a few days, most Kashmiri Hindus left the

Kashmir Valley and moved to other parts of the country, mostly to the refugee camps in the Jammu region of the state.

The ensuing days saw a collapse of normal life—schools were shut; cinema halls were either shut or burnt down. Abductions started happening irrespective of religion and faith and it became a class war. Hooligans took over the chairs of the officers, mostly Muslims, and coerced them to marry off their daughters to them and demanded money openly. Public transport vanished and people needing medical attention were stranded. The medical college and SKIMS became havens for militants and the mujahideen. Those who could travel to Jammu, Chandigarh, or Delhi left with their ailing ones, braving tremendous risks. My uncles and their families left Hawal village and those in the city also packed up and moved to Jammu or Delhi. A few of them came and stayed with us. Meanwhile, their children got jobs and took flats on rent in Jammu, Delhi or Gurgaon and settled there. Most of them sold their immovable property in Kashmir at throwaway prices.

I was a faculty at AIIMS during this time and very few people in the valley knew me. My conscience awoke from slumber when I saw them queuing up at the counter of the Cardio-Thoracic Centre. I always was Kashmir-centric and wanted to do my bit in this time of crisis. I went out of my way in shortening their waiting period for OPD appointments and getting investigations like angiography and procedures like angioplasty and surgeries done. I got the OPD timings extended so that as many of them could be accommodated. One of the incidents I recall is while waiting outside my room, a patient got very sick with heart pain and a heart attack was imminent. I took the patient to the cardiac cath lab straight away for angioplasty and managed to save his life. The phenomenon of patients from the valley coming in large numbers continued for several years. By now, word had spread regarding my soft corner for Kashmiris. This attracted more patients and I came to be known as U. Koul. Most Kashmiris prefer to write Koul rather than Kaul, a spelling which my father had decided upon when he changed his surname from Khan to Kaul.

One of the serious issues faced by these patients was their ignorance of the working of referral hospitals like AIIMS. They would often come without enough cash for their treatment. One such middle-aged gentleman Habibullah Naikoo had come from Shopian, a place close to my native village, with spells of fainting in 1993. He had a pulse rate of only 30 per minute, and in my presence he fainted with eyes rolling over. He clearly needed a pacemaker implantation as a life-saving device. I got him admitted immediately and put in a temporary pacemaker. This had to be followed by a permanent implant. His son, who was accompanying him, had very little cash. There was no method of credit cards then and bank transfers were not known to them. There were no mobile phone services those days either.

I reassured them and got the gentleman a pacemaker from my savings, had it implanted and discharged him within a few days. The family of course paid me the Rs 45,000 which I had spent, once they got it from their home. I could see tears of affection and gratitude flowing out of his eyes. He embraced me and since that day, the Naikoo family has become a part of my household. He came to my home before returning and spent a lot of time with my mother narrating stories of Pandit-Muslim brotherhood in Shopian and surrounding areas.

On one of my visits with my family to Srinagar several years later, they came to see us and insisted that we visit their home. We did go and were treated royally with a *wazwan*, consisting of several delicacies of mutton. The entire neighbourhood of their lane came out to receive us and see us off. My daughter and son received several gifts and both were amazed at the respect their dad got from this family.

Habibullah Sahab would always see me for follow-up visits. In fact, during the ensuing three decades, he got all the replacements of the pacemaker done by me in Delhi. This was in spite of the fact that these could have been done easily in Srinagar hospitals. Recently he developed cancer of the colon, which was diagnosed in Srinagar and had unfortunately spread all over. In spite of the family having been told that his days are limited, they brought him to me for admission under my care and for whatever could be done to make him comfortable. I did that, and consulted my oncology colleagues. He passed away in the hospital. A few hours before he breathed his last, he held my hand and kissed it. It was a really emotional moment for me.

The dislocation of Pandits who had to leave their homes was a very pathetic situation and heart-rending. I used to meet many such members of my community. I did try and get many young men employment, using my contacts with companies whose products we were using to treat our patients. One such company Micronic Devices in Rajinder Nagar, New Delhi, really helped me and I was able to get reasonable jobs of sales executives for at least three of my acquaintances. They worked very hard and honestly and got regular promotions. One of them Sanjay Raina, who I got a job there, moved to several companies, which included some big names. He later moved as the vice-president of a Surat-based company making coronary stents, and lately he has become the CEO in a new stent manufacturing company.

The enterprise and accommodativeness of Kashmiri Pandits is phenomenal. I remember one Veerji Bhat, a boy from my village Hawal, who was doing laboratory technician training in 1988 from Srinagar. He approached me, and I rang one of my students Dr Bhalla who got him a job in a West Delhi private hospital, where he worked for a few years. He was not happy there with the odd hours of work and felt he was being treated as if he was living on charity. He confided this to me, and I made a request to Mr D.V. Batra, vice-president of Batra Hospital, and he was employed in the administration of the hospital as a clerk. He would always help and guide Kashmiri patients coming to the hospital. He continued there till 2015. He finally moved back to the valley and is presently working with the medical team of the Governor of Jammu and Kashmir at the Raj Bhawan as a laboratory technician. He is always very appreciative of my efforts to help Kashmiri Pandits who had to migrate to Delhi.

Batra Hospital, New Delhi, a trust hospital, belongs to Ch Aishi Ram Batra who was a resident of Jammu and Kashmir and owned several petrol pumps in the state. The president of this hospital, A.L. Batra gave jobs to several doctors who had migrated from Srinagar during this period. One of them was Dr Vijay Kumar Hangloo, who after his MS in General Surgery migrated to Delhi in 1990. He was taken in and became very popular because of his friendly nature and producing good surgical results. He is now the HOD of surgery in the same hospital. Dr Ravinder Pandita, again a migrant Pandit, also was taken in 1993 and is still working there. Both of them have excelled in their speciality and are continuing in the same hospital for more than three decades, an unusual phenomenon with doctors these days.

The period between 1990 and 1997 has been the longest period in my life when I could not visit the valley, which had become out of bounds for most Pandits. I would look at persons coming from there as my kins who were lucky enough to be accepted there. One of them is Abdul Majeed Kaboo, a resident of Handwara, in North Kashmir. He owns apple orchards there and now also has a petrol pump in Srinagar. He was flown to Delhi in 1997 after a serious heart attack and taken to Batra Hospital. His father-in-law Haji Rafique Sahab, who owned a petrol pump in Srinagar, knew Mr A.L. Batra, president of the hospital. He was referred to me and needed an angioplasty, which I performed and his heart recovered rapidly. He became a great friend and we continue to have very close family relations till date.

My first visit to Srinagar after the exodus was in 1997. I went there and stayed with a friend Dr V.K. Misri, who was the physician to the

Governor and had a hut in the Chashma Shahi complex on the road which leads to Pari Mahal. Both these places are well-known resorts perfected by the Mughals. The area was surrounded by forests and high mountains, overlooking the majestic Dal Lake. Dr Misri, a very careful man, never allowed me to visit the city of Srinagar despite my pleadings to visit the city in a state government vehicle, which he had. My only contact with the city was Kaboo, who used to come and see me in Dr Misri's hut. On one occasion I did sneak out with him and went to the city and spent a few hours at his residence. When I returned, Dr Misri was very upset and stared at me with anger. I do not blame him because he would not understand my emotions since he was born and brought up in Poonch (in Jammu division) and not the valley.

Mufti Mohammed Sayeed

In 1995, Mufti Mohammed Sayeed, who had heard about my name as a cardiologist, called on me at my residence to get a medical opinion about himself. Following this, he used to meet me and consult me periodically regarding his health. While visiting my home in Delhi, he suggested that I should come to Srinagar at least once in a few months and see patients in a building on Gupkar Road, which was constructed for a nursing home during the government of Sheikh Abdullah. I accepted and started going to see patients there from April 1997 onwards, once a month. My accommodation was always arranged at the Circuit House near the cricket stadium. It was a very gratifying experience—seeing patients from all walks of life and suggesting treatment. There were no investigations available except an ECG. I was advised by staff and colleagues to stay put in the Circuit House and at best take a stroll inside the compound, which was spacious enough but had a barbed wire with gunmen in military uniform guarding the gate.

However, I could not be caged and every evening, after finishing my work in the OPD, I used to go to different directions of the city—from Dalgate to Habba Kadal to Karan Nagar. I found the buildings standing there, some of them burnt, providing a sense of uneasy calm which was very different from what I could feel before 1990. Pandit houses and streets had a ghastly silence even if many had been occupied, mostly bought by their neighbours. In the Ganpatyar area which has a lot of temples, this was abundantly clear. Compared to the hustle and bustle of previous years, it was quite desolate. The roadside hawkers, who used to have their carts full of seasonal vegetables at all times, had very small quantities with them. It was the Pandits who used to consume vegetables in plenty, unlike Muslims who would relish mutton and other non-vegetarian stuff. All this gave me a queasy feeling.

However, when I went to Kanikadal, where my *masi* used to live, the moment I entered the lane, I was greeted by men of my age and many younger than me. They would not leave me unless I went to their homes, have tea and asked about all my cousins who used to live there. All of them used to talk about the good old days of harmony. But nobody had any hopes or any positivity. The general opinion of the Kashmiri Muslims was that Governor Jagmohan was the causative factor in facilitating the exodus of the Pandits so that the security forces could take ruthless action against people belonging to the majority community. They would avoid talking about the targeted killing of Pandits which spread the fear precipitating their exodus. I can imagine the mental state and plight of the Pandits who had to leave their ancestral homes and properties in a rush.

12

Exposure to Himachal Pradesh

During the years 1990 to 1996, visits to Kashmir for me and my family were not possible, because of militancy in the valley and the Pandit exodus of 1990. This led me to visit the mountains in Himachal Pradesh—in both the Shimla region and in Palampur district. This became possible because some of my students at AIIMS were from Himachal. They facilitated these vacations for me and my family. In the meantime, the then chief minister of Himachal Pradesh, Raja Virbhadra Singh, became my patient. He was operated on and treated by me at AIIMS. Interestingly, when Singh was out of power and the BJP took over, the then Chief Minister Mr Prem Kumar Dhumal became my patient. These important acquaintances not only helped me visit the hills, which I was missing, but also facilitated the construction of a small house in Kandbadi, a small village in Palampur district. I got a special permission to buy land in the state. Dr Ram Kumar Sood, a good friend, facilitated the construction of the house.

I had treated him for a serious cardiac condition at AIIMS and this built our good relationship. Dr Ram had specialised in treating leprosy. There is still a leper home in Kandbari where old patients now cured but with deformities are living. He took the responsibility of getting my house made and it was ready by 2000. Over the years, he has become like a family member. My uncle, Mr B.L. Dhar, liked my house and the surroundings very much and decided to settle there. He lived there for more than 12 years, and later when he became sick he moved to live with me in Delhi. He was a bachelor and he treated me like his son. The people of Himachal, especially from smaller towns and villages, are very simple and honest. I developed a good bond with them. A number of patients from there still come to me for advanced treatment of their heart problems.

Despite my frequent visits to several tourist spots in Himachal, and owning a house there, I always thought that it was a poor match to Kashmir. The tourist spots are very small and do not stand a chance when compared to the beautiful Kashmir Valley. Besides, Kashmir is very easily accessible with several flights operating from every metro city of India.

I did visit Himachal extensively during those years. My acquaintance with doctors there got me invited for several guest lectures and also a prestigious oration in the name of Dr Devi Chand. My family would often accompany me to Shimla and Palampur. Amita and Samir, my children, became friends of the children of my friends Drs Atul and Gayatri Mahajan, both belonging to Dharamshala. They are still good friends and after all these years continue to meet each other whenever possible. In fact, my children always prefer Himachal over Kashmir because they cannot speak Kashmiri and are not comfortable with the Kashmiri ideology of separatism. Our last family vacation in Himachal was in the summer of 1995. We went to a place called Sarhan near Rampur via Shimla. Once back, in July 1995, the routine of teaching and clinical work had to be resumed. The memories of the vacation and the hills always make you feel good and energetic.

This was the time my absence from the hospital was felt by the department, especially by the chief of Cardio-Thoracic Centre, Professor P. Venugopal, who although my senior by more than six years, was a good friend and an admirer of my work. He was a workaholic and had become the chief at a young age of 40 years and succeeded the legendary cardiac surgeon Dr P. Gopinath. He used to call me often and tell me not to waste my time in holidays. He always used to keep challenging cases for me and would support me in planning non-surgical treatments for them. That is how we started percutaneous cardiopulmonary bypass in our country. It is a technology in which a patient's heart and lung function is taken over by a machine, while he is conscious and the tubes are passed through the thigh vessels.

Professor Venugopal was a hard taskmaster and was very dedicated to his patients. He had a colleague of his seniority, Professor I.M. Rao, who is a very talented paediatric cardiology surgeon and also hails from Andhra Pradesh. The two, however, did not get along too well. Professor Venugopal, popularly nicknamed Venu, was a graduate of AIIMS and did his training in surgery from PGI Chandigarh before returning to AIIMS for cardiac surgery training under the legendary Dr P. Gopinath, credited with initiating the cardiac surgical programme in India. Venu had his higher training in the USA and Australia. It was he who established the regular programme of open-heart surgery at AIIMS, under the guidance of Dr Gopinath, and built an excellent team, many of whom are heading various national and international centres now. He was the first person to have performed a successful cardiac transplant operation in India and has received many honours. I have learnt a lot from him and acquired some of his habits, like working hard and selflessly, and calling a spade a spade.

13

Visits to Pakistan and China

It had always been my keen desire to visit Pakistan. This was because being a Kashmiri, I knew that Pakistan always claimed its right on Jammu, Kashmir and Ladakh since its inception in 1947. Kashmir has also been a very debatable issue with three wars being fought between the two countries on this vexed problem. As known to all of us, a portion of Jammu and Kashmir is under Pakistani administration and is called 'Azad Kashmir' by them and 'Occupied Kashmir' by us. The capital city of Pakistani Kashmir is Muzaffarabad.

During several of my international meetings, I would meet Pakistani cardiologists and exchange notes. Some of them like Dr (Col) Mujeeb from Lahore, Dr Shahbaz Qureshi, Professor Shaukat Malik and Sania Nishtar from Islamabad, and Professor Mansoor from Karachi had become good friends. I got an invitation from the Pakistan Cardiac Society to deliver a lecture in one of their annual meetings in Rawalpindi in April 1996, while I was working in AIIMS. The travel, boarding and lodging were provided by the conference secretariat. I was really excited to get the invite which I considered was way more thrilling than any of the European and US invitations. I had to take permission from the Health, Home and External Affairs ministries before applying for the visa to visit Pakistan. All this took one month. Finally, I went to the Pakistan High Commission and submitted my visa application to visit Rawalpindi for four days. The visa was granted for visiting only Rawalpindi and had a rider that I would have to present myself at a specific police station in the city once a day. I was told it was a reciprocal rule for visitors from both sides.

There was a flight to Lahore operating every day in the evening from New Delhi and I was booked on that along with another fellow cardiologist Dr K.K. Sethi from G.B. Pant Hospital. We were good friends. Finally, the day arrived and we boarded the Pakistan International Airways (PIA) flight, which was a green and white plane. The flight was to take us to Lahore only and we had to change to another flight of PIA for going to Rawalpindi. The flight got delayed by an hour because of some technical snags. Charming air hostesses dressed up in *salwar* and *kameez* with green dupattas greeted us. It was a short flight of less than an hour, the distance being the same as that to Amritsar. We got down at Lahore's Allama Iqbal Airport and got through their customs. On reaching the PIA counter, we were informed that the Rawalpindi flight won't operate because it is late and that airport does not have a landing facility at night. We looked at each other but very courteously we were informed that our stay will be looked after by PIA.

Both of us were taken to a motel located in the countryside. On our way, we saw a lot of greenery, and flowers lined the streets. The shops had their boards written in Urdu. Most people we heard were speaking in very chaste Punjabi language intermixed with Urdu. At the motel, we were allotted two nice rooms with TV and reasonably good facilities. Since it was only early evening, both of us, after changing clothes, went to the reception and sat there. It was too early for dinner so we went to the receptionist, a burly Pathan with a big moustache. Dr Sethi asked him if we can get some beer. He stared at us and very curtly told us, '*Aisee baat na kariye yahan* (Don't ask such questions here). It is an Islamic country.' We apologised and sat down to watch some local serial running on the TV. The silence of the place was broken when we saw two gentlemen sitting on a balcony with stairs from the lobby side repeatedly asking for ice, water and fried fish. As time went by, we could hear their voices becoming louder and they were slurring a bit. We now knew what was going on. This made us very confident in approaching the Pathan receptionist and asking him if we could also sit on the balcony at a different table.

The receptionist mellowed down and told us to go to our room and asked us what liquor we would prefer. At the same time, he cautioned us that we will have to pay for it in US dollars. We agreed since we were carrying a reasonable foreign exchange with us. We ordered a few bottles of beer. It was nice in taste and was a product of Dyer Meakin Breweries, in the Murree hills. These hills, I remembered, are close to Rawalpindi on the original route to Kashmir before the Partition of India. We, thus, had a nice evening followed by a sumptuous Punjabi, non-vegetarian dinner and also fried Lahori fish. The next morning, we went to the airport and reached Rawalpindi by 10 a.m. We checked into the Pearl Continental Hotel, which is a chain in all the major Pakistani cities.

The conference was starting the next day. We went for a look at the twin cities of Rawalpindi and the capital city of Islamabad along with a resident doctor sent by our friend Dr Mujeeb Ul Haq, who was one of the organisers. The old city of Rawalpindi was like any other city of India, bustling with people, and vegetables and goods being sold on wooden carts called *rehri*, along with the presence of a few ordinary-looking parks and gardens. Islamabad, on the other hand, being a newer city seemed well planned and had some semblance to Chandigarh, which is a much larger planned Indian city. This region has been a very important area of the ancient civilisation of South Asia from the Neolithic era. The Pakistan Parliament and the Supreme Court, the very impressive Faisal Mosque, the Margalla Hills, a few lakes, and fancy restaurants adorned the city like in any metropolitan.

The next day, the scientific meeting kept us busy for the entire day. There were a few European and American faculty invitees. The local speakers started their talks by first reciting *Bismillah i Rahman i Raheem* (In the name of Allah, the most gracious and the most merciful, I start). When my turn to give my lecture came, I also recited it since I was very familiar with the pronunciation being from Kashmir. The lecture on 'Treatment of High BP in South Asians' was well received. The chairpersons asked a few relevant questions. I remember a few of the delegates got up and commented that all this had been narrated by the Prophet in his teachings and a true Muslim should know all this. Nobody responded to these comments and the session ended. Later, a few friends from Pakistan and an invited faculty from the UK told me privately that these kinds of comments mixing religion with modern pharmacology are inappropriate. The three days passed comfortably. The reporting at the police station was handled by our hosts and they got us the sealed paper certifying our visits.

Before leaving, we went to a mall for some shopping of local things like onyx stones. This area is known for these coloured stones that looked like marble and are supposed to bring good luck and keep you healthy. We got a few to be kept at homes as souvenirs. We also went to a store selling tee shirts and were introduced as guests from India. We were welcomed, given a cold drink before the salesman showed us the products. I bought three of them and paid. The shopkeeper insisted that I choose one more of my choice as a gift from them.

It was very touching to see this wonderful hospitality, which is still etched in my mind. This brief visit to Pakistan made me realise that the two populations are so similar and such exchanges should be encouraged. I found that the people were very friendly and hospitable. While talking to commoners on the street like sanitary workers and hotel helpers and waiters, it was interesting to notice their interest in India and its people. Interestingly, many of them had their forefathers coming from Indian cities like Ajmer, Bhopal and several cities of Uttar Pradesh. None of them had any bitterness regarding their country having been divided by the 1971 Liberation of Bangladesh, erstwhile East Pakistan. But while talking to more educated people in smaller circles, the ill feeling on that aspect was quite palpable. Invariably, the Kashmir dispute would crop up and knowing that I came from there, it would start with a friendly debate which used to conclude by saying that it has been a politician-made issue. They would be happy if people from both countries could visit each other. This made my resolve to visit Lahore and other cities stronger.

It just happened that the Pakistani High Commissioner in India, Shahid Malik, sought an appointment with me in 2012 while I was working at Fortis Escorts Hospital. He came to my office for a general check-up and spent some time with me. I found him to be a very pleasant gentleman who showed interest in my work and would often call me directly or through the medical attaché to the High Commission. One day, I received a message from a multinational pharmaceutical company Serdia for visiting Pakistan to deliver a lecture on high blood pressure and related problems, keeping a focus on one of their products. I showed my interest and asked them to go ahead. It was to happen in March 2012 and the lecture tour would involve Lahore, Faisalabad, Islamabad and Karachi. I informed Shahid Malik about this development and he was very pleased to help me with the visa process. I got the visa without visiting the high commission through an official who took my passport and documents for a day and came back with a visa for all the cities, and I was exempted from reporting to the police stations. Since no flights were operating between the two countries at that time, the choice was to either fly to Dubai and come to Lahore or go on a foot visa via the Wagah border near Amritsar. I chose the latter route and informed Serdia officers who had to look after me. I flew from Delhi to Amritsar a day prior to my crossing over to Pakistan from the land route. I spent the night in a hotel after visiting the Golden Temple complex which I had never visited before. It was very impressive and one gets a good spiritual feeling there seeing a large number of devotees and listening to the Gurbani from the Guru Granth Sahib being recited on the loudspeakers, near the sanctum sanctorum, the Harmandir Sahib.

I was instructed to start very early because the border is open till only noon. My hosts took me to the Indian side of the immigration, about 25 km away from Amritsar near Attari, which is the last village on the Indian side, and bid me farewell because only the visa holder could enter. It was a big and very spacious pink-coloured building with an Indian flag hoisted atop it. Mobile phones do not work in that area for security reasons. It appeared only a few persons were crossing over that day—me and a few Pakistani guests who had come to India for a family wedding in Delhi. The procedure was simple—checking of the forms and identity, several stamps put on the papers and the customary stamp of departure from India. An Indian porter, attired in navy blue, carried my suitcase and we boarded a bus till the 'no man's land' of the border. Here we crossed the gate and upon looking back, I saw Mahatma Gandhi's enlarged picture and India written in English and Bharat in Hindi along with the Indian Tricolour.

On two sides were stands from where visitors can watch the closing of the gates ceremony which happens every evening at sunset. This is a colourful parade of the tall BSF (Border Security Force) personnel on the Indian side and equally smart soldiers from the Pakistan Ranger's side. Both sides gesture each other with stamping of their thick leather boots and finally bring down the flags to be kept in safe custody for the night. There were stands with chairs for visitors on both sides. The gate on the Pakistan side was of similar dimensions depicting a large picture of Muhammad Ali Jinnah (founder of Pakistan), the green and white national flag with a crescent, and Pakistan written in English and Urdu.

The 'no man's land' led to a building which was Pakistan's immigration office at Wagah, a bordering village complex on the Pakistan side of the border. The building was smaller in dimension and the porter from Pakistan, who carried my luggage after getting down from the bus, took it inside. I met the officers sitting at the desk and greeted them and presented my papers and the passport. They asked me to wait since there was a power breakdown and their computers were not operational. In the meantime, while scanning my papers, one of the officers asked me if I was a medical doctor and if so, what is my speciality. Once he came to know I was a cardiologist involved in angioplasty procedures, he became very friendly. He himself was a patient with two stents put in by Lahore doctors. He showed me his prescription and had many queries resolved. I also met a money changer, who offered to change Indian currency to Pakistani one at better rates. As per the rules, it is only foreign currency (US dollars or Euros) that can be exchanged officially. Meanwhile, power was restored and I could complete my formalities and get out. I was met by two Serdia senior executives, Dr Rizwan and Qauum, who had come to pick me up. We got into their car and drove to Lahore.

On the journey, we saw the Ichogil Canal and its fortified bund which was built by Pakistan to protect Lahore from an Indian invasion. This was in the news a lot in 1965 during the Indo-Pak war which I remembered was a battlefield for a few days. Being a sensitive issue,

I did not ask any questions beyond confirming that it was the same canal. We reached Hotel Pearl Continental, the place of my stay. I noticed that it was a typical five-star hotel when I checked in. My hosts left me and came back in the evening to take me around. We went to the historic Lahore Fort built by the Mughals with some resemblance to the Red Fort of Delhi. It is much bigger with many sections, including the Diwan-e-Aam and Diwan-e-Khas, and fine designs and carvings on the walls and ceilings. They had hired a guide, Alam Khan, to show me the historic places. I was more interested in talking to him regarding his life and his family. We became friends and continued to chat via Facebook for some time after my return. Towards the end of the fort tour, we also saw the additions made by Maharaja Ranjit Singh whose dynasty succeeded the Mughals, before the British took over Punjab. Maharaja Ranjit Singh's portrait is there, and his mummified warhorse Laili is also preserved there in a museum. The tour of the fort really was very impressive and narrated the history of that era. It was like getting a practical exposure to what we had read in the history books during our school days.

It was getting late in the evening and I was recommended to accompany them to Food Street, which was very close to the fort. This area had recently been renovated by the Pakistan government and is a very sought-after food street in Lahore. I found several buildings with Punjabi and Hindu names there—a few had idols of Hindu gods. Most of these buildings had been converted into restaurants. We took an outdoor table on a balcony facing the fort. The selection of food was a very difficult exercise given the choices in the chef's recommendations. I had a scrumptious meal consisting of 'mutton handi' and Lahori fish with Lahori paratha. On our way back, we went through Anarkali Bazaar, my father had mentioned it as the place for books. It was very crowded and the books available did not interest me so we came back for the night's sleep and preparations for the two lectures scheduled for the next day. The first lecture was at the Punjab Institute of Cardiology. It is a big 347-bedded tertiary care unit caring for heart patients and has facilities for advanced treatments of angioplasty, bypass surgery, valve replacements and a paediatric unit for young children and infants. The director of the institute and the head of the cardiology department welcomed me and introduced me to the gathering of medicos before I gave my talk. The talk was followed by good interactive questions and comments. The evening talk was in a five-star hotel and was well received. The audience during the post-lecture dinner told me that they liked my way of speaking and preferred me over the European speakers, who used to be sponsored by the industry and were coming there frequently. They found a familiarity with me.

The remaining part of the lecture tour was spent in Faisalabad and Islamabad. Faisalabad was new to me as I had not been there before. This city was earlier called Lyallpur after the name of its founder, Sir James Lyall, who was the Lieutenant Governor of Punjab from 1887–1892. Its name was changed in view of the collaboration of Pakistan and Saudi Arabia and to acknowledge the contribution of King Faisal. I found it to be a bustling city with Punjabi as the predominantly spoken language. We saw many textile mills while driving through to the venue of the lecture at Pearl Continental Hotel. The city is also called 'Manchester of Pakistan' for this reason. I had a good lecture and interaction with doctors of the city. They were all very courteous and friendly.

From Faisalabad, we again drove to Islamabad. I found the inter-city roads very good with a lot of Korean buses plying between the cities. I hired a local taxi. My taxi driver was a Punjabi and very talkative. When he came to know that I am from India and that too from Kashmir he became quite inquisitive. Assuming that I was a Muslim, he sympathised with me and asked me about the killings of people in the valley and their abject poverty. On my retorting that things are very nice there with a lot of prosperity and beauty, he did not seem to be convinced. He told me that Pakistani TV shows them everything and people in Pakistan donate money to trusts so that Kashmiris can finally be liberated from the clutches of the *kafirs* (non-believers). Pointing out the new colony, he showed me proudly the development of Pakistan. He, however, conceded that the distribution of wealth is lopsided and should be improved. In general, he thought that military regimens did much more development work than the 18 civilian governments which had been there since the creation of the country. He specially named two generals who ruled Pakistan, General Zia ul-Haq from 1977 to 1988 and General Pervez Musharraf from 2001 to 2008.

I diverted the topic and asked him about Pakistani cricket. He became emotional and said that their boys are the best but local politics and selection process are at times unfair. Imran Khan, according to him, was the best cricketer the world has produced and he got Pakistan the World Cup against England in 1992. Imran, according to him, was the first Pakistani captain to defeat India in a test series in India in 1987. He was, however, sad at the terrorist attack on the Sri Lankan cricket team in 2009 which cost Pakistan cricket dearly, since all international teams refused to visit Pakistan after that. I was amazed at his cricketing acumen and his frank views on Pakistani politics. Once we reached our destination he wished me well and sent his greetings for the 'valiant' Kashmiri people.

Islamabad was quite familiar to me by now. This time, we spent an evening in the Margalla Hills surrounding the city and had dinner in a nice sophisticated eatery, 'The Monal Restaurant'. The beautifully lit up city of Islamabad could be seen from there. My last part of the lecture trip thus was over and we took a flight back to Lahore on our way to the Wagah border, which we crossed before noon the following day as per the protocol. The Indian counterparts of Serdia were waiting to receive me and thus I came back to Delhi from Amritsar.

I got a few more chances to visit Pakistan between 2011 and 2013—once to Karachi and three more times to Lahore. The Karachi visit was organised through Prof. Mansoor for a cardiology summit. Karachi, the port city, was very different from Lahore. It had navy bases and clubs. Being way more cosmopolitan than Lahore, one could see a lot of wealth, contemporary fashion and old colonial buildings of the British Raj times. The harbour was nice and well-lit but I thought Mumbai was of a different class and more glamorous. Prof. Mansoor kept me very comfortable during the stay. The immigration was simple and not as interesting as the 'no man's land' crossing at the Wagah border.

The standard of medicine being practiced in Karachi hospitals was very good. It was in no way inferior to what we have back home. They, however, import most of the medicines unlike us. India itself is a very big producer of generic drugs.

During my last visit to Pakistan in 2013 for another major Pakistani cardiac society meeting in Lahore, besides the scientific component, there was a nice gala dinner preceded by a social event in an auditorium. It was a function of the Pakistan Cardiac Society and as I was an international guest, I also got an invitation. The Indian cardiologists were sitting together and enjoying the deliberations which had a lot of similarities to our meetings. The families of the local cardiologists were also sitting in the audience. Towards the end of their official addresses, the compère invited any representative from India to come to the dais. There was a palpable uneasiness amongst our group, with everybody asking his neighbour to go up. There being no official head of the delegation and seeing my friendliness with Pakistani cardiologists, I was pushed to go. I did not hesitate and went up and spoke from the dais. After the customary pleasantries and speaking about the great hospitality, I told them I come from a beautiful place of the subcontinent, which is the *shahrag* (windpipe) of two neighbouring countries and made an appeal to leave our people alone so that we can look after ourselves better. There was applause from the people sitting around. I also invited the delegates to Kashmir and promised to hold a cardiology meeting there in due course of time. I remember when I came back to my Indian colleagues, they seemed a bit upset and told me, I should not have spoken like that in a country like Pakistan.

During dinner, on the same evening, I met a senior Pakistan army brigadier and we chatted for a while. When he came to know I am in Lahore for one more day, he invited me and a few more international non-Indian delegates for evening tea to his residence. I promptly accepted and the next day I was picked up by his staff. It was a grand bungalow with a very aristocratic drawing room and balconies. After introducing me to other guests, he asked me to accompany him to the basement. It was a grand liquor bar with the choicest brands of beverages and I saw only a few chosen guests there, mostly Caucasian Europeans. While talking about Kashmir, he told me that it is an unnecessary raked-up issue which is ongoing for more than five decades. He also narrated that he, during a casual talk with Rajiv Gandhi, the then prime minister of India, told him that there is no need of being shy of a referendum. There might be more people on the Indian side voting for Pakistan but it will be nullified by the people on their (Pakistani) side.

We also talked about the chequered relationship the two neighbours have had in the past several decades. To sum up in the words of Raj Chengappa, the editor-in-chief of Tribune Group, in 2013, 'India and Pakistan have moved from fighting, to fighting and talking, then fighting about fighting, then talking about talking, then talking and fighting and now back to talking about talking.' The general agreement, however, was that the two countries need to reconcile and move towards development and educating their masses. Wars are not going to lead us anywhere.

The last invitation for visiting Pakistan came in 2014. Everything was organised but a day before leaving for Amritsar, I got an advisory that Imran Khan's march from Lahore could disrupt my visit and the visit had to be cancelled. Since then, it has not been possible to go there because of the deteriorating relationship between the two neighbours. The recent years, post-2014, have seen only deterioration and a total lack of trust between the two regimes. It is a pity that the two neighbours, who have everything in common, cannot see eye to eye with each other. I do hope better sense prevails and both the countries at least become agreeable.

Visiting China

My first visit to China was in 1994 when we had the outbreaks of bubonic plague. On reaching Beijing, I was sent to the health authorities for quarantine but I returned by the earliest flight. I again went in 1996 for a meeting. The road from the airport to the hotel was a dusty track bereft of any vegetation. The airport itself was in a small building, much more primitive in terms of appearance and facilities than the New Delhi terminus of those days. The city was full of cyclists and pavement vendors. These vendors adept at bargaining were selling small trinkets and accepted only US dollars. Besides giving my lecture during the visit, I also saw the Beijing end of the 'Great Wall' and the historic 'Forbidden City'.

My next visit was for a university invitation in 1998, where I saw their public hospitals which reminded me of our own hospitals. I did a few heart procedures too. The procedures, being performed for the first time in Beijing, were reported in newspapers there. It was heartening to see how medical techniques and sharing technology can help people. Such exchanges should be promoted more in the interests of science.

My first visit to Shanghai, the densely populated commercial and banking hub of China with a dazzlingly huge Pudong airport, was in 2006. Besides seeing the large malls and the bund, it was amazing to see a large vacant area being transformed into a lush green park with groomed flowers and trees by transplantation in just two days. Building such parks and the construction of skyscrapers in a few weeks is an everyday affair there. I saw a complete transformation of technology in just eight years.

My next visit was in March 2009, seven months after the Beijing Olympics and the venue was the same village. Our stay was in a very spacious hotel just in front of the amazing Bird's Nest Stadium and the soothingly blue Aquatic Water Cube Stadium. Upon driving towards the city, I could see most modern vehicles but no bicycles.

The other conference cities I visited during these years were Shenzhen, close to Hong Kong, and Suzhou, a city near Shanghai. Both the cities are done up very artistically and are a shopper's paradise. In the Suzhou hotel, robots used to respond to the housekeeping calls, rendering a feeling of fantasy land.

During my several visits, the alleviation of poverty in that country was palpably visible. As per the data, it has fallen from 88 per cent in 1981 to 0.7 per cent in 2015. My last visit to Beijing was in March 2019. Their hospitals and healthcare systems have achieved excellence in delivering both modern and traditional medicines. Their skills in minimally invasive procedures and short hospital stays are remarkable. This is totally in contrast to the scene of 20 years ago, when I felt we, in India, were far superior in all these areas. Their medical research is of high quality, reported in high-impact international journals. Even after the Covid-19, which spread from Wuhan, their current progress in making the vaccine and executing large-scale trials is remarkable.

My experience of China has been very striking. It is a country that is comparable to India in terms of population and natural resources although it has a much larger area with different ideologies and systems. Their huge economy is not dependent on a few countries only. India contributes only three per cent to their exports and they have big investments in almost all the countries of the world. Seeing our dependence on their technologies in several sectors, we cannot afford to stop it overnight. It is premature to make public statements regarding boycotting their products. Their expansionist agenda which is deplorable cannot be curbed by these measures. It, therefore, needs a different approach, keeping in mind our different political systems and our past experiences of dealing with them on border disputes.

14

Association with Sathya Sai Baba and Puttaparthi

On one morning of October 1990, our medical superintendent, Professor A.N. Safaya, called Professor Venugopal and informed him that Sathya Sai Baba of Puttaparthi had indicated that Professor Venugopal should participate in his birthday celebrations on 23 November that year. Professor Safaya was a great devotee of Sathya Sai Baba, who was an Indian guru, a spiritual leader and a philanthropist, residing in Puttaparthi, a village in district Anantapur, Andhra Pradesh. He claimed to be the reincarnation of Sai Baba of Shirdi. He purported materialisation of *vibhuti* (holy ash) and several small objects like rings, necklaces and watches for his devotees. Dr Venugopal had never visited his ashram before this although his parents had. He agreed to go to Puttaparthi for the celebrations. While addressing his devotees in the stadium, where he was celebrating his birthday that year, Baba announced that he had decided to make a state-of-the-art super speciality hospital in Puttaparthi near the airport and the inauguration will be done on 22 November in 1991. The hospital will be free of cost for patients irrespective of their caste, creed, religion, gender, etc. Later in the day, Baba sent for Dr Venugopal and a few more devotees from various walks of life and countries. Baba had over 1,200 Sathya Sai Centres (branches) spread over nearly 126 countries. In the meeting, he conveyed to the select group the basic design and the structure of the hospital that appeared to be very different from a routine hospital. Cardiovascular sciences were one of the very important sections of the hospital. Dr Venugopal was given a free hand to set it up with all the modern facilities and the deadline to perform the first bypass surgery would be 22 November 1991. There was no way he could argue about the slated date. He came back to Delhi and called me and told me about the challenge. Finances were not a constraint. We needed to decide regarding the equipment and the training of nurses, technicians and supportive staff.

We held a number of meetings and decided about the equipment based upon all the minutest details of our previous experience of catheterisation laboratories, echocardiography machines and operating room set-ups. With the hospital being set up away from the metro cities, we could not take any chances of missing anything which would hamper our work. All vendors were very cooperative and there was no question of overcharging. We had no part to play in the negotiations. Whatever we asked for was provided much before the deadline.

That year, we were travelling to Puttaparthi every weekend. Our routine was to take a flight to Bangalore on Saturday at 4 p.m., stay overnight in Bangalore, and start in a car for Puttaparthi around 4 a.m. the next morning. We would reach before the *darshan* time of Baba and would sit in front of Prasanthi Nilayam, the abode of Sri Sathya Sai Baba. Thousands of devotees would be already there to have a glimpse of Baba. It was very difficult to predict his route and people close to his route would prostrate and try to touch his feet or at least his robe.

The lucky ones would get him to glance at them and sometimes get *vibhuti* from his right hand. The ritual would be followed by bhajans in melodious voices by the chosen singers for at least an hour. This routine would be repeated in the evenings too.

Larsen and Toubro were the contractors and builders of this very ambitious hospital project. Work was done round the clock to meet the deadline. Lo and behold, the structure including the installation of the equipment was completed by 20 November. I performed a few angiographies and one angioplasty the same day. One of the patients was kept for coronary artery bypass graft (CABG) to be performed on 22 November, the day of the inauguration of the hospital.

The then Prime Minister P.V. Narasimha Rao came to inaugurate the hospital. Everything around the hospital was spotlessly immaculate. Baba had sent his personal limousine to the airport, which was right next to the hospital, to receive the prime minister, accompanied by Baba's closest associates in the Sai Baba Trust. The prime minister entered the hospital from the main portico, which had a dome with a beautiful Italian chandelier. He came to the cardiac cath lab where I was patiently waiting to receive him in my green laboratory attire. I greeted the prime minister with folded hands and he smiled. Then I took him to show the equipment of both the labs through the glass panes. Following this, I showed him the angiograms I had done along with the moving pictures of the angioplasty procedure performed on the previous day. He showed keen interest and asked me questions regarding the life of the stent used and the welfare of the patients, who were still in the ICU. From there, he went to the ICU and also met Professor Venugopal who was waiting there for him. The first cardiac surgery of the hospital had to happen that day.

In the meantime, Sai Baba suddenly made an entry and the staff standing there went forward to touch his feet, which he did not allow. He told them in Telugu to continue with their work. Baba met the prime minister briefly and blessed him by patting him on his back and leaving for his ashram. The ashram 'Prasanthi Nilayam' was two kilometres away from the hospital. Following the inauguration ceremony of the hospital, Mr Rao came again after a few months to the ashram and sat through the entire morning puja. Baba then asked him to come to his chamber. I was told that the prime minister had come to take his blessings for some important personal event.

My visits continued for a few months till the regular cardiology staff joined and the technicians became comfortable. We also worked for the department to get recognition by the National Board of Examinations for PG in cardiology. This ensured the continued availability of well-trained doctors and a teaching atmosphere in the hospital. With time, there was a deluge of patients. It was anyway expected as the hospital was providing first class medical care free of cost along with Baba's blessings. Very few needy people would miss this chance. I wish every state in India had such philanthropists like Baba.

Puttaparthi, anyway, was a great place for learning with several institutions in the town bustling with activity. Prasanthi Nilayam, the small township around Baba's temple, had several small flats owned by devotees. Many of them were residing permanently there, while others visited occasionally. There was also a canteen providing breakfast and meals at designated hours. A very nice bakery shop also was a part of the food court. Besides these, bookshops and small shops were selling Baba's pictures, calendars and souvenirs. All this added to the hustle and bustle of the area during the daytime.

People in the ashram would go indoors after sunset and sleep quite early. The next day's routine darshan of Baba was always the topmost priority. Many elderly people were living in the ashram who, in the evenings after having an early dinner, would narrate stories and incidents in which Baba had performed a miracle to save a human life or helped in getting the livelihood of a family or organised help to get girls married by sending ornaments, and so on. To me all that appeared fictional and imaginary.

After the hospital became fully functional, my visits became occasional. I went only when requested by the medical director of the hospital, Dr Safaya, for some official meeting. During all my visits, it was customary for me to go for Baba's darshan and attend the morning prayer. Baba, a lean and short-statured person, dressed in the customary saffron-coloured attire, would always have a glow on his face. He was always smiling and had jet black curly hair. His aura would command pin-drop silence when he used to walk through the orderly queues of devotees. During these darshans, I would expect his eyes to meet mine. It finally happened one day when during the morning darshan, while returning to the temple, Baba pointed at me, with a mischievous-looking smile, and signalled me to come in along with a few more devotees he had already chosen for the day. Although I was very excited, I did not show any emotion. Not knowing what was in store for me, I went in. Everybody sitting close to me told me that I was very lucky.

Baba came and sat with us. During our conversations, we asked him about his diet, to which he said that he survived only on *raagi* (millet) and fruits. He also named a few dignitaries who had come to see him in the last few days. He also talked about the new management college he was starting soon. He gave us *prasad* (religious offering) and before leaving, he asked me to open my right hand and slipped in a ring, with nine different stones, on my ring finger. The ring fitted perfectly. I bowed and he allowed me to touch his feet, which was customary. He then blessed me by putting his right hand on my head before I left. It was a great moment which is still fresh in my mind. This ring suddenly appearing from his hand which was empty moments ago was no less than a miracle. Was it magic? Was it a well-planned act, enacted by his inner staff? I have no satisfactory explanation. The silence inside

Prasanthi Nilayam is unique and gives peace of mind. No wonder, people with agitated minds throng the place for treatment.

These four years of my association with Baba and Puttaparthi Ashram have left an indelible mark on me and my life. In spite of several controversies that enveloped Baba, it is very clear he never did anything for himself and did lots of good work for that part of India, in irrigation, health services and education. No doubt his rich devotees were using him for getting connections with politicians and important bureaucrats. It was not his fault. Our society is materialistic and can go to any extent and will not even mind maligning well-meaning people to further their greed.

15

Exit from AIIMS and Experience in Private Healthcare

My life at AIIMS continued and I enjoyed and cherished it to the fullest. I used to be one of the consultants to reach the hospital first and usually the last one to drive out from the parking lot. The Cardio-Thoracic Centre came into being in 1982 with a separate building on the campus. I went on with my routine of hard work for the department, established the techniques of balloon angioplasty for coronary artery diseases and trained several colleagues. I also initiated the arrhythmia services, including a radiofrequency ablation programme, for treating rhythm disorders of the heart.

The first cardiac transplantation in India was done on 3 August 1994 and I was one of the cardiologists taking care of the gentleman. The patient's name was Devi Ram, a 40-year-old industrial worker from Delhi. He had cardiomyopathy, a condition of very poor heart function. In the previous year, he needed hospitalisation thrice and was kept in the hospital as a potential candidate for the first heart transplant surgery. The bill to clear the heart transplant also got passed during this period. Meanwhile, a 35-year-old lady who had a brain haemorrhage and was brain dead with a beating heart was selected as the donor. The family agreed to donate the heart for the noble cause of saving a person with an end-stage heart disease. On the night of 3 August 1994, in an operation lasting for hours, Devi Ram received a new heart. He survived for 14 years after which he succumbed to an unrelated brain haemorrhage. These activities that made our department very famous nationally boosted me to work even harder.

I never thought of leaving AIIMS in years to come. In fact, I never got time to even think of such a situation till the time an interview for the post of a professor at AIIMS, New Delhi came my way in 1994. There were two vacancies for the post advertised. We were three candidates that included one very senior doctor, Dr Savitri Shrivastava, who was a paediatric cardiologist. My interview went off very well, and Professor Venugopal, who knew the expert, told me the same evening that the experts had recommended my name. However, I was shocked to learn after a few days that I was not selected. The selection board had an MP on it. I was informed by an insider that the MP insisted that my other colleague should be selected and he did not leave till he got the final list endorsed by the chairman. This was blatant cheating in one of the premier institutions of the country. This incident shook my confidence. I took this rejection very seriously and met the cabinet secretary, who also happened to be my patient. He listened to my grievance attentively and used his influence to get another post of professorship created at AIIMS. I was selected for that. It did give me consolation but the damage was already done. I had become junior to those selected before me. I continued my work but was an unhappy man.

Then came a difficult period in life when my daughter, who was also aiming to become a doctor, did not get through any government college for her MBBS. However, she got admission in a good private medical college in Pune. The admission and yearly fees were high and I couldn't afford them. I had to, for these reasons, join a private hospital. This is when I decided to leave AIIMS and join Batra Hospital and Medical Research Centre (BHMRC), New Delhi. I felt totally dejected when I went to Pune with the admission money in cash borrowed from my father, uncle and a few friends. The family supported my decision because they had seen me slog for more than 15 years at AIIMS and understood my need to leave AIIMS in order to look after my children and their education.

My last day at AIIMS was on 31 December 1996. I conveyed my decision to leave on the preceding weekend to Professor Venugopal, who, though unhappy and sad, remained calm and balanced. He understood my problems very well. I handed over my resignation without the customary three-month notice. My salary of three months was paid to the AIIMS authorities by my new employer, Batra Hospital. It was a bold decision and I had no ill feelings for the institute. In fact, I threw a going-away party for the cardiology department at India International Centre (IIC) and urged my erstwhile colleagues not to arrange for any other party.

Working at Batra and Fortis

Batra Hospital was one of the first private multi-speciality hospitals started in Delhi in 1986. It was, however, a trust hospital run by a group of trustees. The other major private hospitals in the city were Sir Ganga Ram Hospital and Indraprastha Apollo Hospital. Two other well-known private heart care hospitals were Escorts Heart

Institute and National Heart Institute. I chose BHMRC because the chairman of cardiology, Dr N.S. Dixit, was a very understanding cardiologist who had started this speciality. When I met him, I did not spend much time discussing my emoluments but insisted on making the centre a model cardiology centre at the earliest if I would join BHMRC. He promptly agreed and promised to get a new state-of-the-art cardiac catheterisation laboratory along with other equipment, such as intravascular ultrasound and machines for flow measurement in the coronary arteries, besides getting a new CCU. The terms and conditions were very fair though the emoluments were much lower than in other private hospitals. I also wanted to move with a team consisting of two cardiologists, Dr Balbir Singh and Dr Dinesh Sudan, both my students from AIIMS, New Delhi. We also brought in our own catheterisation laboratory technician, who was actually working on daily wages as a nursing aid for a few years. He had learnt how to operate the recorders and imaging equipment during hours when regular staff would go away, because, in a government set-up, they would work only up to 5 p.m.

Dr T.S. Mahant, a very accomplished cardio-vascular surgeon, who would never refuse to operate on the most complex and very sick patients, and his team had also joined BHMRC from Sanjay Gandhi PGI, Lucknow, a year before we joined. Dr Mahant and I had formed a bond at PGI Chandigarh when I went to work there in 1979-80. He was doing his cardiac surgery training there those days before going to Australia, New Zealand and Birmingham, Alabama, USA, for higher training and experience.

The entire team clicked very well and the volumes of both angioplasty and surgeries picked up phenomenally within a few months of our joining. We took in two more senior residents and made them join the Diplomate in National Board in Cardiology (DNB), a two-year course of cardiology training (DNB, cardiology), post MD medicine recognised by the National Board of Examinations (NBE). Both of them really worked hard and we used to teach them every morning from 8 a.m. to 9 a.m. Although the DNB programme existed in BHMRC for several years, this was the first time students started passing to get their degrees. This attracted a lot of good talent and we got recognised for conducting a fellowship in Interventional Cardiology from the NBE. BHMRC thus became well known in the field of academic medicine and volumes of procedures. The management was always supportive. The department started getting clinical trials from major sponsors both from the device and pharmaceutical industries. We became the first centre in the South Asian region to treat patients with acute heart attacks by angioplasty using metallic stents, with very good and acceptable results. This was published by us as one of the first reports in international journals.

Our next step was to do live demonstration courses to teach complex procedures by inviting internationally known operators whom I used to meet in courses all around the globe. The industry really helped us in these teaching activities. Publication in national and international journals was one of our focused areas. This habit which I carried from AIIMS really worked to keep the group in the limelight. We never hesitated in calling colleagues from other Indian centres to help us in carrying out procedures where they had more experience. Likewise, I used to travel to other upcoming centres to start their programmes. By this time, we had the availability of drug-eluting stents which reduced the gap between bypass surgery and angioplasty. My team became one of the first ones to use them and published very good, internationally recognised studies from Batra Hospital and expanded them to several parts of India. I always believed that a good teacher should distribute his knowledge and training and disseminate it.

This trend continued till December 2004 when we started seeing several new private centres coming to the National Capital Region and neighbouring states. Dr Mahant, our great supporter and surgical colleague, was lured by the upcoming Fortis Group, which came up with a big centre in Mohali close to Chandigarh, and he joined them. It also took him closer to Himachal Pradesh, his native state. That was a loss for us. Balbir, my colleague, joined Escorts Hospital around the same time. I was hurt at this act because it was me who had brought him to Batra Hospital to work as a partner. Nonetheless, I took it in good stride as the move would help him enhance his career. While I was in Batra Hospital, my name was recommended by the president of the Medical Association of India for the coveted Dr B.C. Roy Award for developing specialities. This award is given on National Doctors' Day (1 July), which is Dr B.C. Roy's birth as well as death anniversary. I was awarded this coveted recognition, making me feel very happy and proud. Ironically, the other person was Dr Farooq Abdullah, the chief minister of Jammu and Kashmir and he got it for the category of a doctor and statesman.

One development in Delhi which followed my joining Batra Hospital was that several senior doctors started leaving government-controlled teaching hospitals for more lucrative private enterprises. The leading examples were Professor K.K. Sethi, Professor D.S. Gambhir and Professor Mohan Nair, all from G.B. Pant Hospital. The health ministry took cognizance of this fact and hiked the emoluments of the doctors who stayed back giving them an incentive of continuing to work in the teaching hospitals in Delhi, including AIIMS.

The management of Fortis, in the meantime, decided to come to the NCR, built a hospital in Noida and bought a building made for a hospital in Vasant Kunj. At this stage, they approached me and my group to join Vasant Kunj along with a few well-known colleagues from other disciplines like pulmonology, diabetology, nephrology and urology. The set-up was brand new, challenging and with much better emoluments. My group decided to join them much to the disappointment of Batra Hospital that could not match the grandeur or the paying capacity of corporate hospitals like Fortis or MAX groups.

Within a few days of our joining Fortis in June 2005, we came to know that the Vasant Kunj facility had legal issues and would take some more time to start. The Noida hospital which was promoted as an orthopaedics and neurosurgery centre attracted my attention and I persuaded the Fortis management to start a cardiology department there with the equipment ordered for Vasant Kunj. It made sense to them and there was a full floor unoccupied there which was converted to the cardiology department. There were enough operating rooms and surgical ICUs to start cardiac surgery. Within a month, we started interventional cardiology there and took on board one of our former senior residents, Dr Vineet Bhatia, from Batra Hospital, who had done his post-doctoral course in cardiology from Bombay (now Mumbai). There was a cardiologist, Dr Mittal, who was my student at AIIMS, already working there.

My team, consisting of Dr Ripen Gupta, Dr Ranjan Kachru, Dr Vineet Bhatia and myself, started our work in full earnest and did very well. Our department became the highest revenue earner of the hospital within two months. Noida area had only a few good cardiology centres in the neighbourhood. Patients from the Kashmir Valley who used to come in good numbers to Batra Hospital started coming to Fortis, Noida, and the patient numbers really swelled towards the winter months. Patients from the valley usually hesitate to come to Delhi area in the hotter months. I have always had a very soft corner for them. Most of them are very innocent and unaware of the tricks of the medical profession in big cities. I knew that they came all the way travelling a long distance having full faith in me and having limited budgets. There were several instances when they could not pay their entire bill and I used to help them by making payments on their behalf. The hospital billing section was very strict and would never allow the procedure to start unless an advance had been paid as per the tariffs. Invariably, I had to give assurance and undertaking on behalf of the patients for taking them for procedures.

I remember a few of them coming with the balance money to me in my Srinagar OPD, which I used to visit usually once a month. On my refusing to take it, they would not insist but would get me my favourite Kashmiri vegetables, almonds or walnuts instead. We Kashmiri Pandits are very fond of vegetables grown in the valley, especially *haakh* (greens), *sochal*, *nadroo* (lotus stem), etc.

The location of Fortis Hospital at Sector 64, Noida, was a long distance from my home in Greater Kailash and travelling to do emergency cases of acute heart attacks used to be a problem. My colleagues living closer often used to help me on my call days. I, however, distinctly remember one day, 26 January 2006, which was a national holiday. I had to go to the hospital three times during the day driving myself for doing emergency angioplasties. My colleagues had gone out of Delhi that day. The day is also memorable since it coincided with the announcement of Padma Awards of 2006 by the Government of India and I was conferred with the prestigious Padma Shri. Actually, on the evening before the Republic Day, I got a phone call from a family friend, M.K. Razdan, the then CEO of *Press Trust of India (PTI),* who broke the good news to me. I was thrilled but never told about this to anybody except my parents and family. Such gratifying moments do not come every day and are a once-in-a-lifetime event. It definitely bolsters one's self-confidence. Overall, my experience of Fortis, Noida was good and very educative since it was the first time I was involved in setting up a brand new cardiology department where full authority had been given to me and my team.

On 1 June 2006, the Vasant Kunj facility was commissioned. My colleagues who had been chosen for this facility streamlined most of the protocols for the department, especially for the CCU and the cardiac catheterisation laboratories. Dr Ripen and Dr Ranjan moved to Vasant Kunj while Dr Vineet and Dr Mittal continued at Noida. We also took on board Dr Parneesh Arora, who was working at MAX Hospital at that time, to our Noida facility. The technicians and specialised nursing staff were also divided between the two hospitals. I continued to head the department of both the hospitals and divided my days between the two places—however, on most days I used to travel from one place to the other. Both the centres started doing well and we started a few research projects after constituting ethics committees in both the hospitals. Working in two different hospitals at the same time was a new experience. Travelling through the crowded roads of Delhi and getting phone calls from patients was a hassle.

As a Director (Cardiology) in a corporate hospital entailed my understanding the finances and profitability as well. I was a novice in these subjects. In my first meeting with the other HODs and the medical director, the finance head asked me about the EBITA from our department. I looked vacantly towards the HOD of nephrology, Dr Vijay Kher, who was also a Kashmiri and had come from Sanjay Gandhi Hospital, Lucknow. He too was blank. Later in the day, I learnt from a CA that its full form is Earnings Before Interest Taxation and Amortisation, a measure of financial performance. Taking care of the standard of treatment and developing protocols for patients were already big challenges, that too of two different institutions, which were not my cup of tea. The decision of tariffs of procedures was fixed by the non-clinical members of the management without our consultation, which was not fair according to me.

I ultimately sought an appointment with the Fortis owner, Shivinder Singh, and told him my problems. To be fair to him, he called the MD and asked him not to bother me with these details for at least one year. Then I found that the Vasant Kunj and Noida hospitals were also made to compete against each other in terms of EBITA. I found it a very complex world but had no choice. In fact, I once went to Professor Venugopal requesting him if I can be taken back at AIIMS. He talked to the director who said I will have to apply and compete against the candidates, many of whom were my students. This was not acceptable and I had to be content with what I had. I continued to work as a healer and spent long hours working at the Fortis healthcare.

Meanwhile, news arrived that Fortis had acquired the Escorts Heart Institute and Research Centre (EHIRC) for Rs 585 crore. There were three functional Escorts Hospitals—Escorts Heart Institute, Okhla; Escorts Hospital, Faridabad; and Escorts Hospital, Amritsar. The deal made Fortis India's second-largest hospital chain with a capacity of 2,200 beds, which was next only to Apollo Hospitals group's with 7,500-bed capacity.

My past relationship with Escorts, however, had been rather eventful. EHIRC had made a big name in the 1990s with its chief Naresh Trehan (NT), who was a very dynamic and charismatic cardiac surgeon. The hospital marketed itself very efficiently and used to invite many doctors from other cities for continuing medical education programmes (CMEs). They were generally kept in five-star hotels with lavish comforts. The CMEs would involve referring physicians and building a large referral base initially concentrating on North India and then spreading to several other parts of the country. The consultants were compensated adequately but it was NT who mattered, and only his name was known outside the hospital. Patients coming to the hospital would claim that he/she had been treated personally by him and had become his friend and would demand to see him. He had a good team of well-trained cardiologists.

NT and I had a cordial relationship based upon mutual respect and admiration. On many occasions, he had expressed the desire that we should work together. In August 2004, he approached me and we had several meetings upon which we decided that my entire team would join EHIRC. Things were firmed with the HR department and my team's joining was scheduled after I would return from an international meeting in the USA in October 2004. News had spread by that time in the cardiology circles, but on my return, I learnt that the move had been scuttled, much to my disappointment and embarrassment. Later, I found out that the senior consultants of EHIRC protested regarding this proposed move to NT and threatened to leave; he finally buckled under their pressure. Given these developments, I decided to join Fortis in 2005. NT in collaboration with his business partners was making a big hospital complex named Medanta in Gurgaon. His interests, therefore, were divided between the two places.

When EHIRC became Fortis Escorts, the field again changed. Shivinder Mohan Singh personally informed me about the takeover. We were concerned with this news because with acquiring a big and well-known heart centre, the focus on Vasant Kunj and Noida cardiology was likely to be changed. The management, however, kept on reassuring that our fears were unfounded. With NT having 10 per cent stake and his hospital project only in very early stages, things continued as they were. We continued to work hard and brought the departments at Vasant Kunj and Noida to a good standard. By now, Dr Mohan Nair also joined us expanding our expertise. I used to miss my patients of the OPD who could not afford the fees at Fortis. Hence, I took an assignment at St Stephen's Hospital as a professor emeritus. I started going there on two afternoons every week for teaching their cardiology students and conducting a two-hour OPD. This helped me in reassuring myself that I was not only a rich man's doctor.

Meanwhile, the Fortis management was working hard to gain control of Fortis Escorts Heart Institute (FEHI). They seemed to be avoiding a confrontation with NT. It was a peculiar situation where owners were scared of the tenants. The uneasy relationship continued for several months, but we continued to work diligently while enjoying the gossip going around. Shivinder and Malvinder, the owners, used to spend the whole day in the cafeteria of Escorts planning the process of the takeover. Finally, it happened on 19 May 2007. Shivinder Singh, as the managing director, gave a press conference and announced that NT had been terminated as the executive director and he would not be allowed to perform any surgeries henceforth. NT and his loyal doctors went to Escorts and insisted on getting in, which created a commotion. The guards, who till a few days back saluted him, did not allow him and locked the doors. In the meantime, the relatives of the patients who were in the hospital came and protested that their surgeon should be allowed to see his patients. There was a lot of drama with NT and his team going to the media and narrating the alleged inhuman behaviour towards them of being prevented from seeing their patients. The media covered this event extensively. NT was left with no option but to find a new place till his facility in Gurgaon got ready. It looked like a scene out of a Bollywood film when the media shoots were aired. NT and his team were the heroes and the owners—the Singh brothers—the villains.

He finally decided to join Indraprastha Apollo Hospital, New Delhi, as an interim measure. Several of his erstwhile surgical colleagues, such as Dr Meharwal and Yugal Mishra, stayed back at FEHI. Dr T.S. Kler, after remaining indecisive for some time, also decided to stay put at the hospital. There was widespread news that the cardiology facility at Fortis Vasant Kunj would be pruned. Our fears were confirmed when one of the two cath labs of the hospital was shifted to FEHI. It was a very uncertain time for me and my team after seeing comfortable days at Batra Hospital and Fortis before the Fortis Escorts era.

At this stage, the Fortis management met me and persuaded me to join FEHI while continuing my charge at Fortis Vasant Kunj. An arrangement was made whereby I was made the executive director and dean of academics and research at FEHI, while Dr Kler continued as the executive director of clinical services. Under the circumstances, it was a good solution and a good office was created for me at FEHI. I took up this new role with great enthusiasm and passion, galvanising the teaching activities. NT had left a research team which was really feeling orphaned with NT gone and the new corporate team having no clue about this component. Their rooms were also taken away to accommodate offices of the senior management, including the office of Shivinder Mohan Singh. All the signboards and nameplates started changing to the light green colour of the Fortis emblem. I could see the gloom on their faces. Sardar Bhavdeep Singh, meanwhile, joined as the CEO and met me to discuss the way ahead. He was previously working in the USA as a CEO of a marketing chain. Besides other suggestions to improve the footfall and the image of our hospitals, I suggested the launch of an academic and research department. He initially was in a fix but as soon as I explained to him that clinical trials, especially the sponsored ones, bring in good revenue, his response became very positive.

By now, I had understood very clearly the corporate way of thinking and decision-making. A department was thus created and launched in the presence of the media. Since the hospital had no space, we looked for space in the vicinity of FEHI. Eventually, we got it in the OPD block in a residential area by vacating two flats. The first general manager, employed by NT and who took over as administrative head of the research department, was not liked by the medical director because he found him too expensive as compared to the revenue the department generated. He was not given his due increment as he lacked competence. I, however, wanted a smooth transition before I could find a person to replace him. Hence, for a few months, I supplemented his salary. I did not want the department to collapse.

Meanwhile, I looked at the research coordinators of the department.

It was an easy choice—a young charming lady from Manipur by the name of Priyadarshini. She had done her postgraduation in biotechnology. The problem was that there were a few staff members senior to her, most of whom had a background in nursing. After discussing with the management and HR, it was decided to give her a promotion based on her good track record and administrative capabilities. Meanwhile, the Fortis Group went on acquiring hospitals in different parts of the country and abroad. Between me and our research department headed by Priyadarshini, we strengthened the existing research facilities in 17 hospitals in the country. These centres were in the NCR, Punjab, Jaipur, Kolkata, Mumbai, Chennai and Bengaluru. We used to visit these centres to coordinate and train their staff members.

I proposed having a central research department to coordinate activities in other hospitals which were interested and had the infrastructure. This idea of mine was accepted and FEHI became the central department for academics and research. There were several teething problems in administering the department. A colleague, who was given to administer three departments—training, centralised ambulances, and academics and research—in the capacity of a general manager, started interfering in the running of day-to-day affairs without any logic. This only led to delays in getting and implementing new projects. Such appointments of holding multiple charges were common in the corporate way of functioning, but I was not used to the style. Ultimately, my view prevailed and I was given the full charge independently. Between me and Priyadarshini, we brought the department international repute.

By this time, I had become internationally quite well known in the field of interventional cardiology and was invited to several meetings. One of them was the EuroPCR. This meeting was previously called Jean Marco course and was held in Toulouse, southwestern France. This was later co-sponsored by the European Association of Percutaneous Cardiovascular interventions (EAPCI). I found both the meeting and Toulouse very absorbing. I had been a regular visitor to that meeting. The city was also called the pink city as it had terracotta brick buildings and pavements. With the growing popularity of the meeting, the city became very small to accommodate a larger audience. It was eventually moved to the capital city Paris in a big ground close to the Eiffel Tower in a huge tent. Eventually, it was moved to a convention centre, *Palais des Congrès*, in the heart of the city, a walk away from the Arc de Triomphe, a very well-known monument of the Napoleon era. I have visited it several times and lost my way while coming back to my hotel because of the symmetry of all the streets. There are several sculptured images on the pillars of the arc, depicting soldiers of several nationalities. I could recognise the German faces in particular. I used to take many shy Indian delegates along with me to see the arc.

Another landmark of Paris that stands looming across the city is the Eiffel Tower. It is named after engineer Gustave Eiffel, whose company built the tower. While there was initial resistance with critics panning it, the Eiffel Tower has become the cultural icon of France and is one of the most visited and recognisable international structures where people pay to enter. I have been to the top level which is 276 metres above the ground. It is a very majestic sight of the city of Paris from there. The first two levels have restaurants and are always full of visitors. I remember standing in a long queue along with a friend for at least two hours to buy the entrance ticket. Many people standing in the queue had bottles of water which we did not have. Our throats were parched.

The EuroPCR conference is a great learning experience for cardiologists who are involved in the non-surgical treatment of blood vessels and also provide alternative treatments for repairing or replacing diseased valves. Beginners and also seasoned operators attend this meeting, upgrade their techniques and learn new procedures. Typically, it is in Europe that most new devices and methods of treatment are initiated. One of the reasons is that the approvals for use are not as stringent as in the USA. This, however, does not mean that procedures do not pass safety tests and ethical aspects are not taken care of. In fact, it was in Nuremberg, Germany, after the Second World War, that the 'Nuremberg Code' was endorsed. The 10 points which constituted the Nuremberg Code include principles such as informed consent and absence of coercion, formulated scientific experimentation and beneficence towards the subject's participation in the trial. It is thought to have been mainly based on the Hippocrates Oath. It is interpreted as endorsing the experimental approach to medicine while protecting patients' rights. Ethics is a crucial part of clinical studies. Patient's rights are to be protected and nothing starts without an informed consent process.

The meeting had several parallel sessions going on simultaneously. One of the highlights in the main arena is the live demonstration of cases by expert operators from different parts of the world. The cases are done very systematically so that the delegates get all the information of the technique, the hardware being used and the principle behind it. There is always a good interaction between the delegates, moderators, commentators and operators. I personally have benefitted a lot by watching these cases and, on my return to India, have applied the knowledge gained here. I have also taken part in these deliberations as an operator, a chairperson and a moderator on various occasions over the years. Such meetings have done a lot of good to disseminate knowledge and techniques and helped bring angioplasty to the present status. The true masters are those who disseminate their learning to others so that the new methods of treatment grow, flourish and become widely available. Today, all over the world, the number of angioplasty procedures exceeds the number of bypass surgeries. This is even though the trials have shown better long-term results with bypass surgery in several subsets of patients, especially in diabetic ones, who constitute around 35 per cent of patients requiring revascularisation in our patient population. No doubt a non-surgical procedure is always the preferred one because of minimal morbidity, no anaesthesia and blood transfusions, very short hospital stay and resumption of full activities in a few days. The reason for the phenomenal growth of angioplasty is very logical. It has overtaken bypass surgery long back all over the world.

I along with my friends from India and neighbouring countries used to go on long walks to the Arc de Triomphe and Eiffel Tower, having tea or beer at the pavement restaurants. These places are in great demand during the summers, a time when our meeting used to be held. On a few occasions, Priyadarshini, our research manager, had also accompanied us as a delegate for the research sessions. Somehow she was good at selecting red wines from France and we used to enjoy it along with a steak. We have travelled for conferences to many other parts of the globe, including Buenos Aires in Argentina where we saw the Iguazu Falls on the border of Brazil. These exotic places buzz with tourists and a lot of activity and different cultures. Science and conferences I found are real unifiers and make this world a small global village. These activities came to a standstill during the two years of Covid pandemic. It is hoped that international conferences will start again with the same zeal as till 2019.

My professional work continued along with some small research projects. By this time, in 2010, these small projects or single centre studies had lost all flavour and it was time for sufficiently powered studies, which meant including multiple centres. My department was involved in several international multicentric studies but it only meant a very small role and participation. It did make me travel to some international destinations for investigators' meetings, but sitting as a backbencher with very little opportunity to actively participate did not excite me. I had a desire of conducting a pan-India investigator-initiated trial in my field of coronary interventions.

I got an idea of comparing two different drug-eluting stents in diabetic patients to study their safety as well as efficacy. This was a subject of raging controversy in that period—whether paclitaxel was superior or inferior to another drug called everolimus. India being the diabetic capital of the world, we thought that it should be done by Indian investigators only. My department wrote a full protocol for a study of 1,800 patients from 50 Indian centres. It needed good funding. We approached the companies which made either of these stents. There was no problem in selecting the centres. I met Keith Dawkins, an Englishman and the chief of medical affairs of Boston Scientific Corporation (BSC). Keith became a good friend. The scientific and finance teams of BSC worked out the budget and finally agreed to put in Rs 22 crore under different heads for the trial to be completed in three years. The study was named Taxus element versus Xience Prime in a Diabetic Population (TUXEDO), India trial. The money had to come to FEHI, as it was my place of work and I was also the research head. Priyadarshini was appointed as the operations head. This big sum was a windfall for the hospital and they were thrilled and were glad to control this money. Suddenly, we became the darlings of the CEO and the CFO of the Fortis management. The first case was recruited by me in June 2011 and the numbers steadily increased. The study was a regulated one under the drugs controller of Government of India. We faced many obstacles on the way. The recruitment was rather slow at many centres. Being a study of middle-aged and elderly diabetic population, some mortality was expected.

In 2013, in response to reports of unethical research being done in some centres in the country, the Supreme Court of India stopped all human clinical research in the country till the time the health ministry and DCGI (Drugs Controller General of India) formed new guidelines and fair compensation laws for patients getting adverse effects. We were asked to pay heavy compensation for deaths. Our budgeted money faced serious problems. The insurance company started backing out on several issues. The consenting process became very elaborate with audio-visual consenting, scaring patients and further slowing the recruitment process. We, however, continued our determination to complete the trial and a meticulous follow-up. BSC also understood the issue and after an audit, they decided to give an additional Rs 5 crore for completing the study. Finally, the last patient was recruited in March 2014. We had a retention of 98 per cent and got the result that the everolimus-eluting stent was superior to the paclitaxel stent. The trial results were presented by me as a late-breaking trial at the TCT (Transcatheter Cardiovascular Therapeutics) in San Francisco, USA. This is one of the most prestigious international meetings in angioplasty. Simultaneously, the trial was published in *The New England Journal of Medicine,* a medical journal with the highest ranking. It was a moment of great pride for me and the entire family of investigators. Sub-studies of this trial were published in the *Journal of the American Medical Association* (JAMA) and the two years of follow-ups in *EuroIntervention*, a European journal.

The trial also exposed the corporate mentality when it comes to finances. There was a component of the payment coming for the national lead investigator for running the 46 centres in India. The management of Fortis Escorts created all kinds of obstacles and wanted to take two-thirds of the payment. Finally, as per the proverb 'beggars cannot be choosers', my team who slogged for more than three years, got a pittance.

Clinical trials are very important for the advancement of medical treatment of various diseases. The safety, efficacy and ethical conduct of the studies are of paramount importance. In the past, most important studies were done in Europe and Northern America, especially the USA and Canada. The cost of conducting the trials in these countries is, however, exorbitant. On the other hand, populous countries like China, India and far eastern countries, have a large drug-naïve population ideal for being included in trials at much lower costs. The Drugs Controller General of India and his office have a very important role in allowing these trials and being a watchdog for these studies. Adverse events to patients have to be reported to them at the earliest. As per the rules, compensations are to be given to the patients or their families under pre-set regulations. The proof that the compensation amount has been delivered has to be supplied to the DCGI office. I have some experience with their role while conducting a study for an Indian product to be used. While conducting the study, we were asked at very short notice to be ready for an inspection. A very senior person came and checked the details till the team was satisfied. They also made some observations which had to be carried out. By rule, a product which is evaluated and being used on patients cannot be charged. A full consent for it being used in writing has to be taken beforehand. There are several instances of this rule being violated by hospitals. This needed to be looked into and the concerned hospital and the investigator penalised for not following the protocol. Over the years, this process has improved significantly in our country, leading to better quality of research.

16

Experience in Private Cardiology Hospitals

During my 40-odd years of clinical practice in Delhi, I was witness to the changing patterns in patient care by medical and paramedical staff from the pharmaceutical and device industry. Till the middle of the 1990s, things were reasonably in order and the medical fraternity was in general held in very high esteem. The doctor was regarded as 'next to God' by patients and their families. Referral patterns were straightforward and the doctor used to do it in the best interest of the patients without expecting any returns, except for feedback regarding their welfare. The kickback, at best, would be in the form of free registration for a continuing medical education programme or help in the registration and accommodation of students during conferences. Doctors would also distribute free samples of medicines to needy patients.

My first encounter with the changing system was within a year of my joining Batra Hospital in 1997. I was referred to a few patients by a practitioner from Jabalpur, all of whom needed angioplasty. My team and I did it and kept our Jabalpur colleague informed about the outcomes and procedures, including the follow-up treatment. The patients were sent back to him in a few days. A few months later, the doctor called up to say that he was coming to Delhi and would like to meet me. I told him he was always welcome and asked him to come over. He reached my office on the appointed day and we talked about his practice, his city and I asked him if he would be interested in having lunch together. He refused the offer and said, 'No, I just came here to offer my *namaste*.' I was a bit taken aback but still folded my hands and said, '*Namaste*' and stood up to leave. He got up too and said, 'Wait, what about my share?' I turned around and said, 'Share? About what?' Apparently I was a simpleton without any grooming of what happens in the field.

He looked at me arrogantly and showed me a list of five cases he had sent me and demanded a sum of Rs 30,000 as his share. I was stumped for a moment and then became furious. Never in my professional life had I been asked for money in this manner; neither have I ever demanded from anyone too when I referred my patients. I stared at him coldly and said, 'I don't owe you anything. And never, ever disgrace the profession like this. Please leave before I call security.' The colour rose in his face as I said this. Some people had assembled around us too and it was becoming an awkward moment. He looked around and then slunk off to the nearest exit. He never called or referred cases again. This was my first exposure to this new business.

A new hospital had come up in Noida around the same time. The owner was a cardiologist with moderate skills. The hospital started doing very well and secured approved government empanelments, such as the Central Government Health Scheme (CGHS), Ex-Servicemen Contributory Health Scheme (ECHS), etc. I soon realised that our referrals from physicians started falling in numbers. On trying to find out the reason and reviewing our success rates, I got to know that every referred case for angiography and angioplasty used to get a kickback of Rs 5,000 and Rs 15,000, respectively. In fact, seeing this trend, the doctors went a step further and started paying their referring doctors Rs 1 lakh in advance and adjusting it as and when patients came in—an ingenious move.

This menace slowly spread its tentacles all over the medical field, including radiological diagnostics and biochemistry laboratories. For every test ordered, 20 per cent of the bill was given back to the referring doctor. This led to doctors recommending unnecessary tests. The pharmaceutical companies also saw burgeoning business. Acclaimed doctors and specialists were given freebies, such as fancy TV sets, refrigerators, air conditioners and cars depending upon the prescriptions. General practitioners would prescribe unnecessary drugs, multiple kinds of vitamin supplements and specific brands of drugs, and were given returns in cash. Very often, prescriptions were written in codes which could be deciphered only by specific chemists.

Over the years, the priorities of cardiology students also changed. I stood witness to the change happening over the last three decades. Between 1980 and 2000, the number of seats was limited and both consultants and residents were very committed despite the overwhelming clinical work. Punctuality was the rule. Teaching institutions were mainly confined to government medical colleges in Delhi and AIIMS. There was no strict selection criterion and only students interested in learning used to apply for postdoctoral teachings, such as DM in medical specialities like cardiology, neurology and gastroenterology. In surgical specialities, it was cardiothoracic and vascular surgery, neurosurgery and paediatric surgery. Other specialities got added later.

With the growth of specialities, the need for good specialists increased. The selection of candidates for post-MD specialities has become very competitive and there is a robust selection process for getting admission. However, the standards of teaching have been very variable. In general, the teaching institutions like AIIMS and PGI Chandigarh have maintained the standards. Private institutions, in general, do not have the same motivation. The faculty spends very little time in reading and keeping abreast of new developments. The motivation of the postgraduate students has evaporated. They are only reading to pass the examination and are not interested in writing scientific papers and case reports. They try to find shortcuts for making presentations at seminars. The same is true when patients have to be investigated and prescribed drugs. Patients are now known by their bed numbers and not by their names. The consultant's ward round is more often a 'treatment checking' round and it is often revealed that the patients' complaints are frequently not addressed. Residents are only conscious of their duty hours.

There is a definite need for more specialists in various super specialities in the country where the burden of non-communicable diseases has increased to alarming proportions. There has also been a boom in the number of cardiology clinics, echocardiography and cardiac catheterisation laboratories throughout the country. Even smaller cities and towns have these centres. While Delhi has more than 100 invasive cardiology centres, neighbouring places like Faridabad, Narela, Karnal, Sonipat, Panipat, Hissar, Rohtak, Mathura, Agra, etc. have these facilities too. Gurgaon (now Gurugram), Ludhiana, Jalandhar, Pathankot, Amritsar have become hubs with several big cardiology centres. Most of them are private enterprises and are doing quite well. The downside is that there is no auditing, no appropriateness criteria stipulated by authorities, and it is a general impression that unnecessary and uncalled for procedures are being performed. These not only include diagnostic angiographies but also angioplasties and putting stents in non-critical cases which only need good evidence-based medical treatment. The same is true of device implantations like permanent pacemakers. These uncalled for procedures are not only ethically wrong but sometimes cost the life of the subjects because of clotting of stents and infection of devices, and lead to a lot of morbidity for these unfortunate subjects.

I know from personal experience that patients were being charged for coronary stents when no stent had been implanted. One such case was referred to me by a state government for verification. The patient was subjected to angiography and following that his relatives were told that one of his three arteries has a critical blockage. He was advised immediate angioplasty and putting in a stent. It was a government hospital and the doctor took money for the stent in cash. He went ahead and seemingly did a procedure in the laboratory. Following the procedure, he also handed over the box of the used stent to the family. However, the news leaked out of the lab that no stent was put in. The patient's family complained to the medical superintendent. The cardiologist defended himself and maintained that he had put in the stent. The case was referred to me a few years afterwards. The original angiography records from the hospital went missing under mysterious circumstances.

I decided to do an angiography. Normally a stent is visible in angiography. I could not see any. In spite of this, I did a procedure called intravascular ultrasound (IVUS) to make sure because some stents are very thin and not well seen. IVUS also confirmed the absence of a stent. In spite of my written report, no action was taken against the doctor. He took long leave and went to the USA. The patient ultimately filed a case in court and I was summoned as a witness a few years ago. The doctor pleaded that it was an absorbable stent and hence was not visible. However, absorbable stents had come in the market after several years of this procedure. These arguments still didn't lead to any action being taken, even 20 years after the incident. Obviously, the doctor was very well connected with the high-ups. These incidents can only go scot-free in our part of the world. We need to have serious and rapid redress of such important issues.

There is an unmet need of having more trained cardiologists in our country. As per the figures from the Cardiological Society, we have 4,000 registered cardiologists with a paltry ratio of one per 300,000 population as compared to 23,000 in the USA, giving a figure of 43.8 per 100,000. The other issue is the quality of training, which varies a lot. It depends upon the institution which is imparting the training. The authorities imparting training are the universities offering post-doctoral programmes called Doctor of Medicine (Cardiology) and the hospitals without attached medical colleges were recognised by a Central government body called the National Board of Examinations (NBE) and were allowed to pursue a post-doctoral degree course called Diplomate of National Board (DNB) which is equivalent to DM in a speciality. Both are after postgraduation in medicine or paediatrics. The training of DM cardiology is more thorough and focusses on all the aspects. However, the focus of DNB imparted in private institutions invariably is on procedures like echocardiography, angiography, angioplasty and device implantations. Cardiology is much more than this.

An important issue which came up around 2014 was the exorbitant prices of stents for patients who needed an angioplasty. The number of such patients was around 500,000 per year with an annual increase of around 30 per cent. The reason for the high prices was that there were several intermediaries in the stent supply chain between the manufacturer and the hospital authorities, especially in the privately owned ones. The average cost of an imported drug-eluting stent exceeded its real price by at least 60 per cent. In the absence of any organised insurance system, most patients had to pay this money from their pockets in addition to the cost of the procedure.

This was taken up by a lawyer from Haryana, Birender Sangwan, whose friend had to pay Rs 126,000 for his father who underwent angioplasty in a Faridabad hospital. He filed a case in the Delhi High Court to include heart stents in the National List of Essential Medicines (NELM) in 2014. The court directed the government to get it included in the NELM. However, it took three years and a number of contempt petitions by the lawyer before the government finally relented and handed over this pricing debate to the NELM. It worked and it was realised that the cost was being escalated several folds and left to the institutions at times and there was no maximum retail price written on the container boxes. Finally, in February 2017, a price cap of approximately Rs 30,000 was mandated. It was a substantial reduction of at least Rs 90,000 for the imported drug-eluting stent for the patient needing it. Many private hospitals seeing the loss in profits started hiking up the procedure costs and promoting reuse of the hardware during the procedure, a practice which is banned in Europe and the USA. Such unhealthy practices need to be stopped by the hospitals and those found guilty need to be penalised.

The Focus on Profits

I continued looking after patients and conducting academic and clinical research at FEHI and Fortis Vasant Kunj. The management always looked at research as a money-earning proposition since they had a taste of it from our previous studies. The CEO and the CFO started organising meetings with big clinical research organisations (CROs) like Quintiles and started setting for me incremental targets of earnings from research, but without extending the facilities, manpower or support to strengthen what we had created at the Fortis Escorts Hospital. At one time, I suggested they move the central research department to Fortis Memorial Research Institute (FMRI) in Gurgaon. The MD of the hospital, however, was lukewarm to the idea since it would mean for him to give space on the campus. Meanwhile, the corporate office of Fortis had come up very close to the FMRI. At the same time, my contract with Fortis was only till the end of June 2017 and had to be reworked by the management if they wanted to continue with me. After a series of meetings with me, they started talking to me regarding moving to Fortis Corporate office in Gurgaon as the central research head while continuing my clinical work at Vasant Kunj and Okhla hospitals. A room in the corporate office was allocated to me, which I used to visit off and on since I had my clinical affiliations with Fortis Escorts and Vasant Kunj facilities. This went on till the beginning of June 2017. When the time for renewing my contract came, they wanted me to minimise my clinical work and concentrate on getting business by way of bringing in sponsored research. They wanted to fix targets of revenue earned by me. They also wanted to give me the designation of the head of clinical research of the Fortis group with minimal clinical engagement in the Gurgaon hospital. This was also the time when news of the Fortis group's plan to sell their hospitals to IHH Healthcare, a predominantly Malaysian group, was making the rounds. In fact, a senior partner of the group met me in Delhi and wanted to know my thoughts about the Fortis group. It was very clear from the discussions that clinical research was not their priority. Taking all these happenings together, I did not want to agree to the offered terms and conditions and renew my contract with them, and decided to leave the Fortis group respectfully on 30th June 2017, ending my association of 12 years with them.

I then decided to go back to my previous hospital where I had very good innings of eight years. The president of Batra Hospital and Medical Research Centre promptly offered me the post of chairman at Batra Heart Centre and made me the executive director and dean of academics and research. He also agreed to immediately start the Department of Academics and Clinical Research and appoint staff of my choice and emoluments. I accepted the offer and joined BHMRC on 1 July without taking a day's break.

For my part, it was a sort of homecoming without any interruption. Within one month of my joining, the key persons of the research department at Fortis headed by Priyadarshini and her deputy Yumnam Diana resigned and joined me at BHMRC. I was allotted a decent office space and the secretarial staff of my choice.

I found that during the last 12 years, when I was working at Fortis, the working of Batra Hospital had not matched with the working of the corporate hospitals of the NCR and the processes and quality control had not changed much. This had resulted in a decline in the number of self-paying patients coming to the hospital. The hospital was mainly banking upon empanelled patients' business. The beds in the new block were closed down. The staff had poor enthusiasm to work and the atmosphere did not look bright in general. The cardiology department had only one functional cardiac catheterisation laboratory and no modern equipment for intravascular imaging or physiological studies. The clinical research had been stopped after the 2013 Supreme Court ruling and not restarted after the formulation of new guidelines by the DCGI.

Now that we had re-established the academics and research department, we started resuming all the activities in a phased manner. A memorandum of understanding (MOU) was signed with Amity University, Noida, which helped us in starting PhD programmes. In addition, a number of multi-centric and investigator-initiated studies were started. One of these studies was presented at an international meeting in Seoul, South Korea, as a late-breaking trial. Another large investigator study, which will eventually compare new-generation coronary stenting in diabetic patients with a multi-vessel disease with coronary bypass surgery, was planned to start in 70 Indian centres. The study has started and is making good progress.

On the equipment front, the department has been upgraded with another catheterisation laboratory and equipment for intravascular imaging (OCT) and physiological studies (FFR). We have been doing live-case demonstrations for both national and international meetings. Many procedures, such as the non-surgical Transcatheter aortic valve replacement (TAVR), have been started. The plan is to make it a centre at par with any international centre taking care of patients with heart diseases.

On the social front, we carried out a pilot study in a slum area of South Delhi (Sangam Vihar). We evaluated the coronary risk factors in a cohort of 500 subjects who claimed to be fit and healthy. The study, conducted on people below the age of 45 years, found that nearly half of the population was either overweight or had high blood pressure, and unreported diabetes was present in 8 per cent of the subjects with total cholesterol levels of more than 200 mgs in 17 per cent. The data obtained from this study is the first-of-its-kind, as it used predictive analytics using artificial intelligence (AI) to understand the patterns and processes contributing to the lurking epidemic of cardiovascular diseases in a setting of the cross-sectional community.

This concerning data and the trend has prompted us to plan this study in a larger population in the NCR, focusing mainly on slums and low socioeconomic areas. It is aimed at applying interventional treatment to aggressively treat the risk factors in the high- and intermediate-risk patients in a segment of the population, and compare the outcomes with a demarcated population on usual treatment. All these efforts are in the direction of improving the healthcare model in the NCR and following it up with plans to extend it to various parts of the country in collaboration with the Ministry of Health and Family Welfare.

17

Relationship with Mian Bashir Ahmed Larvi and the Wangath Experience

In 1995, one day I was asked by D.V. Batra, the joint owner of Batra Hospital, to visit his residence to see an important patient from Kashmir. I went and saw an old but very graceful person by the name of Mian Bashir Ahmed Larvi. His son Mian Altaf and other family members were there too. He had cardiac problems and needed a bypass surgery followed by implantation of a pacemaker. He made a good recovery. Our relationship, however, transformed into a family friendship, full of mutual regard and trust, in the years to come.

Besides being a politician and a minister initially of the Indian National Congress and later of the National Conference of Jammu and Kashmir, he was also a Caliph of the Islamic Sufi order (Naqshbandi, Majadadi, Larvi) in Jammu and Kashmir. He was born in November 1923 in Wangath, near Kangan, Kashmir. He is one of the most revered religious leaders of the Bakarwal community. They constitute around 8 per cent of the population of Jammu and Kashmir, mainly settled in the hilly areas like Rajouri, Poonch and Kupwara. Bakarwals mainly are nomads because they have to be on the move in search of pastoral lands to feed their animals, which are mainly sheep.

Wangath is a beautiful part of the valley off the main road on a steep climb before Kangan town. Kangan is in Ganderbal district en route to Leh, about 40 km from Sonamarg, and is known for its glaciers. Wangath is also close to Naranag, a tourist village with a spring and an ancient Hindu pilgrimage site. The place is well known for its ancient but pillaged ruins of ancient Shiva temples. It is also the starting point for going up to Gangabal Lake, one of the most beautiful and revered places for Kashmiri Pandits just like Haridwar. Reaching there entails either trekking or a horse ride, passing through exotic places and strikingly beautiful wild flora. The nomadic tribes of Gujjars and Bakarwals add an extra dimension to the trekking trail of Gangabal.

I have had the good fortune to stay at Wangath with the Mian family and enjoyed their generous hospitality on a number of occasions. An annual function is held there around the first week of June when thousands of Gujjars from the state throng the place, cut the dried grass for fodder and stay there. A special *langar* (feast) is organised on those days and, usually, the weather is at its best at the beginning of the summer.

Mian Bashir Sahab's ancestors came to this place in the last century and set up the Darbar Lar Sahab Sharif which is one of the most sacred places for the Gujjar, Bakarwal and Pahari people of Jammu and Kashmir. Baba Ji Sahab, Mian Bashir Sahab's grandfather, was actually born in Balakot (now in Pakistan) and was a deeply religious person from his childhood, who had left his family and spent years meditating in the areas close to the Khyber Pakhtunkhwa area. His spiritual master (Peer) was Naqshbandi Nizam-ud-Din Kayani

Sharif of Muzaffarabad. In 1893, he migrated to Wangath along with his followers and bought a piece of land where he opened his *Dera* in 1895. Here, he started the traditional *langars*, built a mosque and started preaching the true thoughts of Islam to devotees. A hydropower station near Kangan is built after his name. Mian Bashir Sahab continued the same tradition and expanded the establishment of his forefather. He became a social reformer and brought Gujjars and Bakarwals to the limelight and fought for their rights as they too are a substantial part of the population of the erstwhile state. The family then entered politics and represented their constituency, Kangan. Mian Bashir's father, Baba Nizamudin, he himself and his worthy son, Mian Altaf, never lost an election from that area.

In 1991, Gujjars and Bakarwals were designated as Scheduled Tribes, thanks to the efforts of Mian Bashir. For these meritorious contributions, he was awarded the third-highest civilian award of the country, Padma Bhushan, by the President of India in 2008. He dedicated this award not only to Gujjars of Jammu and Kashmir, but to crores of Gujjars living in 11 states of India. I had been his cardiologist-cum-physician from 1995 till 2021, when we lost him in August 2021. I felt it as a personal loss.

His son Mian Altaf, who is a very good friend, is in active politics from the National Conference Party. In fact, it is because of him and his efforts that allowed me to purchase land and finally construct a house of my own in the valley.

18

My Experience with Covid

During the first wave of Covid-19 around March 2020 in Delhi, the most affected people I saw were those living in the crowded localities and ghettos like Zamrudpur, near Greater Kailash I and Sangam Vihar, a very large South Delhi slum. Persons living in organized and less crowded colonies were in general infected in much smaller numbers although they were very scared and remained indoors.

I had to go for my professional work to the hospital and also perform emergency lifesaving procedures on persons who were not tested for Covid. The result was that I got an asymptomatic infection revealed by a mandatory testing before a proposed air travel to Srinagar in June 2020. I quarantined myself as per the guidelines in a flat, which was my office located close to my residence in Greater Kailash I, all alone. My father and wife along with our maids were living in our home. My daughter from Pune and nephew from Bengaluru used to courier me food items and my routine medicines. This was because no one in our block was prepared to even get the stuff to my doorstep. I became an untouchable with people closing their windows if I dared to come to my balcony to have a glimpse of the outside world. The chemist of our colony also expressed his inability to send me my routine medicines. The Delhi government sent an ambulance to my official address to fetch me to a hospital. I could, however, dodge them successfully by assuring the higher authorities that I am a responsible doctor in a quarantine which could be inspected. The neighbours even complained to the district magistrate and the local police that I am endangering their lives. A police constable came to write a report but when I asked him to come to my flat while maintaining a distance, he too ran away and I was left alone.

I cooked my own meals once a day and kept it preserved in the refrigerator. The isolation period mercifully got over. I got a certificate from the Municipal Corporation of Delhi as my passport to move freely. I felt like a prisoner released from jail after the conviction got over. I decided to finally get a negative certificate and booked an air ticket to Srinagar. I have never been away from Kashmir for so long. However, when I went to the airport, I found my Aarogya Setu app was still red, indicating that I am still showing positive for the virus. I, however, had a certificate from a credible ICMR recognised lab that the test was negative, two days before the date of travel. I could persuade the CISF (Central Industrial Security Force) chief for the terminal somehow and made an entry despite a red mark on the app.

The second and the deadlier Covid-19 wave appeared around March 2021 soon after vaccines had become available. During this wave, a large number of residents of our colony got infected while those living in nearby slums were spared, possibly because of acquiring immunity during the first wave. This time, I became a darling of the neighbourhood and was deluged with phone calls. They wanted me to help them in getting beds in the hospital for treatment, especially for getting oxygen. I tried and got as many as possible admitted to my hospital. Everything including oxygen and common drugs like blood thinners and steroids were in shortage. On one day in our hospital seven patients died because of lack of oxygen. The wave involved the whole of the country. The mortality was significant and the scare enormous. On a personal note, I lost three of my close relations during this horrible wave. Vaccine hesitancy was at its peak but the good thing is that people soon started realizing its importance and started coming forward for both the doses. The vaccination programme of India has really been superb, and kudos to the manufacturers, especially Serum Institute of India and Bharat Biotech, for providing the vaccines and the government for vaccinating people.

As we were getting out of the second wave, the highly transmissible third wave came with the Omicron variant and brought with it an unprecedented surge of infections globally. These variants spread the infection rapidly than the existing Delta variant (of the second wave) with a much faster doubling time. Though the severity of illness was milder with lower hospitalisation requirements, the Omicron variant resulted in very high morbidity in the community though with a much lower mortality. There were many instances where persons who had previous Covid infections and were fully vaccinated got infected. As an example, several key doctors in the health centres the author is involved with were down with Covid, some of them even after taking the precautionary third dose of the vaccine. Entire families getting infected has been a hallmark of the third phase. Knowing the exact numbers of those infected won't be possible because a large population did not get tested. The patients who got admitted and had a bad outcome had been suffering from severe pre-existing illnesses. The future forecast from the WHO (World Health Organisation) is that Omicron will be followed by more mutants of the virus. The next virus is likely to be more transmissible because it has to overtake the present strain. The precise effect on morbidity and mortality is as yet unpredictable.

The responsibility of the healthcare workers, especially doctors, has really been very challenging since the onset of the pandemic in March 2020. From a position of denial to a frightening situation during the second wave when everything was in short supply and treatment algorithms kept on changing, they also faced the anger and ire of the families of very sick patients who were dying in front of them, making them feel helpless. According to a report of June 2021, 1,342 doctors died since the beginning of the pandemic including 594 in the two months of the second wave. Isn't it a supreme sacrifice?

Finally, since there is no indication the virus will leave the human host unscathed, we cannot be complacent, and it is time to make Covid-appropriate behaviour a part of our life. Vaccinations can save us from death and hospitalisation but not from getting infected.

19

Gauri Manzil: A Dream Come True

In the last few years of her life, Amma used to reminisce often about Kashmir. She would watch the Doordarshan Koshur channel most of the time. We would often find her singing along with the Kashmiri songs being telecast. While sitting in the verandah in front of our Greater Kailash home, she would call the Kashmiri shawl vendors and chat with them, enquiring about how things were back in Kashmir. Sometimes, she would be so delighted to talk to people from her homeland that she would offer them tea and the group of vendors would continue gossiping till they wanted to go on their business. At times, she would introduce them to the neighbours who would then call them to their place. Any Kashmiri patient coming to see me would come home frequently before visiting the hospital. She would call them in our living room, greet them and also offer them a cup of tea. She would sit with them and chat for a long time. This gesture of hers is still remembered by them several years after her passing away.

One day, while watching a Kashmiri serial on TV, she said, 'I wish we could have a small place of our own in the valley. After all, it is our real home.' I looked up at her and smiled. I had also been toying with this idea for a while because I hated to stay in hotels on my frequent visits to the valley. None of my family members, especially my father and uncles, who had seen the migration of the Pandits in 1990, encouraged this idea of mine. It would be the usual argument—Kashmir was no longer safe; people were leaving and not coming back; how would I maintain a place over there? These arguments never convinced me, as I never thought I would not be welcomed there. Moreover, my feelings for my place of birth were intense.

My mama Prithvi had once mentioned that Maharaja Karan Singh, who was a good friend of his, had gifted a piece of land to him and Mir Qasim, the then chief minister of Jammu and Kashmir, around 1978. Since he was the principal secretary to Prime Minister Indira Gandhi, he had accepted the land in the name of B.L. Dhar, his younger brother. The land was on Gupkar Road, a prime area on the bank of Dal Lake, but on the side of the Maharaja's palace, now leased to Hotel Lalit Palace. He offered that land to me for building a clinic-cum-residence. He gave me the papers. I got them verified for their authenticity from the revenue department at Srinagar. I even went to inspect the land. There was a wall in between the road and the allotted land. After being gifted the land, Mir Qasim had sent an architect to review the place for utilising it. The gentleman was not given much cooperation to enter the area despite trying a few times. Mir Qasim felt bad and returned the allotted land to the Maharaja, who took it back without any grudge. Likewise, P.N. Dhar's son was also told by Karan Singh's son Ajatshatru that tampering with the historic wall was not possible. The meaning was loud and clear and this plan of having a house in Srinagar on the gifted royal land was abandoned.

The next step was to ask my friends there to look for a piece of land at an appropriate place in Srinagar. Many of them thought I was not serious since I was comfortably living in Delhi. The search continued till one day I got a call from Mian Altaf, in April 2013, that he had seen a place ideally suited for me and had paid an advance too, since the owner had to leave for Dubai. The area was near Srinagar airport in a cooperative colony called High Land Enclave. It was a place which till recently was an almond-growing orchard area with snow-clad mountains visible on all sides. I ensured that the work starts soon. Within a few days, my friend and architect Dileep Thusoo produced the drawing of the house we were planning and my dad flew to Srinagar to do a *bhoomi poojan* in May 2013. Now that things were underway, the family started getting excited about returning to Kashmir, even for a few weeks in a year.

The construction of the house started and by April 2014, it was finally ready. It was a small, two-storied house with three bedrooms, a lawn with seasonal flowers and even a mini kitchen garden. I named the house after Amma—Gauri Manzil. All the supervision, quality control and getting the hardware was supervised by my friend, mentor and a grateful patient Abdul Majeed Kaboo, who too was instrumental in transforming this burning desire into a reality. Liaqat Ali, a gentleman from Rajouri, had joined as a multipurpose caretaker during the construction period. I taught him cooking and today he cooks well and is part of Gauri Manzil for the last seven years. Entering Gauri Manzil gives me profound satisfaction and when I sit on the carpet in my living room with friends, my mother's smiling portrait gives me solace. The place is full of peaceful tranquillity, broken only by the chirping of birds and the occasional helicopter meandering.

The long-term plan for this abode is to shift the office of Gauri Kaul Foundation, which I will talk about next, and keep one room as a gallery of my mother's pictures with other family members for posterity.

20

Gauri Kaul Foundation and Genesis

One fine evening, in July 2020, while sitting at Gauri Manzil with my friends, Azaz Rashid, Nasir Lone and others, I mentioned that I have never visited North Kashmir and the much-talked-about Lolab Valley. I proposed that we take a day trip the next day. I was told that the visit should be for at least two days and a night. Since time was short, we decided to go the next month. We kept our resolve and went to Kupwara. There we saw the famous Kalaroos (Qila-e-Roos) cave and a giant rock called Satbaran (a stone with seven doors for different routes to Russia). One of the caves is called Tramkhan, a crimson-coloured copper mine cave. These secret caves which mythologically are supposed to connect to Russia have been explored extensively and it was found that they end after a short distance, and a few of them have been blasted by the armed forces to prevent them from being used as hiding places by extremists. Many believe that Satbaran was a temple in the ancient era where the Pandavas used to worship.

After seeing these caves, we went to Nasir's ancestral home in Sogam, Lolab, which was a rather deserted multi-storied building, and spent the night there. We also coaxed him to get it cleaned and white-washed so as to make it liveable. He came from a family of popular politicians of the National Conference party in that area, and we knew he could actually do it and become a successful politician. He heeded our coaxing and stood in the district council elections in 2021. He got elected and is bringing in development plans to Sogam area along with other elected members.

On our way back, we came via Kupwara town and met some people and patients with uncontrolled high blood pressure and diabetes with plenty of heart diseases. We decided to do something good for the community there and came up with the idea of organising a camp. Incidentally, we met the commandant of Rashtriya Rifles 44, who invited us to stay in their premises at Kalaroos hills. We accepted the offer and had a typical military-style immaculate get-together in the evening. We touched base with the chief medical officer of Kupwara and held a medical camp in the District Hospital, which had kept screened patients. Our team consisted of a group of doctors from Srinagar, Dr Aijaz Mansoor, our partner Dr Zubair Saleem and our friend Ajaz Rashid. I learnt that Ajaz's father was a medical officer at Kupwara for many years in the 1970s. For these reasons, Ajaz knew Kupwara very well and liaised with the doctors and the Deputy Commissioner there. All of us together decided to name our project Gauri Healthy Heart Project. The first camp was held on 29 September 2020, which coincided with World Heart Day. More than a hundred patients were seen and their treatment was optimised by giving them cost-effective combination drugs and starting new medicines for diabetes patients, besides counselling them on diet and exercise.

After successfully organising the camp, on our return to Kalaroos, the CO asked us if we had heard about Machil, a sector which gets cut off for five to six months in a year because of heavy snowfall and avalanches. The name also reminded me of the Machil encounters near the LoC (Line of Control). We made a plan to go there too and organised a health camp in the PHC (primary health centre) of Dudi village in Machil. The next morning, on 30 September 2020, we had a half-day camp with the help of a few doctors posted there. During the camp, patients narrated their woes of very poor medical care during long periods of no accessibility to the valley. We also saw patients with out-of-control blood pressure and diabetes with classical symptoms of impending heart attacks. The supply of drugs was very erratic. The dispensary attends to patients from 20 villages of this area.

I was struck by the idea of providing improved healthcare strategies for these people. The population of the area was only 15,000. It made it look feasible for our foundation. With the area being cut off for long periods brought in the idea of extending digital medicine to solve it, under the banner of 'No Heart Attacks Mission'. Our team deliberated about this and also discussed it with Col. Chauhan, the 2IC (second in command) of RR 56, who was incidentally a graduate of the London School of Economics. The unit had laid out a lunch to welcome us. He also showed us a building named posthumously after Major J.S. Sahi, Shaurya Chakra, who got martyred in an encounter fighting gallantly.

The army welcomed the idea and offered to provide internet connection and electricity throughout the year for the project and revamp the building. This area gets intensely cold and cut off from rest of the valley during winter. Such low temperatures can also lead to worsening of the condition of heart patients.

Our monthly district camps continued. From Machil in Kupwara, we went to Krim Shore and Ring Zabal in Tehsil Khan Sahab, Budgam district, Rajpora near my ancestral village Hawal in Pulwama district, Banihal across the Pir Panjal Range in Ramban district, backwaters of Dal Lake in the area of Bahri, Moti Mahal, the Leper Colony, and

Bahrore on the banks of Nagin Lake, Srinagar. We also conducted a healthy heart camp under 'No Heart Attacks Mission' in the migrant township in Jagti in January 2021. This population consists mostly of Kashmiri Pandits who earlier had a harrowing time in several makeshift camps after being forced to leave their hearths in villages of the valley. This exodus had happened around 1990 during the militancy period in the valley.

As one enters the township, one is struck by the sadness and isolation looming large on the faces of its inhabitants. They come mostly from villages of different districts of the valley and only a small number come from Srinagar. Problems like high blood pressure, diabetes and related heart problems were seen in high numbers in the two-day camp we organised. We did not see any working facility in that area or the neighbourhood looking after their health and once again felt the need for a digitally operated preventive cardiology unit like in Machil. The organization and execution of these camps were done by my colleague and CEO of the Gauri Kaul Foundation, Ajaz Rashid, and the Research Department of Batra Hospital headed by Priyadarshini and her coordinating staff.

After returning from these two distant and diverse areas of the Union Territory, we approached several organisations to provide us funding for these projects. The first response came from R.N. Dubey, Deputy GM Corporate Social Responsibility (CSR) wing of Indian Oil Corporation (IOC). He, however, wanted us to submit a novel project, something out of the box. We thought of two telecardiology systems—one for Kashmir and another for the migrants of Jagti township near Jammu. The project was written and submitted. It received the attention of the management of the IOC under their CSR head. M.A. Pathan, former chairman of the IOC, used his extensive experience and good offices to guide us in this endeavour. Our proposal, fortunately, met all their stringent requirements. The

IOC gave us a clear signal to go ahead with these two projects. They also agreed to give us a specially designed ambulance to ferry patients in the Machil area. The army worked at the Sahi Memorial Hospital, in Machil, and trained their personnel to take care of the telecardiology system. The unit was inaugurated on 18 October 2021 and is functional. We are also in the process of seeking cooperation in several projects to improve healthcare in several remote areas of the UT of Jammu and Kashmir.

At this stage, we realised that a large number of patients seen by us in camps were not getting optimal investigations done and the follow-up of those who need special care was far from satisfactory. This led us to plan a service where all the non-invasive cardiology facilities could be kept under one roof. Two cardiologists trained by me in Delhi, Dr Abid Hussain and Dr Muneer Ahmad, agreed to be part of it full-time. That was the beginning of the 'Gauri Heart Centre' in the heart of Srinagar at Chanapora, dedicated to the people of the valley. In this paid facility, besides ECG, echocardiography and doppler studies, stress tests, long-term monitoring of BP and heart rhythm, and a head-up tilt test has been made available. No patient is denied a consultation and investigation for want of finances. Finally, the Gauri Healthy Heart Project was registered as Gauri Kaul Foundation, an NGO, on 10 April 2021, with its offices in Srinagar and New Delhi.

The trustees of this foundation are: M.A. Pathan, former chairman of IOC and consultant to the Tatas, Amod Kanth, former Director General of Police and founder of the NGO Prayas—an organization protecting children's rights, Devaki Jain, a well-known feminist economist and author, Sudhir S. Bloeria, former chief secretary, Jammu and Kashmir government, and Meeraben Shah, a well-known social worker and activist.

We plan to continue our camps with the motto of 'No More Heart Attacks by 2025'. These camps will be organised with the cooperation of local authorities and the army. The aim is to see and investigate 100 to 150 patients having high risk for getting heart attacks; optimise their treatment, wherever possible to provide drugs, and counsel them; and organise a public lecture for inhabitants and an interactive session with physicians. We are being helped by many good Samaritans including through the corporate social responsibility (CSR) funds of many organisations. Reaching to the farthest points of every district is our motto. We are hopeful that the present administration will also appreciate these efforts and strengthen us.

The academics and research component of the Gauri Kaul Foundation is an integral part of our endeavours. It is a separate vertical with a team of trained research coordinators working under our General Manager Priyadarshini. An ethics committee headed by Prof A.H. Zargar has already been constituted. The paperwork as per the ICMR (Indian Council of Medical Research) guidelines has been completed. It would be submitted in the office of the Drugs Controller General of India (DCGI). The Gauri Kaul Research Centre is located in the office of our foundation in Srinagar and was launched on 11 April 2022 in the presence of our trustees.

Afterword

However well you think you know people you met as adults, you never truly get to know them till you get to hear or read about their life stories. Not just as mature grown-ups, but also of their formative influences and experiences in childhood and youth. Only then you get to understand the many elements that moulded their personality, shaped their beliefs, sharpened their skills and positioned them as leaders in their chosen fields. You also get a better understanding of their world view, of people, places and things. That is an education by itself. Reading this fascinating personal narrative by Dr Upendra Kaul has been a revealing and enriching experience in many ways.

I have known Dr Kaul as an accomplished, dedicated and eminent Indian cardiologist who is a Kashmiri by ethnic identity. Before reading this book, I did not clearly recognise that this Delhi-bred cardiologist holds Kashmir dearest to his heart, deeply in love with its land, people and culture. After reading the book, I can see why. Even as I read his evocative descriptions, I felt suffused with affection for the land that has unparalleled natural beauty, rich culture, culinary excellence and pride in its distinct identity. I also shared the author's anguish at the troubled history of this land in recent decades.

I was indeed also unaware of Dr Kaul's talent as a writer who could carry his reader with him with such deep engagement. Having been his colleague in the Department of Cardiology at AIIMS (Delhi), I knew of his ability to publish excellent scientific papers in prestigious medical journals. Those were necessarily impersonal and unemotional. This book is very different. Through its pages, the author carries the reader through the varied experiences of his life with an intimate style that makes the reader visualise every event, experience every relationship and identify with every emotion of the narrator. It is a story that is told with frankness, without masking his reactions to unfair happenings and persons who did not behave well with him. More than the sharp stings of those prickly recollections, the reader is entranced by myriad cherished memories of loving family ties, treasured and enduring personal friendships and valued professional associations.

The book is rich in anecdotes, where you applaud his ability to walk miles to college, smile at his short-lived experiment with charas, and appreciate his ability to cross class barriers to form a firm friendship with a police constable who deals with medico-legal cases at the hospital's emergency department. Such personal vignettes dot almost every page, as the author moves from childhood in rural Kashmir to the status of a celebrated cardiologist in India and abroad. On the way, we meet many individuals, visit diverse lands and share numerous experiences—all of which shaped Dr Kaul and now reshape our understanding of who he is.

As a doctor and cardiologist, I fully identify with his reflections on the professional attributes of a competent and caring doctor and share his concerns on the impersonal disconnect that the technology-driven medical practice is creating between doctors and patients. When he laments that the art of attentive history taking and conducting a thorough clinical examination is fading fast, I know that it is not the generational gripe of an old-school physician but the genuine angst of a technologically adept interventional cardiologist who respectfully views the patient as a human being and not as a tally of test results.

As a cardiologist, I also enjoyed walking through the gallery of physicians and cardiologists, Indian and international, who are profiled in the book. Some have passed on, others are still active. Several I know personally, others only by reputation. They are all introduced through brief pen portraits of both their professional accomplishments and personal attributes. We also learn about how cardiology evolved over the past five decades, to blend the strengths of advancing science and innovative technologies to bring remarkable relief to persons suffering from serious heart and blood vessel diseases. To a current student of cardiology, this book provides a very illuminating introduction to the history of cardiology in India.

The love of cardiology, Kashmir and his mother are blended into Dr Kaul's most passionate project—the creation of the Gauri Kaul Foundation and the Gauri Heart Centre in Srinagar. He may have studied, worked, married and risen to heights of professional glory in Delhi but his heart still beats for Kashmir with a constant cadence of committed love for that land. I hope he will soon be able to celebrate the return of harmony to a land from where his childhood memories carry only messages of love, friendship and peaceful co-existence.

Prof. K. Srinath Reddy
President, Public Health Foundation of India,
Former HOD Cardiology, AIIMS, New Delhi

Index

SOCIO-ECONOMIC PROFILE OF RURAL INDIA (SERIES II)

Volume Five

NORTH AND CENTRAL INDIA

ABOUT THE CENTRE FOR RURAL STUDIES

The Centre for Rural Studies (formerly Land Reforms Unit) of the Lal Bahadur Shastri National Academy of Administration was set up in the year 1989 by the Ministry of Rural Development, Government of India, with a multifaceted agenda that included among others, the concurrent evaluation of the ever-unfolding ground realities pertaining to the implementation of the Land Reforms and Poverty Alleviation Programmes in India. Sensitizing the officer trainees of the Indian Administrative Service in the process of evaluating of land reforms and poverty alleviation programmes by exposing them to the ground realities; setting up a forum for regular exchange of views on land reforms and poverty alleviation between academicians, administrators, activists and concerned citizens and creating awareness amongst the public about the various programmes initiated by the Government of India through non-governmental organisations are also important objectives of the Centre for Rural Studies. A large number of books, reports related to land reforms, poverty alleviation programmes, rural socio-economic problems etc. published both externally and internally bear testimony to the excellent research quality of the Centre.

ABOUT THE EDITOR

Raj Mohini Sethi was Professor of Sociology at the Panjab University, Chindigarh. She has written extensively on different aspects of development studies, covering areas of land reforms and other aspects of rural society especially gender and development. Her earlier works include: *Modernisation of Working Women in India and Turkey; Female Labour in Agriculture: Punjab; Women in Agriculture: A study of Women and Development in Himachal Pradesh;* and *Globalization, Culture and Women's Development.*

She has written several papers and completed research projects in the area of integrated development, and gender studies. She has also written on the legal profession and other socio-cultural issues. She has been a member of the Editorial Review Committee of the *Journal of Contemporary Ethnography and Sociological Bulletin,* and a consultant to the Government of Punjab. She is a resource person for several organizations which include the Indain Council of Social Welfare, Punjab and Chandigarh branches; University Grants Commission, and Centre for Budget and Governance Accountability, New Delhi.

SOCIO-ECONOMIC PROFILE OF RURAL INDIA (SERIES II)

VOLUME FIVE

NORTH AND CENTRAL INDIA

(Punjab, Haryana, Himachal Pradesh and Madhya Pradesh)

Edited by

Raj Mohini Sethi

Published for
Centre for Rural Studies
L.B.S. National Academy of Administration, Mussoorie
By
CONCEPT PUBLISHING COMPANY PVT. LTD.
NEW DELHI-110059

ISBN-13: 978-81-8069-721-0 (Series)
ISBN-13: 978-81-8069-736-4 (Vol. 5)

First Published 2011

Published and Printed by

Concept
Since 1974

Concept Publishing Company Pvt. Ltd.
Regd. Office:
A/15-16, Commercial Block, Mohan Garden
New Delhi-110059 (India)
Phones: 25351460, 25351794, *Fax*: 091-11-25357109
Email: publishing@conceptpub.com,
Website: www.conceptpub.com

Editorial Office:
H-13, Bali Nagar, New Delhi-110 015, India.

Cataloging in Publication Data--Courtesy: D.K. Agencies (P) Ltd. <docinfo@dkagencies.com>

Socio-economic profile of rural India (series II).
v. 5 cm.
Contributed articles.
Includes bibliographical references and index.
Contents: v. 5. North and central India (Punjab, Haryana, Himachal Pradesh and Madhya Pradesh) / edited by Raj Mohini Sethi.
ISBN 9788180697210 (set)
ISBN 9788180697364 (v. 5)

1. India--Rural conditions. 2. India--Economic conditions. I. Lal Bahadur Shastri National Academy of Administration. Centre for Rural Studies.

DDC 307.720954 22

Lal Bahadur Shastri
National Academy of Administration
Mussoorie - 248179 (Uttarakhand) INDIA

Padamvir Singh, IAS
Director & Chairman
Centre for Rural Studies

Foreword

Socio-economic profile of Rural India is a regular publication of the Centre for Rural Studies, LBSNAA, Mussoorie. It consolidates the Village Study reports prepared by the Indian Administrative Service Officer Trainees who undertake detailed village level studies as part of their year long district training.

This publication is the product of these studies covering the States of Punjab, Haryana, Himachal Pradesh and Madhya Pradesh. The State Papers have been enriched by inputs from academics and experts with experience in the study of North and Central parts of India.

I hope this volume will prove useful to academics, administrators and planners alike.

Padamvir Singh, *IAS*

Tel. : (0135) 2632727 (O)
EPABX : (0135) 26332374, 2632489, 2632405, 2632236, 2632367 Fax: (0135) 2632350, 2632720
Website : www.lbsnaa.ernet.in

Socio-Economic Profile of Rural India (Series - I)

Vol. I : SOUTH INDIA
(Andhra Pradesh, Karnataka, Kerala, Tamil Nadu)
Edited by **V.K. Agnihotri** IAS

Vol. II : NORTH-EAST INDIA
(Assam, Manipur, Tripura, Nagaland)
Edited by **C. Ashokvardhan** IAS

Vol. III : NORTH-CENTRAL & WESTERN INDIA
(Himachal Pradesh, Punjab, Haryana, Gujarat, Maharashtra) *Edited by* **Rajendra Vora**

Vol. IV : EASTERN INDIA
(Bihar, West Bengal, Orissa and Uttar Pradesh)
Edited by **C. Ashokvardhan** IAS

Socio-Economic Profile of Rural India (Series - II)

Vol. I : SOUTH INDIA
(Andhra Pradesh, Karnataka, Kerala, Tamil Nadu)

Vol. II : NORTH-EAST INDIA
(Assam, Manipur, Tripura, Nagaland)
Edited by **S.C. Patra & Ashish Vachhani** IAS

Vol. III : WESTERN INDIA
(Gujarat, Maharashtra, Rajasthan)

Vol. IV : EASTERN INDIA
(Orissa, Jharkhand, West Bengal, Bihar and Uttar Pradesh) *Edited by* **C. Ashokvardhan,** IAS & **Ashish Vachhani** IAS

Vol. V : NORTH & CENTRAL INDIA
(Punjab, Haryana, Himachal Pradesh and Madhya Pradesh *Edited by* **Raj Mohini Sethi**

Preface

A continuous evaluation of the rural economy and society in India is necessary in view of the constant changes occurring in it. Ever since the 1950s when a series of reform and rural development measures were initiated to change the face of rural India it has shown both upward and downward swings in its economy, polity, and society. Much has been done and much more could have been done to change the face of rural India. The present volume achieves this object and has made an attempt to gauge the extent of socio-economic changes experienced by rural society of North and Central India especially in view of the agrarian crisis in many parts of Indian society. In doing so, it not only provides the *raison d'etre* for this study but also fulfils one of the major objectives of the Centre for Rural Studies, LBS National Academy of Administration. It also puts forward suggestions for remodelling strategies for change taking into consideration the different social and cultural contextual factors hindering development within the region.

Eminent social scientists and administrators from the states of Punjab, Haryana, Himachal Pradesh and Madhya Pradesh were asked to write a report on the socio-economic scenario within the state and how the state had responded to the different development schemes introduced by the Central and State Governments. The different chapters of the volume give an illuminating account of the social and economic indicators of development, existing infrastructural facilities, land use patterns, agrarian relations, land reforms and farm and non-farm employment opportunities and the major concerns of each state. The information given in each chapter is based on both secondary source data and the empirical studies conducted by the authors themselves and by the I.A.S. Officer Trainees and by other research scientists.

Dr. Raj Mohini Sethi has helped in editing this book based on materials provided by the Centre. We would like to acknowledge the lucid contributions of all the authors and thank them for the tremendous effort undertaken to prepare the state reports and thereafter introduce a series of revisions.

Ashish Vachhani, IAS
Deputy Director &
Coordinator
Centre for Rural Studies
Lal Bahadur Shastri National Academy of Administration
Mussoorie

Acknowledgements

A considerable amount of empirical and theoretical work already exists in the social sciences in relation to the social and economic characteristics of rural India. Periodical evaluation and research on the subject helps in evolving new understanding and suitable research methodology and for devising strategies in accordance with the ground reality. The present volume: *Socio-Economic Profile of Rural India* is a modest attempt in this direction.

I owe a sense of deep gratitude to Shri Padamvir Singh, Director and Chairman, Centre for Rural Studies, LBS National Academy of Administration for handing over the stupendous task editing this volume to me.

I am also grateful to Shri Ashish Vachhani, Deputy Director and Coordinator, Centre for Rural Studies, LBS National Academy of Administration, Mussoorie in giving this volume the present shape through his interactions with the authors and the editor at various stages of the preparation of the volume.

I would also like to acknowledge the lucid contributions of all authors, and IAS trainee officers and thank them for the tremendous effort taken to prepare the state reports and thereafter introduce a series of revisions.

In the end, I would like to thank the Staff of the Centre for Rural Studies and Varunendra Vikram Singh, Research Associate, for the work done by him and for his perseverance because of the endless delays in the editing of this volume.

Raj Mohini Sethi

Contents

List of Tables

Annexure A

List of Boxes

List of the Contributors

Sucha Singh Gill, Professor, Department of Economics, Punjabi University, Patiala.

Padamvir Singh, *IAS*, Director, Lal Bahadur Shastri National Academy of Administration, Mussoorie, Uttarakhand.

H.R. Sharma, Professor & Head, Department of Agricultural Economics, Extension Education & Rural Sociology, CSK Himachal Pradesh Agricultural University, Palampur, Himachal Pradesh.

Virender Kumar, Senior Scientist, Department of Agricultural Economics, Extension Education & Rural Sociology, CSK Himachal Pradesh Agricultural University, Palampur, Himachal Pradesh.

S.N. Chaudhary, Professor, Rajiv Gandhi Chair in Contemporary Studies, Barkatullah University, Bhopal.

Introduction

RAJ MOHINI SETHI

Social and economic development in Third World societies is one of the most widely discussed subjects in social sciences. The nature of underdevelopment and poverty in these countries is complex and varied and its solutions quite challenging as it requires a good grounding and knowledge of basic and peculiar features of social and economic conditions in each state and its constituents. Like all other phenomena rural social and economic profile has also been undergoing a change since time immemorial. This change has sometimes been imperceptive and slow and sometimes quite rapid showing visible signs of rural social transformation. Information gathered from various research studies by social scientists such as economists, sociologists and anthropologists reveal the role of variety of factors, in conjunction or alone, in this transformation. These studies also bring out the several institutional and other details of rural social and economic life and the changes that have occurred over time in the developing societies. Such periodical assessment helps in understanding the nature of change and development taking place if any in a society and the changes that are occurring in its social profile.

The pre-independence Indian economy which was overwhelmingly rural was marked by a period of stagnation. The growth of aggregate real output of Indian economy during the first half of the twentieth century was less than two per cent a year and the per capita output was less than half a per cent. The hallmark of the predominantly agrarian economy comprised 'village republics' practicing traditional agriculture and which had very low productivity. Illiteracy was as high as 84 per cent, mass communicable diseases had a widespread. And the problems of poverty, ignorance and disease were further aggravated by inequalities in the distribution of resources between groups and regions (Vaidyanathan, 1984: 947-948). After Independence, from the mid-sixties onwards the social and economic scene in rural India has been rapidly changing from stagnation to growth, from isolation to interconnection and from dependence to self-sufficiency in food grains. The reasons for this change were many but the most important were the modernization of agriculture, introduction and implementation of land reforms and the provision of infrastructural facilities such as all weather roads, easy access to credit and markets and other related development measures. State intervention in agriculture and rural society as a whole did not aim only at changes in agrarian relations only but also extended to the provision of public investments in education, health, irrigation, land improvement and agricultural research and extension apart from investments in farm subsidies. Increased agricultural production has mainly been achieved by intensification of agriculture and the introduction of high yielding varieties. The accelerated growth of agricultural economy has been instrumental in raising the income levels of agricultural workers and the per capita incomes rose around 40 per cent. All these factors taken together were responsible for the change in the overall social and economic profile of rural India. However, the rate of growth in non-farm sectors such as, manufacturing and services was far greater than that of the agricultural/rural economy as a whole. Such differential growth in different sectors of the economy has resulted in the loss of gross domestic product in agriculture from 57.7 per cent in 1950-51 to 20.8 per cent in 2004-05 but its share in the total employment market has declined only marginally (Bhalla, 2007:2).

This imbalance in agricultural and non-agricultural occupations and employment has deepened the intra-rural as well as the rural and urban divide in many parts of the country. During the first three Five Year Plan periods, that is between 1950-51 and 1964-65, the overall GDP grew at the rate of 3.94 per cent per annum and the per capita income growth was at the rate of 1.86 per cent per annum. The contribution of agriculture to this income was 2.54 per cent while that of the secondary and tertiary sectors was 6.88 per cent and 4.76 per cent per annum respectively. Between 1967-68 and 1979-80 there was a significant decline in GDP and per capita income. The overall GDP declined to 3.44 per cent and in agriculture, secondary and tertiary sectors it declined to 2.05, 4.23 and 4.54 per cent per annum respectively; while per capita income declined to 1.23 per cent. Between 1981-82 and 2003-04 the overall GDP increased considerably to 6.10 per cent but this increase was highly visible in secondary (6.29 per cent) and tertiary sectors of the economy (8.22%). The GDP in the agricultural sector increased substantially between 1980-81 and 1990-91 (3.08%) but registered a significant decline between 1992-93 and 2003-04 and the GDP came down to 2.38 per cent (Bhalla, 2007: 55-60 also see Table 0.1).

Table 0.1: Growth Rates of GDP and per capita Income at 1993-94 Prices

Years	*GDP*	*GDP Agric.*	*Secondary Sector*	*Tertiary Capita*	*Per Sector Income*
1950-51—1964-65	3.94	2.54	6.88	4.76	1.86
1967-68—1979-80	3.44	2.05	4.23	4.54	1.23
1981-82—1990-91	5.62	3.08	7.10	6.72	3.50
1992-93—2003-04	6.10	2.38	6.29	8.22	4.21

Source: Bhalla, G.S., *Indian Agriculture since Independence*, National Book Trust, 2007: 59. Also see Sivasubramanian, 2000, and National Accounts Statistics 2004.

While the transformation of Indian society from the sixties onwards was quite impressive in leading the Indian economy out of a state of stagnation to sustained growth and diversification, however, the overall pace of this development failed to match the standards set by other developing countries both in terms of industrial and agricultural growth. Resultantly, there were shortfalls in the growth of per capita real incomes during the different plan periods and between the objectives of the different Five Year Plans and the achievements of the Indian economy during the period. The main reason for this mismatch was attributed to the rapid growth of population accompanied by a decline in mortality rates because of the control of communicable diseases. Apart from that because of the introduction of liberalization and economic reforms, the post reform period (from the 1990s onwards) witnessed a significant decline in agricultural growth rates both at the all India and state levels. Though this slowdown was experienced by all the states, its impact was more on the relatively prosperous states barring the states of Maharashtra and Gujarat. Agricultural growth between 1980-81 and 2003-04 came down from 9.9 per cent to 6.0 per cent. In Punjab increase in per worker annual agricultural growth rate between 1993-94 and 1999-2000 was only 0.85 per cent; while in Haryana it was 2.08 per cent, and in Himachal Pradesh it was 1.90 per cent (Bhalla, 2007:54-95). The main reasons for this slowdown in agricultural growth were the liberalization of the economy in the early 1990s, India's membership of W.T.O. and the resultant change in the food policy discourse in India. The immediate impact of the new policy was the acute shortage of wheat within the country while it continued to export the same (Shergill, 2008:5-6). Food security has once again become a major problem in agriculture. Another fallout of this slowdown in agricultural economy was the decline in the demand for labour in rural areas and significant increases in the number of unemployed and a decline in rural incomes and savings which dampened the incentives for private investment in agriculture. Moreover, the increased provision of subsidies during and after the eighties made a dent into the available surplus for public investment on agriculture and rural infrastructure (Rao, 1994:20-21). Institutional sources of credit have not been able to meet the total credit needs of the farming community. Around 42.3 per cent of their credit needs are met by non-institutional sources of credit which charge exorbitant rates of interest (GOI, 2005). The overall impact of the agrarian crisis can be seen in large scale indebtedness of the peasantry resulting in suicides in many parts of the country. Large sections of small and marginal farmers and landless labourers today have become vulnerable to extreme levels of anxiety and stress because they are unable to get out of the debt trap and often resort to suicides (IDC, 1998:45-46).

It was quite clear in the seventies that the strategy of economic growth that helped in the maximization of GNP was not enough to minimize poverty. For the removal of poverty, it was felt, a direct approach of rural development with a special focus on specific rural groups required urgent consideration. This idea gave birth to new schemes of development that were anti-poverty in focus such as small industries, minimum needs programme, SFDA, MFAL, IRDP, NREP, RLEGP and JRY. While framing the target group approach it was not, however, visualized that a uniform policy which ignored the overall regional disparities in development and institutional frameworks and also the divergence in cultural patterns would not be a viable solution.

It was incumbent on the planners and policy makers to understand that the developed and underdeveloped regions required different strategies of development to overcome the problem of poverty (Rao, 1994:105-156). Research in social sciences and state reports presented in this volume reiterate these variations in the incidence of poverty and the proportions of BPL households as well as the response of the people to these schemes. They show how the existence of a favourable institutional framework and labour intensive "wage-goods" friendly agricultural economy helped in a better sharing of the benefits of growth with the poor in the states of Punjab and Haryana. Similar has been the experience of Himachal Pradesh which resorted to eco-friendly diversification in cropping patterns and institutional reforms. In Madhya Pradesh where the institutional framework has been adverse and agricultural growth has been slow, the benefits of growth have not percolated to the level of the poor to the extent they have in the northern states. For such states, poverty alleviation programmes, especially the schemes of Jawahar Rozgar Yojana and the Rural Labour Employment Guarantee Programme, have more relevance and have been instrumental in increasing the income and living conditions of the poor in spite of leakages and inefficiencies at the level of implementation which is bound to happen in a top down approach. Political institutions such as decentralized planning involve local level institutions or panchayats in planning and implementation of development strategies and in ensuring egalitarian sharing of benefits of development (Rao, 1994:195). In India, the processes of social development have been painfully slow in spite of several well thought of poverty alleviation schemes because of several fault lines in the functioning of political institutions and bad governance in making decisions, identifying beneficiaries, and implementation and supervision of development schemes.

Agrarian reforms such as land redistribution and security of tenures and higher crop shares for share croppers are other factors that help in a more inclusive growth. A progressive land reform policy helps to translate relatively small advantages in landholding into effective social dominance only if it is accompanied by involvement in new forms of capital and commodity markets. Institutional sources of credit for productive purposes provide the farmers some protection against unscrupulous money lenders and their unfair practices. The creation of an alternative institutional source of credit on easy loan payments helped the farmer to take capital intensive risk especially in the case of Punjab and Haryana where peasant proprietorship coupled with relatively small size of landholdings and consolidation of holdings contributed to investments of capital and innovative farm practices by the average landholder. In Himachal Pradesh on the other hand, in spite of the fact that surplus land has been redistributed among the landless reducing significantly the proportion of landless households, capital investments and innovative technologies suitable for hill areas, have largely remained out of reach of the poor landowning households (Sethi, 2004:1-26). A contrary picture emerges from Madhya Pradesh where the agrarian structure shows the predominance of absentee landholders and is highly skewed, and capital investments in agriculture have not been made. Resultantly, notable achievements in agricultural growth and the condition of the rural poor are not really visible.

Such differential growth in rural India raises the crucial question as to what is the current rural social and economic profile of North and Central India. What has been the history of development within this region? How have the government policies and programmes affected the lives of rural people and how have the people responded to them and which sections among them have benefited from rural social transformation and why? And in what manner have institutional reforms and other state interventions contributed to this transformation or even retardation? The present volume attempts to answer these and related questions in the context of three prosperous states of North India, that is, Punjab, Haryana, and Himachal Pradesh and another a 'BIMARU' state from Central India, Madhya Pradesh. The state papers discuss the performance of peasant society in the globalizing world by bringing together theory and experience at each level. The study was commissioned by the Centre for Rural Studies, Lal Bahadur Shastri Academy of Administration at Mussoorie. The state reports have been compiled by eminent academicians from each state. The authors provide an insight into the social and economic conditions of rural society within the state from a macro perspective with the help primarily of secondary source data and bring out the specificities of each state with the help of primary source data of micro studies done by IAS probationers or by the academicians themselves. The aim of the state reports is to provide an overall view of the state's performance in rural socio-economic development.

The state of Punjab was the first to experience the green revolution and in providing a lead to the country in rural development up till the beginning of the decade of the eighties. Between the sixties and the eighties it recorded the highest per capita income and its net State Domestic Product from agriculture rose to 33.6 per cent while rural poverty was reduced to 16.37 per cent. It acquired the best agricultural marketing system and achieved hundred per cent electrification and connected all villages to market towns with metalled link roads. All this was possible because of the early introduction of the community development programme, coupled with consolidation of holdings, extension of irrigation facilities, and research and extension back up of agricultural university. Sucha Singh Gill highlights the acute agrarian crisis confronting the state of Punjab today in spite of these impressive achievements. The crisis is not only in terms of high levels of unemployment because of non-diversification, stagnation and decline of economic growth, but also because of the fast deterioration of its social and cultural fabric and the rise of social inequalities. The relatively large component of urban population of the state (33.95%) is unable to absorb the growing numbers of unemployed in the rural and urban areas. The state has been undergoing a steady process of marginalization of the small and marginal farmers because of leasing out, sale and mortgage of land to the large land holders and rural indebtedness. Farmer's suicides have become a common occurrence while the rural social institutions have decayed and other support structures and social capital are virtually nonexistent. The state's performance on social indicators such as sex ratios, levels of literacy, especially female literacy rates, is dismal while the change is more visible in the urban areas. The reasons attributed to this lopsided development are many but the core ones are administrative preoccupation with the restoration of law and order as basic functions, along with official apathy and lack of political will of the ruling elite towards meaningful development in the state. Anti-poverty programmes and other centrally sponsored schemes have not been implemented and grants under these schemes have remained almost unutilized or underutilized because the state has not been able to provide the matching grants from its own kitty. Development schemes such as RLEGP provide very low wages which are not acceptable to most unemployed as agricultural wages in the state are quite high because of the use of hired labour. Development functions and the requisite finances have not been transferred to Panchayati Raj Institutions. Panchayat bodies have become highly politicized and elections to these bodies are a costly affair. Sucha Singh Gill poses serious questions on the mismatch between economic and social growth on the one hand and lack of vision and will of the ruling elite in giving a forward push to the state's economy and society on the other. The paper also raises the issue of the introduction of state or region specific development policies.

In his paper on Haryana, Padamvir Singh has effectively spelled out the changes occurring in the rural society of Haryana. His analysis is based on the socio-economic surveys of nine villages conducted by IAS probationers during 1994 and 2002; and he introduces the reader to district and village level differentials in agriculture, animal husbandry and agrarian structure and relations. Apart from these, variations in social and demographic indicators such as education, health and other socio-cultural practices have also been spelled out vividly. The author further looks at the state's performance on government interventions such as poverty alleviation programmes and political institutions such as the panchayats. The overall profile of Haryana is a success story because of substantial increases in productivity of food grains and ushering in an era of green revolution between the years 1966-67 and 1993-94 through the use of intensive agricultural practices such as fertilizers and tractors. The average size of the operational holding in the state is much larger (2.13 hectares) than the national average. The average size of the operational holdings varies from 1.44 hectares in district Faridabad to 3.15 hectares in district Sirsa (Statistical Abstract of Haryana 2001-02). The peasant cultivator mode of production has made the agricultural holdings progressive and highly productive. In addition Haryana also has a rich stock of productive livestock and the average milk yields are quite high. Agricultural growth in Haryana is reflected in the steep rise in per capita income, accelerating the growth rate of Net Domestic Product, and overall reduction of poverty over the years. The state's location on the outskirts of the national capital region has helped it to create a dent in the secondary and tertiary sectors as well. However, the state of Haryana lags behind in its performance on social indicators, especially at the level of literacy, health and sex ratios. The social and cultural ethos continue to remain orthodox and traditional and which continue to pose a big challenge in alleviating the status of women and weaker sections of society. Panchayati Raj Institutions have deepened the caste/class divisions and fissures while the parallel functioning of '*Khaap Panchayats*' resists all change. Poverty Alleviation Programmes have not made a significant dent in the state because of low income limit of these programmes and the *ad hoc* nature of their functioning. The author suggests that greater emphasis needs to be placed on overall development plans such as Haryana Urban Development Authority to achieve better results in removing poverty than the existing poverty alleviation schemes. This suggestion can be contested since it is doubtful that such efforts alone would help to bridge the gap between the rich and the poor. The village case studies are informative and bring out the social and cultural specificities of each district. However, the state report would have become far more informative and rich in analysis if the impact of New Economic Policy and / or the agrarian crisis, if any, faced by the state had also been included.

H.R. Sharma and Virender Kumar highlight how the least developed state of Himachal Pradesh was able to transform its socio-economic profile by adopting development strategies that took into cognizance the geo-physical and agro-climatic differentiations within different regions of the state. The state today presents a picture of holistic and balanced growth and development as compared to the neighbouring states of Punjab and Haryana. In terms of economic growth the state accounted for only 0.1 per cent of the total very poor households and 16.7 per cent of the total poor and has helped in diminishing social inequalities to a large extent. This is evident from the proportions of landless agricultural labour to cultivators and also the assets owned by the poor households. This has been possible because of the diversification of the cropping pattern and growth of high value crops suitable to specific agro climatic regions which has further helped in the regeneration of trade and business and related non-farm activities giving a boost to the economy and absorbing both skilled and unskilled labour. Other factors that contributed towards agrarian development were effective implementation of land reforms and the establishment of an effective institutional backup. The state has achieved remarkable success in the provision of infrastructural facilities such as roads, electricity, safe drinking water, apart from the facilities of education and health. On the level of social and demographic indicators also the state's performance is highly commendable in terms of sex ratios, female literacy, fertility and infant mortality rates and in the reduction of social inequalities. However, regional and inter-district variations are paramount at all levels—social, economic and infrastructural. The authors rightly point out that because of liberalization and globalization the state faces the challenge of competition with foreign markets which it can overcome only if it expands the public sector of employment by creating ultramodern infrastructural facilities for attracting new industries and by checking the downward slide of its fiscal health.

The profile of Central India is represented by one of the largest and also sick states of India—Madhya Pradesh which comprises 48 districts and most of them have very high percentage of the poor. Some districts like Jhabua, Burhanpur and Sagar have more than fifty per cent of the population living below the poverty line. Landlessness is quite acute in the state and the proportion of marginal farmers is as high as 37.33 per cent. The process of redistribution of land to the poor is slow, arbitrary and the quality of distributed land is poor and so small that it is unfit for cultivation or for making any improvement on it. Land reforms have been a failure and absentee landlords (30.9%) continue to hold large tracts of land above the ceiling limit. The state which has a rich wealth of forests, minerals and traditional handicrafts could have made giant strides in development during the last sixty years but administrative apathy and lack of political will has led to unchecked deforestation, non-provision of irrigational facilities, and non-introduction of modern technology and also improper implementation of development schemes. For these and other reasons the state today represents a picture of overall deterioration and near total neglect of the agrarian economy and society. Lack of interest in improving rural community life and half hearted implementation of Anti-Poverty Programmes has left visible imprint on the social indicators of the state as well. Madhya Pradesh has the highest IMR (Infant Mortality Rate) and maternal mortality rate is the third highest in the country while 80 per cent of the children are vulnerable to preventable diseases and female literacy rate is very low and shows wide gap with the male literacy rate. The paper on Madhya Pradesh by S.N. Chaudhary brings out these and other facts quite vividly. However, if the author had provided some more information on indicators of economic growth in relation to overall growth rates in India and other states and also inter-district variations within the state the report would have become more meaningful. Also data on the reach of Anti Poverty Programmes at the village and district levels would have provided a better understanding of the nature of social and economic development occurring in the state.

The emphasis on agrarian society in North and Central India helps in reconceptualising the existing agrarian structures, the shifts occurring within these structures and the manner in which they affect other processes of change. It shows how structures of rural industry, trade and commerce help to promote or retard agricultural activity within a region. The present volume looks at the growth in agriculture and also its deceleration in later years leading to the present agrarian crisis, and the rising imbalances in economic and social sectors of development and the importance of people's agency in development and processes of cultural change. It further emphasizes the need to devise state and region specific policy initiatives.

REFERENCES

Bhalla, G.S. (2007): *Indian Agriculture since Independence,* National Book Trust, New Delhi, India.

Government of India (2005): *Draft final report of the task force on revival of co-operative credit institutions,* Ministry of Finance, New Delhi.

Institute for Development and Communication, (1998): *Suicides in Rural Punjab.* The Punjab State Co-operative Bank Ltd., Government of Punjab, Himalaya Press, Chandigarh.

Rao Hanumantha, C.H. (1994): *Agricultural Growth, Rural Poverty and Environmental Degradation in India,* Oxford University Press, Delhi.

Sethi, Raj Mohini (2004): "Land Property and Reform: A Study of Gender, Discriminatory Practices in Himachal Pradesh" in *Gender Discrimination in Land Ownership in the Context of Total Status of Women's Empowerment,* Lal Bahadur Shastri Academy of Administration, Mussourie.

Shergill, H.S. (2008): *Economics of Food Self-Sufficiency,* Institute for Development and Communication, Chandigarh.

Sivasubramonian, S. (2000): *The National Income of India in the Twentieth, Century,* Oxford University Press, New Delhi.

Vaidyanathan, A. (1970): "Indian Economy since Independence (1947-70)", in *The Cambridge History of India,* edited, Dharma Kumar, Vol. 2:947-995, Orient Longman: Cambridge University Press.

Appendix I

LIST OF TRAINESS WHOSE STUDIES ARE INCLUDED IN THIS VOLUME

Punjab

Sl. No.	Author	Village	District	Year
1.	Avhad, Nilkanth	Bhamabadi	Sangrur	2001
2.	Bhandari, Rahul	Jogipur	Patiala	1999
3.	Bhandari, Rakhee Gupta	Akbarpura	Patiala	1999
4.	Garg, Bhawna	Malian	Jalandhar	2001
5.	Garg, Vikas	Dhapai,	Gurdaspur	2000
6.	Gurjar, Sumer Singh	Akol	Sangrur	2000
7.	Kaur, Dilraj	Abhipur	Ropar	2002

Haryana

Sl. No.	Author	Village	District	Year
1.	Shyamal Misra	Kasumbhi	Bhiwani	1996
2.	A.K. Gupta	Silakhari	Faridabad	1994
3.	Deepak Tayal	Ransika	Gurgaon	2000
4.	Brijendra Singh	Kherki Daula	Gurgaon	1999
5.	Panka Aggrawal	Sikarpur	Hisar	2001
6.	Nitin Yadav	Bibipur	Karnal	2002
7.	D. Suresh (U.T. cadre)	Guskani	Rohtak	1997
8.	Rakesh Gupta	Kakana Bhadri	Sonepat	1999

Himachal Pradesh

Sl. No.	Author	Village	District	Year
1.	Anuradha Thakur	Movi Seri	Mandi	1994
2.	Onkar Chand Sharma	Rehlu	Kangra	1994
3.	Bharat Khera	Guruwala	Sirmour	1995
4.	Rahul Anand	Baidi	Kangra	1996
5.	Subhasish Panda	Khala Kiar	Sirmaur	1997
6.	Pushpendra Rajput	Hadal	Kangra	1999

(Contd.)

(*Contd.*)

Sl. No.	*Author*	*Village*	*District*	*Year*
7.	Amandeep Garg	Nahan	Sirmour	1999
8.	Madhup Vyas	Kasarvarnem	North Goa	2000
9.	R. Selvam	Nerti	Kangra	2001
10.	Nandita Gupta	Salogara	Solan	2001

Madhya Pradesh

Sl. No.	*Author*	*Village*	*District*	*Year*
1.	Nidhi Chibber	Purasani	Gwalior	1994
2.	Hari Ranjan Rao	Nayapura	Hoshangabad	1994
3.	Manoj Kumar Pingua	Kathautia	Shahdol	1994
4.	Sanjay Kumar Shukla	Ichkela	Raigarh	1994
5.	Vivek Aggrawal	Susera	Gwalior	1994
6.	Richa Sharma	Rajkudi	Durg	1994
7.	Rajkamal	Sankara	Durg	1994
8.	Rashmi Arun	Agasod	Sagar	1994
9.	Smita Gate	Ambachandan	Indore	1994
10.	Pallavi Jain Govil	Multhan	Dhar	1994
11.	Ravindra Telang	Dapka	Hoshangabad	1995
12.	Amit Rathore	Kosamdih	Bilaspur	1996
13.	Niteshkumar N. Vyas	Bhadakya	Dhar	1996
14.	Faiz A. Kidwai	Midkulnar	Bastar	1996
15.	R.K. Singh	Kamthi	Hoshangabad	1997
16.	Sukh Veer Singh	Patthar Khan	Bilaspur	1997
17.	Subodh Kumar Singh	Pipariya	Mandal	1997
18.	Manish Singh	Kamdevkurushpal	Bastar	1997
19.	Geetha M. Pingua	Belaji	Sagar	1997
20.	Beela Rajesh	Belaur	Bhojpur	1997
21.	Gulshan Barma	Amarpura	Jhabua	1997
22.	S. Karuna Raju	Pathapur	Chhatarpur	1998
23.	Mukesh Chand Gupta	Telikhamhi	Bilaspur	1998
24.	Akash Tripathy	Cheerakhan	Dhar	1998
25.	Pawan Kumar Sharma	Mawaijar	Mandla	1999
26.	Anil Yadav	Piplya	Ratlam	1999
27.	E. Ramesh Kumar	Kolawa	Mandsaur	1999
28.	Vivek Kumar Porwal	Chiklya	Dhar	2000
29.	Shobhit Jain Satbhaiya	Kharpai	Jhabua	2000
30.	N. Nawin Sona	Misrod	Hoshangabad	2000
31.	Sandeep Yadev	Kanknar	Sagar	2000
32.	Navneet Mohan Kothari	Richha Bachha	Mandsaur	2001
33.	Parikipandla Narahari	Karei	Chhindwara	2001
34.	C. Namdeo Borkar	Surgaon Joshi	Khandwa	2002
35.	Ajeet Kumar	Chiraidongri	Mandla	2002
36.	M. Selvendran	Bamori	Dewas	2002

1

Punjab

SUCHA SINGH GILL

INTRODUCTION

Rural areas continue to be the major place of residence of majority of population in India. The state of Punjab, in spite of being more urbanized compared to all India, also continues to be dominated by population living in the rural areas. 2001 Census data show that 66.05 per cent of the total population lived in rural areas of Punjab compared to 72.22 per cent in India as a whole. In spite of green revolution, a large section of people in the rural Punjab are in difficult situation. Labour absorption capacity of agriculture is declining for the last two decades and more. Agricultural labourers, small and marginal farmers are facing problem of underemployment on a massive scale. The tiny farms of many cultivators have become non-viable with modern technology and the existing farm management pattern. Manufacturing and service sectors are not showing signs of their vibrant existence in the rural areas. The rural areas of state are facing a host of new problems caused by falling water table in major parts of the state and rising water table in the south-west Punjab. The depletion of soil caused by its over utilization and excessive use of chemical inputs along with pollution of air caused by burning of paddy and wheat straws, are accompanied by pollution pushed out towards rural areas by burgeoning urban centres. The villages of the state economically, socially and ecologically are faced with deterioration. Many villages are stinking and are fast becoming unlivable for decent living.

In view of a large proportion of population living in the rural areas, deteriorating quality of life, little participation of ruralites in modern occupations due to blocked mobility process, rural development deserves a better attention and positive consideration of policy makers.

The rural areas of state are fast becoming afflicted with suicides of the poor cultivators and other poor sections. These sections are not only facing the problems of downward socio-economic mobility but are fast deprived of social support system. There is a decline in investment in the rural areas for the last two decades. The reduction in social capital in the form of collective social support and concern, decline of institutions and values of human concern has virtually broken the back of valiant rural population of the state. They are losing confidence in themselves and a very few of them are hoping for bright future. The desperation among them is either pushing them towards self-destruction or out of the villages preferably outside the country where they are no longer welcomed.

If development in the state, already facing deceleration, is to be sustained it will have to based on rural areas of the state. It is through regeneration of the rural areas and particularly the dynamism of the rural people that Punjab can hope to regain its losing glory at all India level. The core problems of growing inequality, desperation, and unemployment find their origin in the stagnation and often retrogression of economic life in rural areas. The disturbed decade of 1980s has contributed much to growing woes of the rural people. They were caught in the crossfire from the militants and the security forces. The state was primarily concerned with restoration of law and order, therefore, whole development process went in the background from the agenda of policy makers. The orientation of the administration shaped during this decade continues even today, a decade after the militancy has been over. In fact in the era of liberalization, the state is withdrawing from economic activities. Faced with financial crunch many rural development programmes are either not implemented or implemented in half hearted ways.

Todaro and Smith (2003: 452-54) has formulated three propositions which constitute the necessary conditions for the realization of a people oriented agricultural and rural development in the developing countries. They are:

(i) Farm structures and land tenure patterns need to be adopted to the dual objectives of increasing food production and promoting a wider distribution of benefits of agrarian progress.

(ii) The full benefits of small scale agricultural development cannot be realized unless government support system are created that provide the necessary incentives, economic opportunities and access to needed inputs.

(iii) Rural development encompasses (a) improvements in levels of living including income, employment, education, health and nutrition, housing and a variety of social services; (b) a decreasing inequality in the distribution of rural incomes and in urban-rural imbalances in income and economic opportunities; and (c) the capacity of the rural sector to sustain and accelerate the pace of these improvements over time.

These propositions are based on the imperative that the agriculture's role in economic development is no longer passive and supportive. It is viewed as the dynamic and leading element in any overall strategy. Rural development, therefore, is identified with overall national development. In terms of quality of life and human development index, the gap between rural and urban areas have to be bridged. The rural areas must experience expansion and diversification of income and employment involving production, processing and marketing activities. At the same time social attributes of quality of life such as health, education, sanitation, water supply and other amenities of life must grow at the pace they are growing in urban centres, if the rural people are to be partners in economic development.

HISTORICAL BACKGROUND OF RURAL DEVELOPMENT

Rural development in Punjab in the first phase started with number of policy initiatives taken by the State and the Union governments. Community Development Programme was launched in India in October 1952. This programme was launched as a part of planned development in the country. Rural development attracted considerable attention under the Community Development Programme started in Punjab in 1952. The objective was to bring change in mental outlook of the people and create a spirit to strive for better living. At the same time, attempt was made to create and promote feeling of co-operation and collective effort at community/village level to improve rural infrastructure. The consolidation of land holdings which accompanied Community Development Programme gave further boost to rural development. The process of consolidation enabled village community to demarcate areas for common use of the village. A circular path around each village was created, and area for village link roads was demarcated, a piece of land near the village was earmarked for future use such as a school, dispensary/rural hospital, veterinary clinic, stadium etc. The occasion of consolidation of landholdings was used to persuade all the farmers to contribute to the pool of village common land in proportion to the land held by them. This (common) land was kept at the disposal of the village Panchayat on behalf of the whole community. This created a base for development and consolidation of rural infrastructure where land was required. Since consolidation of landholdings could not be achieved in states other than Punjab, Haryana, this provided a great advantage for undertaking of programmes of collective rural development.

Rural development picked up very fast with the extension of canal irrigation in the state. With inauguration of Bhakra Canal, the irrigation facilities became available in the dry areas particularly arid zone in the southern Punjab. The productivity of various crops began to increase with availability of canal water for irrigation. This also increased cropping intensity along with increase in area under cultivation. The hard work of farmers and agricultural labourers brought some signs of prosperity in the rural areas.

The achievement of consolidation of holdings and construction of network of canals placed Punjab in a position of advantage in relation to other states in the matter of rural development. This created favourable conditions for further development in the rural areas.

The second phase of rural development began in early 1960s. Following the recommendations of Balwantrai Mehta Committee report in 1958, the Government of India decided to introduce three-tier Panchayati Raj Institutions in the country. The institutional structure consisted of Gram Panchayat at village level, Block Samiti at block level and Zila Parishad at district level. The task of rural development was handed over to these institutions with the pivotal role of Block Samiti to direct and supervise the community development. This scheme was introduced in Punjab in 1961. The basic principles underlying the community development programme were:

(a) The motive force for development and improvement should come from the people themselves. A vast unutilized energy lying dormant in the countryside should be harnessed for constructive work for the benefit of the community as a whole.

(b) The co-operative principles should be applied in its varying forms, for solving problems of rural life.

(c) Organized efforts should be made to construct works of common benefit to the community such as village roads, school buildings, health centres, pavement of streets, construction of *pucca* drains, disposal of sullage water and drinking water supply. An awakening amongst the people was to be created for improving their socio-economic lot (Government of Punjab, 1978: 1-2).

In the changed scheme of things the *Gram Sewak* or village level worker (VLW) was made key figure for community development. Gram Sewak was expected to act as development secretary of the village panchayat or Panchayat Samiti within his/her circle which was not to exceed four thousand persons. Along with the construction of works of common benefits, the VLW was to encourage people to form multipurpose co-operative societies for the village or group of villages. VLW was a link between the village people and block samiti for promotion of rural development and creation of spirit of collective self-development in the rural areas.

During this phase, the centrally sponsored scheme of rural development was supplemented by efforts of Punjab Agriculture University (PAU), Ludhiana and agriculture department of the state government. PAU was set up in 1962 as a specialized university wholly devoted to teaching, research and extension work for development of agriculture and allied activities. PAU with its main campus at Ludhiana along with Regional Research Centres established in various parts of state concentrated on development of high yielding varieties (HYV) of seeds, their multiplication and distribution among the farmers. At the same time the university was involved in extension work for adoption of new seeds, mechanical and chemical inputs, market and storage practices etc. The university also made pioneering role in training of human resources for agriculture extension and research. The technical manpower in the departments of agriculture, horticulture, dairying and animal husbandry of Punjab are trained by PAU.

The efforts of PAU were supported by agriculture, animal husbandry and horticulture departments in extension work for adoption of new technology and farm practices in the field. The government support in market infrastructure and purchase of wheat and paddy at minimum support prices (MSPs) provided great impetus for agriculture and rural development of Punjab.

Along with institutional support in agricultural research and extension, the government played a significant role in development of irrigation in the state. The rainfall in Punjab is not adequate and many times is not timely for crop cycle in the state. But the state is richly endowed with surface and ground water which has been harnessed for developing agriculture on sound footing in the state. As early as 1950-51, the percentage of gross cropped area irrigated was 52.30 (against 17.11 per cent at all India level). Because of massive public investment in subsequent years the area under irrigation increased from 55.90 per cent in 1960-61 to 74.70 per cent in 1970-71 and 85.48 per cent in 1980-81. Irrigation and power remained a priority area in the five year plans of the state. From the First Five Year Plan to Fifth Five Year Plan, this head accounted for more than 51.0 per cent of total plan expenditure of the state. After partition, Punjab started from a scratch and per capita power generation and consumption was much below all India average. But from the beginning of the sixties, power generation and per capita consumption shot up in the state. Between 1965-66 and 1982-83 power generation increased by 328.0 per cent in the state. This was comparable to all India growth. But power consumption in the state increased by 241.0 per cent compared to 138.0 per cent in India as a whole. A large part of the total power has been consumed by agriculture in the state. After achieving 100 per cent electrification in mid-seventies, the agriculture sector became a largest consumer of power. By 1982-83, 41.0 per cent of it was consumed by agriculture in the state. Another important infrastructure is related to provision of co-operative credit for agriculture. The number of co-operative agricultural societies increased from 9845 in 1950-51 to 11,243 in 1965-66 and member from 5,18,000 to 12,07,000 and loans disbursed increased from Rs. 2.20 crore to Rs. 19.84 crore during this period (Chadha, 1986: 96).

Role of rural education in achieving modernization of agriculture has been discussed by many scholars (Schultz, 1964; Chaudhari, 1979; Hendrix, 1981). The state government took a keen interest in promotion of rural education. Further, the programme of construction of link roads made considerable impact on pace of transportation and contact with urban marketing and manufacturing.

The introduction of three-tier PRIs along with state government's several measures of infrastructure development like Intensive Area Development Programme made a success and laid foundations for enactment of green revolution in state in 1965-66. Subsequently, Integrated Cattle Development Programme, Small Farmers Development Agencies and Marginal Farmers and Agricultural Labourer Agencies were started for specific purpose and sections of rural population. The model village scheme for improving civil amenities through pavement of streets, construction of drains and disposal of sullage water etc. was started in 1969-70. Initially 970 villages were selected and each village was provided Rs. One lakh for this purpose.

The Jayanti Village Scheme was the second scheme under individual village approach to develop rural areas. One Jayanti Village was selected in each block and a sum of Rs. 50,000 was allotted per village for the pavement of streets, construction of drains and street lights etc. The aim was to improve the physical environment in the village and improve the infrastructure. But, the amount was provided on *ad hoc* basis and was insufficient to complete the contemplated works under the scheme.

The schemes of rural development including centrally sponsored schemes for small farmers, marginal farmers and agricultural labourers (1970), IADP etc. addressed themselves only to specific issue/problem for section of the rural population who remain isolated from the general development activities in the state.

Third phase of rural development started in 1978-79 with introduction of Integrated Rural Development Programme. It was felt in the country that a large number of programmes have been operating in the country aimed at improving the condition of the rural poor. None of these programmes covered the whole country, though a large number of blocks had more than one programme operating for the same area and for the same target group. The territorial overlap and different funding patterns created many difficulties in effective monitoring and accounting of these programmes. At the same time objectives of the programme were also got blurred and they fell short of lifting out of poverty a large number of people living below poverty line. With a view to remove the weaknesses of existing programmes and tackle rural poverty seriously, a new programme known as Integrated Rural Development Programme (IRDP) was launched in 1978-79. The basic change in this programme over the earlier programmes was to provide the target groups the income generating assets and access to credit and inputs to empower them to remain out of poverty in the sustained way. To achieve the twin objectives of raising income and generating employment were to be achieved through investment in agriculture and ancillary occupations, cottage and small scale industries and any other viable economic activity suiting beneficiary family.

When the programme was launched the rural poverty was an issue in Punjab but not as serious as at all India level. In 1977-78 the proportion of rural households living below poverty line in Punjab was 16.37 per cent compared to 53.07 per cent in the country as a whole (Planning Commission, 1993: 40).

The fast growth in agricultural production and per acre yield following green revolution had made a considerable dent in rural poverty in the state. The proportion of such population declined from 28.21 per cent in 1973-74 to 16.37 per cent in 1977-78 (Planning Commission, 1993: 39-40). While operationalizing the IRDP, the Punjab Government felt that while continuing to fight rural poverty the emphasis of this programme had to be on increasing production, productivity and gainful employment. It was further felt that in spite the remarkable increase in agricultural production, a sufficient scope existed for increasing agricultural production. The following objectives were set for IRDP in Punjab (Government of Punjab, 1978: 5-6):

- (i) to provide full and gainful employment;
- (ii) to achieve at least 50 per cent increase in agricultural production;
- (iii) to revive/intensify traditional industries and trades;

(iv) to facilitate development of cottage and small scale agro-based and ancillary industries;

(v) full development of local resources; and

(vi) to ensure that weaker sections of rural society are enabled to participate in the development process.

For achievement of these objectives under IRDP a strategy of establishment and development of growth centres/focal point was planned. Under this strategy no village in the state was to be more than 5 kms from a focal point. The state was divided into 500 units with an area of 100 sq. kms each. In each unit, 20-25 villages were included. In the first instance, a cluster of five contiguous villages in each of 117 (at that time) blocks in the state were taken as a unit for planning and development. In each cluster, one village was selected as a focal point. The selection was made on the basis of geographic location in relation to other villages and capability to ignite development activities in the area. This strategy was based on the proposition that multi-sectoral investment and activity at the focal point would lead to generation and dispersal of economic development in the surrounding clusters of villages. It was decided to provide certain infrastructure facilities (including economic and social services) to achieve integration of agricultural and non-agricultural activities. In the first phase these included:

(i) banking and credit facilities;

(ii) agro service centre;

(iii) retail outlets for essential commodities and agricultural inputs;

(iv) marketing yard;

(v) diesel/petrol pump;

(vi) post office with telephone facilities;

(vii) veterinary hospital; and

(viii) civil hospital.

In the second phase, more facilities were to be provided at these focal points depending on the needs of the area. These included setting up of godowns and cold storage, research and training facilities, larger units of agro based industries. Other facilities like a stadium, open theatre/cinema, rural water supply, community centre-*cum*-library etc. were also to be provided at the focal point. The setting up of such complexes were also expected to generate job opportunities for skilled, semi-skilled and unskilled persons, assure fuller utilization of local sources, add some elements of urbanism into the rural sector and help to discourage the movement of people towards towns and cities.

In the completion of 117 clusters through focal point strategy, the scheme was to be gradually extended to other clusters covering the entire state within five years. On an average, each block was to have five focal points and then one or two major focal points to be developed into an urban estate providing housing facilities, commercial centres and an industrial estate. There was a proposal to set up a Rural Development Council for 5-6 villages consisting of representatives from punchayats of each village and other people like ex-servicemen, progressive farmers and representatives of weaker sections.

The IRDP was to be co-ordinated in the Community Development Department at the state level under the Development Commissioner assisted by Joint Development Commissioner. At the district level the programme was put under the charge of Deputy Commissioner assisted by Additional Deputy Commissioner with other concerned officers attached to the Additional Deputy Commissioner. The Additional Deputy Commissioner was made responsible for the implementation and supervision of the scheme. At the block level, the Block Development and Panchayat Officer was made incharge of the scheme. At the focal point one Agriculture Inspector and one Co-operative Inspector was to be appointed and in each of the villages of the selected cluster one Agricultural Sub-Inspector, one Cooperative Sub-Inspector and two VLWs were to be appointed. The persons appointed at the village were to be responsible for implementation of the programmes while inspectors at focal point were given the responsibility to supervise the development work in all villages attached to focal point.

As per time frame of the strategy starting in 1977-78, by 1981-82 it would be possible to entirely cover two groups of 117 clusters each, the third group would be covered to the extent of 3/5th, the 4th group to the extent of 2/5th and 5th group to the extent of 1/5th. Thus the intensive development of 3rd, 4th and 5th groups were to be taken after 1981-82 over a period of 4-5 years. However, with the elections held in 1980, there was a change to the government in the state. The new government decided to abandon the micro level strategy of focal points but continued with IRDP as envisaged at country level under the charge of Additional Deputy Commissioner (Development). The specific character of Punjab IRDP was replaced by IRDP pattern at all India level. IRDP was to cover all development blocks with emphasis on providing substantial assistance to the beneficiaries living below poverty line so that they cross the poverty line. The programme implemented in Punjab was essentially anti-poverty in nature rather than a general development programme. It was essentially intended to provide additional gainful employment to unemployed and underemployed in the rural areas, creation of durable assets and infrastructure for rural development and improvement of nutritional status of persons living below poverty line.

For implementation of this programme a survey for identification of weaker sections was conducted during September-December 1980—by Economic and Statistical Organization, Punjab. A family with income from all sources less than Rs. 3600 per annum was identified as belonging to weaker section and was issued a Yellow Card for availing of various facilities provided to weaker sections in the state. There were a number of problems in survey conducted for identifications of weaker section, consequently many deserving families could not get Yellow Cards while non-deserving persons got such cards (Government of Punjab, 1987). After 1980 no such survey has been conducted for fresh enlisting of the poor families.

A survey conducted by Government of Punjab in 1985-86 to evaluate the working of this programme found that against the Government of India guideline for eligible beneficiaries with income from all sources less than Rs. 3500 and cultivators with less than 5 acres of land, in Punjab, Yellow Card holders with income from all sources up to Rs. 3600 were identified as target groups. The banks which were supposed to finance IRDP were not consulted for identification. The capabilities and abilities of the persons to maintain assets created under IRDP were not assessed. The survey based on sample households from three districts of the state came to following conclusions:

> "Improper identification of beneficiaries had resulted into inclusion of many who were not poorest and the exclusion of several really poor families from the programme. The failure to identify properly the beneficiaries had been attributed partly to lack of preparatory work to determine the number of the families below the poverty line and the hurried manner in which the programme was extended to cover all blocks in the country and in the states without toning up the administration to deal with the job. Besides, there was no attempt whatsoever to involve the Gram Panchayats in the job of identification. One of the major weakness of the programme had been the tendency to overlook the differences in the level and incidence of poverty in different blocks/districts within state.
>
> A common allegation against IRD Programme is that the assets received by the poor are worth much less than its book value. Hence, they are not satisfied with the present procedure of IRDP implementation. It was reported by the beneficiaries that they were not getting assets of their choice. They emphatically said that unwanted assets were thrusted upon them resulting into poor returns. Hence, the very purpose of IRD Programme to pull all poor families above poverty line was defeated, and bank money is frozen and Government money wasted..." (Government of Punjab, 1987: 68).

Besides IRDP, the National Rural Employment Programme (NREP) began its operation since October 1980. The three departments, viz. Rural Development and Panchayats, Forest Department and Irrigation Department are implementing this programme. Though, this programme demonstrate better results yet it has its own problems of implementation and co-ordination. NREP was merged with Rural Landless Employment Guarantee Programme (RLEGP) in 1989 and named as Jawahar Rozgar Yojana. Another centrally sponsored programme in operation in the state since 1982 is Development of Women and Children in Rural Areas (DWACRA).

The major difficulty with the various rural development programmes (both state and the Central), along with the operational, monitoring and implementation flaws in 1980s, was related to break down of law and order in the rural areas due to militant insurgency. The prolonged problem of insurgency led to long period of President rule in the state (1982-1985 and 1987-1992). During this period orientation of the state administration changed from development to restoration of law and order in the state. The priority to restore order and efforts to win over various sections of population, the administration resorted to granting of concessions (under populist policy) and avoided strict tax compliance and widening of tax base. This created financial crisis of unprecedented scale in the state. When democratic process was restored in 1992, the state was already on the verge of financial bankruptcy. The successive governments could not overcome this crisis for the period exceeding last one decade. At the same time, orientation of the administration could not be shifted back towards development activities. Many centrally sponsored programmes are either not implemented or implemented half way due to difficulty of arranging matching share of the state government's financial resources.

The decade of 1980s was lost, in case of Punjab, in implementation of rural development programmes and more so in case of any experimentation on this count. When Punjab was engulfed by political turmoil, the states of Karnataka, West Bengal and Kerala were engaged in new initiatives and experimentation of rural development. In these states the attempts were being made to decentralize the process of rural development and free it from the clutches of cynical bureaucracy. Karnataka passed a new legislation on the model of Ashok Mehta Committee recommendation in 1983 which helped the state go forward with boldest decentralized planning. 20 per cent of the plan outlay which was earlier devoted to district schemes were devolved to zila panchayats as lump sum grants and criteria for inter-district allocations and devolution from districts to mandal panchayats were clearly laid down. The district plans formulated by zila panchayats were incorporated in the annual state plans. In West Bengal, though the involvement of panchayat started in implementation of land reforms during 1978-1983 for detection of illegal landholdings, identification of the share croppers, their rights and distribution of land yet their participation in decentralized development started in 1985 when three tier planning machinery was constituted. The District Planning Committee headed by Zila Parishad chairman with district collector as the member secretary was made effective constituted as planning machinery at the district level. West Bengal's decentralization of planning with active involvement of PRIs made significant contribution in implementation of land reforms, rural development programmes and rejuvenation of agricultural growth. Kerala plunged into this experiment in mid 1980s through Special Component Plan and Tribal Sub-Plan for district plan. But the formulation of the Eighth Five Year Plan was based on proposals submitted by District Development Council prepared in consultation with Block Planning Committees and the Gram Panchayat Committee. The government decided to earmark 35-40 per cent of plan outlay for local self-government institutions (Thomas Isaac, 2000: 8). Due to the creative experimentation in 1980s the states of West Bengal, Karnataka, Kerala, Maharashtra and Gujarat were better placed in implementing 73rd Amendment to the Constitution of India. In this amendment 29 departments included in the Eleventh Schedule and related to rural development are transferred to the PRIs.

Seventy third Amendment to the Constitution brought PRIs into the centre of socio-economic development of the rural area in India. In pursuance of this amendment, the Punjab Panchayats and Municipalities Act, 1994 was passed by the State Legislative Assembly. The Governor of Punjab constituted a Finance Commission on April 22, 1994 to review the financial position of panchayats and municipalities and to make recommendations. The Commission submitted its report in December 1995. The recommendations of the Commission remain buried in the files of the government and no action had been taken on them. The rural development continues to be governed by earlier ways without any involvement of people.

The Government of Punjab in 1997 involved all the Universities (including Panjab University at Chandigarh) and research institutes in the state to get a technical support for decentralized planning. Work on plans for 23 development blocks was commissioned with emphasis on decentralized development based on strategy of focal points. These reports/plans became available by mid 1998 but the state government did not take any initiative for rejuvenation of rural development. In fact the whole process of economic development remained paralyzed due to lack of political will, acute financial crunch and cynicism of the bureaucracy. Consequently, no new experiments/initiatives are to be seen in spite of several technical reports/studies. The traditional mode of rural development through implementation of centrally sponsored schemes continues in half hearted and disinterested ways.

STATUS OF RURAL DEVELOPMENT

The rural population of the state has been considerably higher than urban population. The share of rural population was 78.3 per cent in 1951 and that of urban population was 21.7 per cent. Over the years the share of rural population has been declining and reached to 66.05 per cent in 2001. In spite of declining share of rural population and rising share of urban population, the rural population is still nearly double of the urban population of the state (Table 1.1). At the same time the share of the urban population of the state has been higher than all India average as well as that of our neighbouring state of Haryana. The rate of change of share of urban population has been higher in Punjab compared to this rate of Haryana as well as in the country as a whole (Table 1.2). But the rural population of the state has been quite open to innovations and technological advances. At the same time, it has been very enterprising and hardworking. Braving the brunt of partition and two wars with Pakistan, the rural people continue to cultivate land in the villages situated on international border. The hardworking nature, openness to technical change and spirit of enterprise have contributed to reconstruction of rural Punjab.

Table 1.1: Distribution of Rural-Urban Population in Punjab (1951-2001)

(*in percentage*)

Year	*Rural*	*Urban*
1951	78.30	21.70
1961	76.90	23.10
1971	76.30	23.70
1981	72.30	27.70
1991	70.50	29.50
2001	66.05	33.95

Source: Director of Census Operations, Punjab, *Provisional Population Totals* paper 2 of 2001, Chandigarh, p. 27.

Punjab led the country in rural development till 1982-83. The state achieved 100 per cent electrification of the village by the mid 1970s. There are 8,29,114 energized tubewells (2002) providing assured irrigation to the agriculture. This has enabled on the average 6.7 electric tubewells per village and one tubewell for 5.15 hectare of land. 97.3 per cent of the total villages were connected to towns

Table 1.2: Distribution of Rural-Urban Population in India, Punjab and Haryana

(*percentage*)

	1991		*2001*	
	Rural	*Urban*	*Rural*	*Urban*
India	74.28	25.72	72.22	27.78
Punjab	70.45	29.55	66.05	33.95
Haryana	75.21	24.79	71.00	29.00

Source: Director of Census Operations, Punjab, *Provisional Population Totals*, paper 2 of 2001, Chandigarh, p. 27.

and villages by 1982-83, with metalled link roads. As early as 1977-78, 85.35 per cent of villages of the states had all weather metalled link roads. Between 1982-83 and 1991-92, the proportion of villages having link roads remained unchanged but this proportion increased

Table 1.3: Percentage of villages linked with roads in Punjab

Sl. No.	*District*	*1977-78*	*1982-83*	*1991-92*	*2001-02*
1.	Gurdaspur	88.87	96.5	96.65	98.06
2.	Amritsar	69.27	98.7	98.91	98.67
3.	Kapurthala	85.61	85.5	85.88	100.0
4.	Jalandhar	88.59	97.3	98.12	100.0
5.	Nawashahar	—	—	—	100.0
6.	Hoshiarpur	69.91	97.9	99.87	99.57
7.	Rupnagar	94.60	97.2	97.31	98.98
8.	Ludhiana	94.12	100.0	100.0	98.78
9.	Firozpur	70.85	92.9	92.94	98.24
10.	Faridkot	99.65	100.0	100.0	100.0
11.	Mukatsar	—	—	—	100.0
12.	Moga	—	—	—	100.0
13.	Bathinda	100.0	99.6	99.62	98.23
14.	Mansa	—	—	—	100.0
15.	Sangrur	99.86	100.0	100.0	99.86
16.	Patiala	95.21	99.4	99.37	99.25
17.	Fatehgarh Sahib	—	—	—	100.0
	Punjab	85.35	97.3	97.76	99.24

Note: District of Nawanshahar, Mukatsar, Moga, Mansa and Fatehgarh Sahib were created after 1991-92 respectively from districts of Jalandhar, Faridkot (Mukatsar and Moga), Bathinda and Patiala.

Source: ESA, *Statistical Abstract of Punjab* 1978, 1983, 1992, 2002, Government of Punjab.

to 99.24 per cent in year 2001-02. Table 1.3 shows that inter-district variation in link roads is very low, The lowest proportion of villages having link roads is 98.06 per cent. The state is having 33, 838 kms of link roads. All weather link roads ensure regular and easy connectivity of villages to towns and cities for marketing activities. The metalled roads enable fast and motorized transport of commodities and human resources from villages to cities and back to villages. The fast and sustained road communication has made villages of Punjab as extension of towns and cities. At the same time this has enabled many people to live in villages and work in towns and cities.

The connectivity of villages with link roads to market towns and cities was supplemented by the expansion of the regulated markets in the state. The number of regulated markets (Table 1.4) increased from 88 in 1966-67 to 108 in 1975-76, 123 in 1981-82, 143 in 1989-90 and 144 in 1996-97 and stays at that level till this 2001-02. These markets are regulated under Punjab State Agricultural Produce Market Act, 1961. There are 144 market committees established for regulation of these markets. They are responsible for development and maintenance of marketing yards, construction and maintenance of village link roads and supervision of marketing operations in the state. There are 144 principal marketing yards, 514 sub-yards and 491 procurement centres. Punjab State Marketing Board (at state level) has established one of the best agricultural marketing system in the country. There are adequate arrangements for marketing, procurement and storage of agricultural produce for principal crops (such as wheat, paddy, cotton, sugarcane, etc.) in the state (Raul, 2001: 123-52). The cultivators are able to dispose of very quickly these crops at minimum support price announced every year. This has sustained the agriculture production and cropping pattern in the state.

Table 1.4: Regulated Markets in Punjab

Year	*Number of Regulated Markets*
1966-67	88
1976-77	108
1981-82	123
1989-90	143
1992-93	144
2001-02	144

Source: *Statistical Abstract of Punjab*, 1978: 168; 1983: 174; 1994: 212; 2002: 224; Government of Punjab, Chandigarh.

The expansion of irrigation network in Punjab has been a major factor in rural development. This provided one of the essential conditions for successful launching of green revolution in the state. The total irrigated area more than doubled in the state between 1960-61 and 2001-02. The area irrigated increased from 20,20,000 hectares in 1960-61 to 40,57,000 hectares in 2001-02. In 1960-61 government canals contributed 58.07 per cent of the total irrigated area and tubewells and wells share was 41.04 per cent. The share of canals progressively declined to 41.07 per cent in 1990-91 and to 24.33 per cent in 2001-02. The share of tubewells in total irrigated area has grown over time to make it a dominant mode of irrigation. The share of tubewells and wells has increased from 41.04 per cent in 1960-61 to 75.62 per cent in 2001-02 (Table 1.5). Compared to canal irrigation, the tubewell irrigation is better assured. This has happened with achievement of 100 per cent electrification of villages initially and later on free supply of electricity to tubewells between 1997-2003. The availability of assured irrigation and 100 per cent electrification of the villages played a major role in the success of green revolution. At the same time, electricity and road connectivity brought the rural life closer to that of towns and cities. The durable consumer goods such as T.V., refrigerators, fans, coolers, jeeps, motor cycles, scooters etc. are found with large number of households in the rural areas. In fact agriculture has been the largest user of electric power in the state. This sector was using 38.00 per cent of the total electricity consumed in 1970-71 and used 43.66 per cent in 1980-81 and 42.87 per cent in 1990-91. After this, the share of this sector has been declining and touched all time low of 27.49 per cent in 2001-02. Agriculture, now, has been replaced by industrial sector as the largest consumer of electricity accounting for 42.11 per cent of the total electricity used in the state during 2001-02 (Table 1.6). The electricity has not only lighted the houses, energized the tube wells but also brought enlightenment with introduction of initially radios and later on T.Vs. It also brought comforts of urban life associated with use of durable consumer goods (Kaur, 2004: 137).

The structure of rural economy is undergoing fast changes in Punjab. Traditionally rural economy in post-Independence period have been dominated by agriculture both as a source of income as well as employment. Between 1971 and 1991 roughly 76.01 per cent to 78.43 per cent of the workforce had consisted of cultivators and agricultural labourers. All other seven industrial categories of workers

Table 1.5: Net Irrigated Area in Punjab by Source

('000 Hectare)

Year	*Government Canals*	*Tubewells/ wells*	*Other sources*	*Total*	*Irrigated area as percentage net sown area*
1960-61	1173 (58.07)	829 (41.04)	18 (0.89)	2020 (100.00)	54
1965-66	1288 (56.91)	921 (40.70)	54 (2.39)	2263 (100.00)	59
1971-72	1364 (46.16)	1554 (52.59)	37 (1.25)	2955 (100.00)	72
1975-76	1366 (43.80)	1742 (55.85)	11 (0.35)	3119 (100.00)	75
1980-81	1430 (42.28)	1939 (57.33)	13 (0.38)	3282 (100.00)	81
1985-86	1412 (38.27)	2274 (66.63)	4 (0.11)	3690 (100.00)	88
1990-91	1567 (41.07)	2233 (58.52)	16 (0.42)	3816 (100.00)	90
1996-97	1620 (40.14)	2408 (59.68)	7 (0.17)	4035 (100.00)	95
2001-02	987 (24.33)	3068 (75.62)	2 (0.05)	4057 (100.00)	95

Note: Figures in parentheses are in percentage of total.

Source: *Statistical Abstract of Punjab*, 1976: 175; 1978: 175 and 2002: 237, Government of Punjab, Chandigarh.

have absorbed less than 24 per cent of the workforce in the state. Between 1991 and 2001 there is a major shift of workforce employed by agriculture and non-agricultural activities in the state. The share of agricultural cultivators and agricultural labourers has declined from 76.01 per cent in 1991 to 53.5 per cent in 2001. The share of other services (factory employment, construction, trade and commerce, transport and communication and other services) has increased from 25.79 per cent in 1991 to 43.4 per cent in 2001 (Table 1.7). Among these services which category has gained, as yet break up of census data are no available. But this is a major structural change which has occurred in the last decade of the 20th century, in the rural Punjab.

This change has been observed across all the districts of the state. Though census data and NSS data are not comparable yet some answer

Table 1.6: Consumption of Electric Power in Punjab by Users

(Million K.W.H.)

Sl. No.	Category of Consumption	1970-71		1980-81		1990-91		1999-2000		2000-2001		2001-2002 (P)	
		Consumption	%age of total	Consumption	%age of total	Consumption	%age of total	Consumption	%age of total	Consumption	%age of total	Consumption	%age of total
1.	Domestic	119.1	9.77	497.39	11.74	1619.9	13.60	3779.5	18.06	4224.1	22.02	4380.7	22.47
2.	Commercial	63.7	5.22	139.29	3.29	325.8	2.74	799.2	3.82	911.4	4.74	965.8	4.96
3.	Industrial	438.6	35.96	1613.40	38.09	4317.6	36.26	7697.8	36.78	8047.1	41.95	8208.6	42.11
4.	Public lighting in bulk	134.7	11.05	136.51	3.27	539.1	4.53	420.7	2.01	467.6	2.44	486.2	2.49
5.	Agriculture	463.4	38.00	1849.75	43.66	5104.5	42.87	5233.1	39.33	5534.3	28.85	5451.9	27.49
	Total	**1219.5**	**100.00**	**4236.34**	**100.00**	**11906.9**	**100.00**	**20930.3**	**100.00**	**19184.5**	**100.00**	**19493.2**	**100.00**

Source: *Statistical Abstract of Punjab*, 2004: 258-259, Government of Punjab, Chandigarh.

is found from NSS data of 55th round pertaining to the year 1999-2000. If we compare the NSS data of 1999-2000 with 2001 census data it is found that agriculture employees 62.7 per cent of the total workforce in rural Punjab whereas 2001 census put this figure to 53.5 per cent, i.e. the gap of 9.2 per cent. But 1999-2000 NSS data gave details of distribution of workforce in the state across nine industrial categories (Table 1.8). A comparison of 1991 census data with NSS 1999-2000 shows that the categories which have gained are manufacturing from 6.36 per cent in 1991 to 7.9, construction from 3.95 per cent to 7.4 per cent, trade and commerce from 2.47 per cent to 8.0 per cent (this includes restaurant), transport and storage from 2.47 per cent to 5.3 per cent (transport alone). Since a large number of vacancies in the government are not filled (since 1991) when incumbents retire, this would obviously lead to decline in the share of government services in the employment. The end result of

Table 1.7: Percentage Distribution of Rural Workforce (Main Workers) of Punjab (1971-2001)

Sl. No.	*Industrial Category*	*1971*	*1981*	*1991*	*2001**
1.	Cultivators	53.64	46.11	44.39	31.5
2.	Agricultural Labourers	24.79	31.82	31.62	22.0
3.	Allied Activities	1.06	0.92	0.65	—
4.	Mining and Quarrying	0.02	0.01	0.01	—
5.	Manufacturing				
	(a) Household industry	3.42	2.23	1.15	3.1
	(b) Other than household industry	3.23	4.71	5.31	43.4 (items 5(b)–9)
6.	Construction	1.54	1.42	1.81	
7.	Trade and Commerce	3.17	3.64	3.95	
8.	Transport, storage and Communication	1.28	2.12	2.47	
9.	Other services	8.48	7.00	10.24	
		100.00	100.00	100.00	100.00

* Nine industrial classification of workforce in 2001, census is not available.

Source: *Census of India*, Punjab, Economic Tables, Part II-B-Series 1971, 1981 (pp. 122-25), 1991 (pp. 185-86), 2001 *Primary Census Abstract* (p. 1).

the structural change in the workforce across economic activities in the rural areas demonstrate that it is following urban economy to move away from agriculture. This can be explained in terms of long term structural changes which accompany economic development (Kuznets, 1956: 41-75; Chenery, 1979: 5-45).

Table 1.8: Distribution of Working Rural Persons in the Principal Status of Broad Industry (1999-2000)

Sl. No.	*Industry division*	*Per cent Distribution*
1.	Agriculture	62.7
2.	Mining and Quarrying	0.0
3.	Manufacturing	7.9
4.	Electricity, Water, etc.	1.1
5.	Construction	7.4
6.	Trade, Hotel, Restaurant	8.0
7.	Transport	5.3
8.	Financial Services and Business	0.5
9.	Public Administration, Education and Communication	7.2
	Total	**100.00**

Source: NSS, 55th Round, *Employment and Unemployment Situation in India*, Vol. I, Report No. 485, Govt. of India, New Delhi, 2001, p. 114.

Though Punjab has shown considerable lead in terms of per capita income and changes associated with it yet the state's performance in social indicators and particularly in the rural areas tell a different story. In literacy rate Punjab is ranked at 16th position among the states and Union territories (Table 1.9). The major states which are considerably ahead of Punjab (69.95 per cent) are Kerala (90.92 per cent), Maharashtra (77.27 per cent), Himachal Pradesh (77.13 per cent) and Gujarat (69.97 per cent). Except for Maharashtra, all other states ahead of Punjab have considerably lower per capita income. Literacy rate of the state, though, higher than all India average, is not matching with state's position in terms of economic resources.

Literacy rate in the rural areas of the state has been growing over time. It has increased from 27.60 per cent in 1971 to 35.20 per cent in 1981, 52.77 per cent in 1991 and 65.16 per cent in 2001 (Table 1.10). Literacy rates in the rural areas have been lower than overall literacy rate but considerably lower than urban literacy rate. Among

Table 1.9: States and Union Territories Ranked by Literacy Rate (2001)

Rank	*States/UTs*	*Literacy Rate (Percentage)*
1.	Kerala	90.92
2.	Mizoram	88.49
3.	Lakshadweep	87.52
4.	Goa	82.32
5.	Delhi	81.82
6.	Chandigarh	81.76
7.	Pondicherry	81.49
8.	Andaman and Nicobar Islands	81.18
9.	Daman and Diu	81.09
10.	Maharashtra	77.27
11.	Himachal Pradesh	77.13
12.	Tripura	73.66
13.	Tamil Nadu	73.47
14.	Uttaranchal (Now Uttarakhand)	72.28
15.	Gujarat	69.97
16.	Punjab	69.95
17.	Sikkim	69.68
18.	West Bengal	69.22
19.	Manipur	68.87
20.	Haryana	68.59
21.	Nagaland	67.11
22.	Karnataka	67.04
23.	Chhattisgarh	65.18
24.	Assam	64.24
25.	Madhya Pradesh	64.11
26.	Orissa	63.11
27.	Meghalaya	63.31
28.	Andhra Pradesh	61.11
29.	Rajasthan	61.03
30.	Dadra & Nagar Haveli	60.03
31.	Uttar Pradesh	57.36
32.	Arunachal Pradesh	54.74
33.	Jammu and Kashmir	54.46
34.	Jharkhand	54.13
35.	Bihar	47.53
36.	India	65.38

Source: Director Census Operation, Punjab, *Provisional Population Tables*, paper 2 of 2001, Chandigarh, p. 50.

the rural areas, female literacy rate has been considerably lower than the male literacy rate. The gap between male-female literacy rate has stayed within the range of 14 per cent to 17 per cent during 1971-2001. Rural female literacy rate in 2001 was nearly 14 per cent lower than male literacy rate (Table 1.10). It is a sign of gender discrimination and social backwardness.

Table 1.10: Progress in Rural Literacy Rate in Punjab

(in percentage)

Year	Person	Male	Female
1971	27.60	34.55	19.58
1981	35.20	41.91	27.63
1991	52.77	60.73	43.85
2001	65.16	71.70	57.91

Source: *Statistical Abstract of Punjab* 1978 (p. 42), 1986 (p. 56), 1996 (p. 68), 2004 (pp. 74-75), Government of Punjab, Chandigarh.

Further, there is a considerable inter-district variations in rural male-female literacy rates. There is a clear divide between northern and central districts and southern districts. The northern and central districts consisting of Gurdaspur, Amritsar, Kapurthala, Jalandhar, Hoshiarpur, Nawanshahar, Rupnagar, Fategarh Sahib, Ludhiana and Patiala have literacy rate higher than the state average. The literacy rate in these districts varied between 69.96 per cent (Patiala) and 81.40 per cent (Hoshiarpur) in 2001. The southern districts consisting of Moga, Firozpur, Mukatsar, Faridkot, Bathinda, Mansa and Sangrur have literacy rate lower than overall literacy rate of the state. This ranged from 52.50 per cent (Mansa) to 63.94 per cent (Moga) in 2001. The same pattern is followed in rural and urban literacy rates and between male-female literacy rates (Table 1.11).

The data reveal that rural literacy rates are lower than urban literacy rates. The gap is lowest in Hoshiarpur district (6.59 per cent points) and highest in Mansa district (23.67 per cent). Similarly, female literacy rates are lower than male literacy rate in all districts of the state both in rural as well as in the urban areas. The gender discrimination is higher in the rural areas compared to urban areas in the matter of literacy rates.

Literacy rates among the rural Scheduled Castes are lowest in the state. Against the overall literacy rate of 58.51 per cent in 1991, the literacy rate among the rural Scheduled Castes was 39.55 per cent, a gap of 18.96 per cent point. It is further revealed that literacy rate is lowest in Bathinda district (including Mansa district in 1991) and highest in Hoshiarpur district. Amongst Scheduled Castes, women have lowest literacy rate. Against the overall female literacy rate of 50.41 per cent in 1991, the Scheduled Caste female literacy rate was 29.20 per cent. There is a considerable variation in

Table 1.11: Literacy Rate in Punjab by Residence and Sex (2001)

(percentage)

Sl. No.	District	Total			Rural			Urban		
		Persons	Male	Female	Persons	Male	Female	Persons	Male	Female
1.	Gurdaspur	74.19	80.44	67.31	70.96	77.70	63.58	83.43	88.16	78.11
2.	Amritsar	67.85	73.58	61.41	60.65	67.83	52.69	78.37	81.84	74.39
3.	Kapurthala	73.56	78.66	67.90	70.57	76.27	64.41	79.63	83.30	75.33
4.	Jalandhar	77.91	82.37	72.93	74.41	80.14	68.17	81.74	84.73	78.29
5.	Hoshiarpur	81.40	86.97	75.75	80.09	86.11	73.87	86.66	90.30	82.62
6.	Nawanshahar	76.86	83.67	69.52	75.99	83.15	68.27	82.26	86.84	77.30
7.	Rupnagar	78.49	84.43	71.74	74.51	81.39	66.71	86.60	90.63	82.01
8.	Fatehgarh Sahib	74.10	78.85	68.60	71.71	76.86	65.83	80.22	83.87	75.67
9.	Ludhiana	76.54	80.19	72.11	72.88	78.32	66.73	79.42	81.58	76.66
10.	Moga	63.94	68.40	58.96	61.18	65.93	55.87	74.84	78.05	71.20
11.	Firozpur	61.42	69.55	52.33	55.75	64.78	45.78	71.22	82.58	71.03
12.	Mukatsar	58.67	65.94	50.59	54.10	61.84	45.49	71.93	77.78	65.40
13.	Faridkot	63.34	68.92	57.09	58.58	64.18	52.27	72.71	78.35	66.49
14.	Bathinda	61.51	68.31	53.76	55.30	62.46	47.16	75.96	81.88	69.19
15.	Mansa	52.50	59.12	45.07	47.56	54.27	40.03	71.23	77.56	64.14
16.	Sangrur	60.04	65.97	53.29	55.86	61.93	48.98	70.12	75.67	63.76
17.	Patiala	69.96	76.13	62.94	63.34	70.40	55.29	81.99	86.52	76.84
18.	Punjab	69.95	76.63	63.55	65.16	71.70	57.91	79.13	82.97	74.63

Source: Director of Census Operations, Punjab, *Provisional Population Totals,* paper 2 of 2001, Chandigarh, pp. 51-52.

the inter-district female literacy rate among the rural Scheduled Caste women. It was highest (51.60 per cent) in Hoshiarpur district and lowest in Bathinda district (10.20 per cent). Thus, the rural Scheduled Caste female of Bathinda and Mansa districts are lagging behind their counterparts in other districts and the females in the urban areas (Table 1.12).

Table 1.12: Literacy Rate of Rural Scheduled Castes in Punjab (1991)

(*in Percentage*)

Sl. No.	*District*	*Persons*	*Male*	*Female*
1.	Gurdaspur	46.32	55.98	35.39
2.	Amritsar	31.01	39.74	20.83
3.	Kapurthala	46.16	55.50	35.66
4.	Jalandhar	56.26	65.91	45.37
5.	Hoshiarpur	63.82	74.74	51.60
6.	Rupnagar	56.21	67.62	42.86
7.	Ludhiana	51.40	61.33	39.37
8.	Firozpur	21.68	29.57	12.57
9.	Faridkot	21.91	28.99	13.67
10.	Bathinda	17.61	24.01	10.20
11.	Sangrur	26.18	34.99	15.85
12.	Patiala	36.83	46.87	25.16
13.	Total (Punjab)	39.55	48.54	29.20

Source: *Statistical Abstract of Punjab*, 2002, Government of Punjab, Chandigarh, p. 70.

The record of Punjab in adverse sex ratio is well known and in 2001, the state was ranked at 29th position among the states and Union territories in the country. The only state which was ranked below Punjab was Haryana. Compared to Kerala and Pondichery (with favourable), Punjab had very unfavourable sex ratio of 874 females per 1000 males. It is interesting to note that this ratio has become adverse during 1991-2001. It has declined from 882 females per 1000 males in 1991 to 874 females per 1000 males in 2001 (Table 1.13). This decline is felt in the overall population and both in rural as well as in urban areas. The change is more pronounced in the urban areas compared to the rural areas.

The rural urban differences in terms of health indicators show poor quality of life in rural areas. The birth rate remains higher in rural areas compared to urban areas. The same is the case of death rate. But decline in birth rate is at higher rate in the urban areas

Table 1.13: Ranking of Districts by Sex Ratio—Punjab, 1991 and 2001

Rank in 2001			*State/District*	*Sex Ratio (Number of females per 1000 males in 2001)*			*Sex Ratio (Number of females per 1000 males in 1991)*			*Rank in 1991*		
T	*R*	*U*		*T*	*R*	*U*	*T*	*R*	*U*	*T*	*R*	*U*
(1)	(2)	(3)	(4)	(5)	(6)	(7)	(8)	(9)	(10)	(11)	(12)	(13)
—	—	—	Punjab	874	887	848	882	888	868	—	—	—
1	1	3	Hoshiarpur	935	947	888	924	932	890	1	1	4
2	2	1	Nawanshahar	913	914	911	900	898	914	3	5	1
3	5	8	Gurdaspur	888	895	868	903	905	895	2	4	3
4	7	4	Mukatsar	886	888	883	880	877	888	11	11	6
5	3	15	Kapurthala	886	907	843	896	910	857	5	2	16
6	6	14	Firozpur	883	893	857	895	898	887	6	6	7
7	8	6	Moga	883	885	873	884	883	889	7	8	5
8	4	13	Jalandhar	882	904	859	897	907	883	4	3	9
9	11	2	Faridkot	881	876	892	883	882	884	9	9	8
10	12	5	Mansa	875	875	878	873	871	881	13	14	10
11	9	12	Amritsar	874	885	859	873	871	876	12	13	12
12	13	7	Rupnagar	870	869	871	870	870	870	16	15	15
13	14	10	Sangrur	868	869	864	870	866	881	15	17	11
14	15	11	Bathinda	865	868	860	884	888	873	8	7	14
15	16	9	Patiala	864	862	868	882	875	899	10	12	2
16	17	16	Fatehgarh Sahib	851	859	832	871	870	873	14	16	13
17	10	17	Ludhiana	824	877	784	844	880	812	17	10	17

T = Total, R—Rural, U = Urban

Source: Director of Census, Punjab, *Provisional Population Totals*, paper 2 of 2001, Chandigarh, p. 40.

compared to the rural areas. In 2000, the birth rate in rural areas was 22.7 per thousand compared to 18.6 per thousand in the urban areas of the state. But the differences in the infant mortality are much more pronounced. In fact mortality rate was 96 per thousand live births in 1980 in the rural areas of the state compared to 89 per thousand in the urban areas. The urban infant mortality rate has declined to 38 per thousand to 56 per thousand in the rural areas in 2000. It shows that the rural areas have achieved nearly the infant mortality rate in 2000 roughly what was infant mortality rate in urban areas twenty years back, i.e. in 1980 (Table 1.14).

This is an indication of poor health infrastructure and its utilization in rural areas compared to urban areas of the state.

Table 1.14: Vital Statistics of Punjab

(per thousand per annum)

Year	*Birth Rate*			*Death Rate*			*Infant Mortality*		
	Rural	*Urban*	*Combined*	*Rural*	*Urban*	*Combined*	*Rural*	*Urban*	*Combined*
1980	30.3	28.3	29.9	9.2	6.6	8.7	96	58	89
1990	28.4	25.6	27.6	8.5	5.8	7.8	66	45	61
1998	23.7	18.5	22.4	8.2	6.3	7.7	58	40	54
1999	22.5	18.6	21.5	7.9	6.1	7.4	57	39	53
2000	22.7	18.6	21.6	7.9	5.9	7.4	56	38	52

Source: *Statistical Abstract of Punjab, 2002*, Government of Punjab, Chandigarh.

The rural areas of Punjab were known for sweet and clean water for drinking purposes. Over years the number of identified water scarcity villages has been increasing at a fast rate. In 1980, 3712 (30.46 per cent) villages were identified water scarcity villages but this number increased to 11849 (95.34 per cent) in 2002 (Table 1.15). This shows that most of rural areas of the state have become water scarce within 22 years. This is caused by fast declining water table accompanied by degradation/pollution of water resources. Consequently, the percentage of the scarcity villages with commissioned water supply has gone down from 83.3 per cent in 2000 to 63.7 per cent in 2002 (Table 1.15).

To sum up in terms of physical infrastructure such as irrigation network, rural electrification, linking of villages with metalled roads, the system of regulated markets and market clearance at MSP for the major crops, rural Punjab is still leaders in the rural development in the country. But rural areas of the state have lagged behind other progressive states in terms of quality of life indices such as literacy rate, infant mortality rate and availability of clean drinking water supply.

Table 1.15: Villages Covered under Water Supply Scheme in Punjab

Year	*No. of Inhabited Villages*	*Identified Water Scarcity Villages*	*Villages Where Water Supply Commissioned*	*Percentage of identified villages with commissioned water supply scheme to identified water scarcity villages 4/3*
(1)	(2)	(3)	(4)	(5)
1980	12188	3712	1945	52.4
1990	12342	6287	3898	62.0
1999	12428	8517	6957	81.7
2000	12428	8518	7092	83.3
2001	12428	10065	7281	72.3
2002	12428	11849	7543	63.7

Source: *Statistical Abstract of Punjab 2002*, as supplied by Chief Engineer, Public Health, P.W.D., Punjab, p. 510.

SOCIAL STRUCTURE OF RURAL PUNJAB

Social structure of rural Punjab is characterized by division of population based on castes and religions. It is a multi-caste and multi-religious society. The major religious groups of India are present in rural Punjab. But rural Punjab is dominated by the Sikhs. The proportion of Sikhs in the rural areas has grown between 1981 and 1991. They constituted 71.30 per cent of the total population in 1981 which increased to 73.97 per cent in 1991. The proportion of Hindu population declined from 26.51 per cent in 1981 to 23.56 per cent in 1991. The Muslim population was 0.88 per cent of the total in 1981 but increased to 1.01 per cent in 1991. The Christian population's share has remained at 1.25 per cent between 1981 and 1991. The other religious groups constituted 0.06 per cent of the rural population in 1981 which increased to 0.21 per cent in 1991 (Table 1.16). The predominance of the Sikh religious groups in the rural Punjab is also confirmed by the reports of the IAS probationers. The multi-religious division of population is not the cause of tension in the rural Punjab.

Different religious groups are living in harmony with each other.

Table 1.16: Religious Distribution of Rural Population of Punjab

Sl. No.	*Year*	*Hindu*	*Sikh*	*Muslim*	*Christian*	*Others*	*Total*
1.	1981	3218391	8656518	107699	151431	7119	12141158
		(26.51)	(71.30)	(0.08)	(1.25)	(0.06)	(100.00)
2.	1991	3366040	10569604	144850	178865	29385	14288744
		(23.56)	(73.97)	(1.01)	(1.25)	(0.21)	(100.00)

Note : Figures in parenthesis are in percentage of total.
Source: *Statistical Abstract of Punjab*, 1992 (pp. 74-77) and 2002 (pp. 80-83), Government of Punjab, Chandigarh.

The religious differentiation is intersected by caste differentiations in the rural Punjab. Followers of both Hindus and Sikhs, the two major religious groups, are divided into different caste groups. Though, caste has no place in Sikh religious principles yet Sikhs are practically caste divided. There are Sikhs of upper castes, backward castes and Scheduled Castes. The division is quite similar to such divisions among Hindus. Census data give only break up of Scheduled Castes and other castes population. The proportion of Scheduled Castes population in the state stood at 24.70 per cent in 1971 increased to 26.87 per cent in 1981 and 28.31 in 1991. Corresponding proportion of other castes population has declined from 73.30 per cent in 1971 to 71.69 per cent in 1991. Compared to other castes, the Scheduled Castes population is less urbanized and concentrated more in the rural areas. The proportion of Scheduled Caste population living in the rural areas was 79.09 per cent in 1991 while share of urban Scheduled Castes was 20.91 per cent. The proportion of SC population living in rural areas (79.09 per cent) is considerably higher than the overall share of the total rural population (70.45 per cent) in 1991 (Table 1.17).

Further, it has been observed that except for the district of Jalandhar and Ludhiana (highly urbanized districts of the state), the proportion of SC population in rural areas is higher than the share of total rural population to total population of the state (Table 1.17). Since Census data do not throw any light on caste division of other population, the data collected by IAS probationers (out of 15 reports, 9 reports give some information) have been used to get some idea of other caste population. These data show that SC population in rural

Punjab was 37.99 per cent (between 1996-2002) compared to their share of 32.06 of the rural population of the state as per Census data of 1991. Table 1.18 reveals that upper caste population largely

Table 1.17: Distribution of Scheduled Caste Population in Rural and Urban Areas (1991)

Sl. No.	*District*	*Rural*	*Urban*	*Total*
1.	Gurdaspur	347822 (80.09)	86484 (19.19)	434306 (100.00)
2.	Amritsar	539609 (76.91)	161973 (23.09)	701582 (100.00)
3.	Kapurthala	152213 (79.91)	38271 (20.09)	190484 (100.00)
4.	Jalandhar	435801 (69.26)	193397 (30.74)	629198 (100.00)
5.	Nawanshahar	182957 (88.35)	24125 (11.65)	207082 (100.00)
6.	Hoshiarpur	383212 (87.21)	56195 (12.79)	439407 (100.00)
7.	Rupnagar	180465 (82.19)	39109 (17.81)	219574 (100.00)
8.	Ludhiana	417077 (70.16)	177361 (29.84)	594438 (100.00)
9.	Firozpur	238453 (77.33)	69919 (22.67)	308372 (100.00)
10.	Faridkot	115134 (72.76)	43099 (27.24)	158233 (100.00)
11.	Mukatsar	198076 (83.07)	40368 (16.93)	238444 (100.00)
12.	Moga	205820 (87.52)	29345 (12.48)	235165 (100.00)
13.	Bathinda	229631 (79.08)	60740 (20.92)	290371 (100.00)
14.	Mansa	146360 (88.05)	19865 (11.95)	166225 (100.00)
15.	Sangrur	370266 (82.12)	80637 (17.88)	450903 (100.00)
16.	Patiala	278953 (82.11)	60793 (17.89)	339746 (100.00)
17.	Fatehgarh Sahib	119794 (86.23)	19204 (13.77)	138918 (100.00)
	Total (Punjab)	4541643 (79.09)	1200885 (20.91)	5742528 (100.00)

Source: *Statistical Abstract of Punjab 2002*, Government of Punjab, Chandigarh, p. 71.

consisting of Jat Sikhs and at some other places of other castes (Brahmins and Khatri-Arora) constitute 44.82 per cent of the total population. There is another major caste group named as Backward Castes (BC) which constitute 17.19 per cent of the total rural population of the state. The probationers report bring out very clearly that untouchability based on caste is not practiced in the rural Punjab. There is no apparent discrimination at public places yet caste based division between upper castes and lower castes (mainly SCs) is very pronounced.

Though no IAS probationer has reported yet there are several reported cases of conflict between upper castes and Scheduled Castes resulting in boycott of the SCs for several days in villages of conflict. The conflict between upper caste Sikhs and SCs (*Adharmis*) led to a major conflict at Talhan village in Jalandhar district leading to violence and imposition curfew in the village and some parts of the Jalandhar city in 2003 (Jodhka and Lauis, 2003).

Table 1.18: Caste Structure of Rural Punjab*

Caste	*Per cent Distribution*
Upper Caste[1]	44.82
Backward Caste[2]	17.19
Scheduled Caste	37.99
All Castes	100.00

* This is based on study of 9 villages two each from Jalandhar, Ropar, Patiala and Sangrur and one village from Nawanshahar districts. These studies were conducted by IAS probationers between 1996-2002 as a part of their training at LBSAA, Mussoorie and they are listed in the bibliography.

1. Upper Castes includes Jat Sikh, Arora, Khatri, Brahmins.
2. Backward castes include Tarkhan, Nai, Kumhar, Mehra (Jheur).

Social Structure of rural Punjab is dominated by the upper castes particularly Jat Sikhs. They own and cultivate land and employ Scheduled Castes and Backward Caste persons as agricultural labourers. They also control common property resources such as *Shamlat* land, *panchayati* land and places of worship. The hegemony of Jat Sikhs in rural Punjab is also found in terms of their dominance in politics of Legislative Assembly and Parliamentary seats and members of Shiromoni Gurdwara Prabandhak Committee (SGPC). Along with the numerical dominance, they control land, the primary source of livelihood. There were 11,16,951 operational holdings in 1990-91 operating 40,33,000 hectares of land divided into various size classes (Table 1.19). Out of these holdings, the number of SC holdings was 54,000 accounting for 4.8 per cent of total holdings. The SC population account for 32.06 per cent (1991 census) of the rural population but account for 4.8 per cent of the holdings and 2.4 per cent of the cultivated area. On the other hand the upper castes mainly own and operate almost the entire area under cultivation.

Table 1.19: Size Class of Operational Holdings in Punjab (1990-91)

Sl. No.	*Size Class*	*Number of holdings*	*Percentage*
1.	Marginal (Below 1 Hectare)	295668	26.48
2.	Small (1-2 Hectares)	203842	18.25
3.	Semi-Medium (2-4 Hectares)	288788	25.85
4.	Medium (4-10 Hectares)	261481	23.41
5.	Large (Above 10 Hectares)	67172	6.01
	Total	**1116951**	**100.00**

Note: Total operated Area = 4033000 hectares
Average size of holdings in Punjab = 3.651 hectares

Source: *Agricultural Census of Punjab 1990-91*, Department of Agriculture, Government of Punjab, Chandigarh reproduced in Statistical Abstract of Punjab 2008, Government of Punjab, Chandigarh.

Further, SC holdings are mainly marginal and small in size. Both these categories account for 66.6 per cent of the total holdings. Another 22.2 per cent holdings are semi-medium in size (Table 1.20). In comparison to this, the marginal and small holdings constitute 44.73 per cent of the overall holdings, semi-medium 25.85 per cent of the holdings and medium and large holdings account for 29.41 per cent of the holdings (Table 1.19). Consequently, the average size of overall operational holdings (3.61 hectares) is more than that of SC holdings (1.76 hectares). Most of the SC households are landless and those among them who own/operate land are operating tiny holdings which do not ensure them enough income to survive. Therefore, SC households are dependent on wage labour on the farms of upper caste farmers or seek employment outside agriculture. The majority of them fall on the bottom of the rural society both in terms of social as well as economic status. This is also confirmed by village study reports of IAS probationers related to different districts of Punjab. The households described in distress belong to Scheduled Caste category. This is also reflected from the type of houses they live in and the lower social status they enjoy in their interaction with other sections of population.

Table 1.20: Size Class of Scheduled Caste Operational Holdings in Punjab (1990-91)

Sl. No.	*Size Class*	*Number of holdings*	*Percentage*
1.	Marginal (Below 1 Hectare)	24000	44.4
2.	Small (1-2 Hectares)	12000	22.2
3.	Semi-Medium (2-4 Hectares)	12000	22.3
4.	Medium (4-10 Hectares)	5000	9.3
5.	Large	1000	1.9
	Total	**54000**	**100.00**

Note: SC holdings as percentage of total holdings in Punjab = 4.8
Percentage of total operated area by SC holdings in Punjab = 2.4
Average size of SC holdings= 1.76 hectares

Source: *Agricultural Census of Punjab 1990-91*, *op. cit.*, p. 208.

PANCHAYATI RAJ INSTITUTIONS AND RURAL DEVELOPMENT

Panchayati Raj Institutions (PRIs) have a lot of potentials in promotion of rural development. They are institutions of democracy at grassroots level and instruments of empowerment of the people at local levels. At the same time these institutions can identify projects at local level, prepare plans, arrange part of resources and implement-plans efficiently and in a transparent way. They can harness collective energy and resources for constructive purposes.

In the post-Independence period panchayats were organized in Punjab through the Punjab Gram Panchayat Act, 1952. This Act provided for mandatory constitution of village panchayats through universal adult franchise. Later on in 1962-63, Punjab state decided to introduce three-tier system comprising Gram Panchayat at village level, Panchayat Samiti at block level and Zila Parishad at district level under Panchayat Samiti and Zila Parishad Act, 1961. The elections to Gram Panchayats had been regularly held in Punjab (1952, 1957, 1962, 1968, 1973, 1978, 1983, 1992, 1998 and 2003) with exception of 1988. But Block Samitis and Zila Parishads functioned as representative bodies up to 1970 and between 1975 and 1978. They remained dissolved between 1970-75 and 1978-1994. Under the Punjab Panchayati Raj Act, 1994, elections to 138 Panchayat Samitis and 14 Zila Parishads were held in 1994 and again Panchayat elections were held in 1998 and elections to Panchayat Samitis and Zila Parishads in June 2002, though they were due in 1999. Recently elections to Panchayats have been held in 2003. In 1998 there were 12369 panchayats with 87842 elected members (panches and sarpanches). Out of these representatives 2485 members of Panchayat Samitis (140) and 281 members of Zila Parishads (17) were elected in 2002.

Under the new Act (1994), the reservation has been made for sarpanches for SCs and women have also been given 1/3rd reservation separately for the post of sarpanches. In 1998, there were 2854 women sarpanches from general category and 1260 women sarpanches from SC category. The total number of SC sarpanches (both male and female) was 2499 in 1998 (Kesar Singh *et al.*, 2002). This has also been continued in 2003 election to Panchayats.

At present panchayats are performing three development functions: (a) Community works such as brick lining of village streets and drains, construction of Panchayat Ghar, Dharmsala etc., (b) help to individuals in getting old age pension, widow pension and other benefits decided by the state from time to time, and (c) help in identification of beneficiaries under IRDP and execution of some programmes.

Twenty nine subjects listed in the Eleventh Schedule to the Constitution are not as yet transferred to Panchayats in Punjab. At the same time, the government has not transferred the requisite funds as recommended by First Punjab Finance Commission. The Commission submitted its report in December 1995 and was accepted by the Punjab Government with effect from January 1, 1997. The Commission had recommended for transferring of 20 per cent of the net proceeds to PRIs and Urban Local Bodies (ULBs) from five taxes: stamp duty, Punjab motor vehicles tax, electricity duty, entertainment tax and entertainment cinematograph show tax. The amount due to these bodies over five years 1996-97 to 2001 was Rs. 607.29 crore. The actual amount transferred was Rs. 155.67 crore. Additional Rs. 150.98 crore due to PRIs and Rs. 102.41 crore to ULBs had been withheld by the Punjab Government. Thus, as yet Punjab Government has neither transferred the functions nor the finances to PRIs to perform functions and duties assigned to them under 73rd Amendment to the Constitution.

If the functions and duties under Eleventh Schedule to the Constitution are transferred along with the requisite funds by the state government, would the Panchayats successfully perform? This needs some examination. The reports of the IAS probationers throw some light on this question. The two reports (Vikas Pratap, 1996: 46-47; Hussan Lal, 1997: 44-45) bring out that elections to panchayats have become costly affair for contestants particularly for the post of sarpanch. This includes expenditure on organization of *langer* (community meal) for many days before elections as a part of campaign. The use of liquor and other intoxicants have become very common to win over the requisite support. After elections, an elaborate party for celebrations has also become a common practice. Thus contesting of elections for the position of sarpanch involves expenditure of several lakhs of rupees. In the recent years, particularly after 1992, the Panchayat elections have become politicized. The ruling party and main opposition (both Congress and Akali-Dal) sponsor elections of panches and sarpanches to expand electoral mass base (Abhi and Singh, 1997). This happened in 1992, 1998 and 2003 panchayat elections. This process has created a lot of factionalism at village level and marginalized the non-rich/poor people from contest of sarpanch elections. This has introduced two elements in functioning of panchayats. One, there are large number of cases of misappropriation of panchayat funds and resources. Two, objectivity in functioning of panchayat has been eroded and supporters of the sarpanch are favoured in execution of panchayat works, identification of beneficiaries and in pursuance of cases of old age pension, widow pensions etc.

The participation of the poor and the women has been ensured through reservation of seats for SCs and women. It has been brought out by reports of IAS probationers. Leaving one or two exceptions (Ajay Sharma, 2001: 25; Vikas Garg, 2000: 14) women sarpanches and panches participation vary from non-existent to negligible in panchayat affairs. Their husbands and other male relatives effectively perform functions on their behalf. This undermined the very purpose of 33 per cent reservation of seats of sarpanches and panches for women. The same is the case with most of SC sarpanches and panches. The reports of villages studied bring out that either SC sarpanches and panches are inactive or work under the guidance of Jat Sikh land owners, the persons with resources. Consequently, the working of the panchayats does not reflect priorities of the village poor nor gender bias has been rectified as yet.

The women participation in the panchayat affairs is limited due to gender bias against them in rural society of Punjab. This is reflected by adverse sex ratio (which has become more adverse during 1991-2001) and low literacy rates in the female population. In case of SCs, the literacy rates are lower and lowest among the females. At the same time, their lower social status and lack of ownership of land and other productive resources place them at lowest economic status in the rural areas. Their daily struggle for survival hampers their participation and limited capability excludes them from participation in the affairs of the panchayat.

These handicaps can be partly overcome by empowerment of the SCs and the women through greater emphasis on their educational attainments and entitlement of productive resources. In the short term, those elected to the position of panches and sarpanches, effective training programme can create necessary awareness of their rights and duties and sensitize them for participation in the affairs of panchayats. This would require involvement of existing training institutes and establishment of new ones for training of elected representatives of panchayats. For this purpose financial and academic inputs are required. The state is found wanting on both these counts. Between 1998 and 2002 (14th August) 4198 representatives of PRIs could be given short duration training out of the total 90568. If all of them are to be given two days training Rs. 10.97 crore are required (Kasar Singh *et al.*: 163). For adequate training at least effective ten days duration training programmes need to be organized. The increase of duration of training and rising price index would raise fund requirements many folds (may be Rs. 30-40 crore). Given the tight financial position, the state government has not been able to arrange its matching funds to draw funds from the Union Government.

The handicaps of growing fractionation caused by politicization of PRIs and money based campaigning in elections along with tendency to misappropriate resources are more difficult to handle. They are connected with present political culture in the state and can be handled jointly by political parties involved in managing the affairs of the state. At present there is no social movement within and outside these parties to rectify the malady. This would make the task of PRIs more difficult if the 29 subjects are transferred to them for administration and developments.

The long term solution to make effective role of PRIs requires wider participation of people in local political process. This demands greater involvement of women and weaker sections in the affairs of panchayat. As yet this is not happening for want of necessary awareness, sensitization and entitlement of productive resources with women and SCs. Consequently, the spread of quality education beyond literacy in rural areas is of prime importance. The present trend of schooling, non-functional public funded schools for the poor and private funded (costly) schools for the rich do not provide solution to the problem. The proper handling of the elementary education towards quality education for everyone, both for rich and poor at the same place, is required. This is beyond the present policy framework in the state and the country.

ANTI-POVERTY PROGRAMMES AND CENTRALLY SPONSORED SCHEMES

India has many years experience of implementing anti-poverty programmes in the rural areas. It started with setting up of Small Farmer Development Agency (SFDA) and Marginal Farmers and Agricultural Labour Agency (MFALA) in 1970-71. These agencies were set up for specific target groups, i.e. small farmers and marginal farmers and agricultural labourers. These target groups were extended loans with some components of subsidy for purchase of productive assets or setting up of economically useful activities. These agencies were set up at district level in Punjab also as centrally sponsored programme. These agencies provided financial help to meet credit requirements and extend other facilities such as marketing facilities for the project sponsored to small and marginal farmers and agricultural labourers. Area specific programmes were started in the form of Draught Prone Area Programme (DPAP) and Tribal Area Development Programme (TADP) in 1970s for weaker sections and economically depressed areas. These programmes were expected to tackle rural poverty by helping weaker sections to increase their income through promotion of self-employment and increased wage employment. The Minimum Needs Programme (MNP) was also launched to supplement income generating efforts by providing civil amenities and facilities in the rural areas. In 1978-79 these programmes were merged into Integrated Rural Development Programme (IRDP) for providing income generating assets and promotion of self-employment in the rural areas.

There was an understanding that for rural poverty alleviation, gainful employment promotion for target groups has to be an essential element in the strategy. A series of special employment generation programmes were started in the seventies. These included: Rural Works Programme (RWP); Crash Scheme of Rural Employment (CSRE); Pilot Intensive Rural Employment Projects (PIREP); Employment Guarantee Schemes (EGS); Food For Work Programme (FFWP); National Rural Employment Programme (NREP); and Rural Landless Employment Guarantee Programme (RLEGP). In April 1989, ongoing NRE and RLEGP were merged into single rural employment programme and named as Jawahar Rozgar Yojana (JRY). For larger and efficient use of human resources for poverty alleviation, reduction of inequalities and a reasonable high pace of economic growth, Employment Assurance Scheme (EAS) was launched on October 2, 1993. JRY was merged into EAS scheme from January 1, 1996. This scheme covers all the blocks in the country and aims to provide assured employment of 100 days of unskilled manual work in a year to the rural poor in need of employment and seek it too. At the same time this programme intends to create economic infrastructure and community assets for sustained production. A maximum two adults (between 18-60 years) both male and female per family can get benefit in this programme. From April 1, 1999, the Jawahar Gram Samridhi Yojana (JGSY) has been started for development of rural infrastructure at the village level replacing EAS.

The Swarnjayanti Gram Swarozgar Yojana (SGSY) has been started from April 1, 1999 along with JGSY. This has been started as a comprehensive self-employment programme for the rural poor in view of weaknesses and the strength of earlier programmes such as IRDP, Training of Rural Youth for self-Employment (TRYSEM), Development of Women and Children in Rural Areas (DWCRA),

Supply of Improved Toolkits to Rural Artisans (SITRA), Ganga Kalyan Yojana (GKY) and Million Wells Schemes (MWS), which are no longer in operation. SGSY is a holistic scheme of micro enterprises covering various aspects of self-employment like Self Help Groups (SHG) of rural poor, capacity building, training, planning of activities clusters, infrastructure building, technology, credit and marketing.

All these centrally sponsored schemes have been in operation in Punjab. The actual expenditure incurred on these programme is shown in Table 1.21. The expenditure on rural development as a percentage of total plan expenditure has increased from 2.78 per cent during the Sixth Five Year Plan to 5.53 per cent during the Ninth Five Year Plan. Though the share is increasing slowly yet it remains a very small proportion of the total expenditure of five year plans. The impact of expenditure on the overall development of rural areas is bound to be low.

In the centrally sponsored scheme, Punjab has seen underutilization of funds for the Ninth Five Year Plan period. This has varied between minimum of 74.62 in case of Pradhan Mantri Gramoday Yojana (PMGY) and maximum of 91.06 per cent in case of Swarnjayanti Gram Swarozgar Yojana (SGSY).

The average utilization of these funds as percentage of funds available from the four centrally sponsored schemes has been 87.46 per cent (Table 1.22). The state government has been facing acute financial crisis during 1980s and 1990s and crisis continues even today. The government has been unable to arrange requisite matching funds from its resources, leading to underutilization of funds made available by the Union Government. Obviously, there has not been full achievement of targets in employment generation among the target groups and their poverty alleviation.

The data provided by Joint Development Commissioner (RD), Government of Punjab reveal that with utilization of these funds 35167 beneficiaries received assistance under Swarnjayanti Gram Swarozgar Yojana during the Ninth Five Year Plan (up to February 2002). Per beneficiary assistance given amounts to Rs. 11,382.83. The employment created under Jawahar Gram Samridhi Yojana is reported to 51.86 lakh mandays during the Ninth Five Year Plan with annual average employment of 10.37 lakh mandays. This is just 83.44 man days annual employment generation per village. This does not meet

Table 1.21: Rural Development under Five Year Plans

Sl. No.	*Sub-Head*	*Actual Expenditure (Rs. lakh at current prices)*					
		7th Plan (1985-90)		*8th Plan (1992-97)*		*9th Plan (1997-2002)*	
		Actual Expenditure	*Percentage to total*	*Actual Expenditure*	*Percentage to total*	*Actual Expenditure*	*Percentage to total*
1.	IRDP	3043.45	30.84	2977.24	12.55	1770.45	3.38
2.	National Rural Employment Programme	1667.35	16.89	—	—	—	—
3.	JRY	—	—	1705.34	7.19	4575.77	8.74
4.	Other Rural Development Programmes including Community Development Progamme	2813.02	28.50	13436.46	56.65	23172.39	44.27
5.	Rural Development Fund	—	—	—	—	13773.00	26.31
6.	Kandi Watershed and Area Development Programme	2247.00	22.77	5405.99	22.79	8961.74	17.12
7.	Integrated Rural Energy Programme	97.60	0.98	193.53	0.82	94.04	0.18
	Total Rural Development	9867.82	100.00	23718.54	100.00	52347.39	100.00
	Total Plan Expenditure	354716.55		681933.76		976711.33	
	Percentage of Rural Expenditure to total Plan Expenditure		2.78		3.48		5.53

Source: *Statistical Abstract of Punjab*, 2002 (pp. 324-27), Government of Punjab, Chandigarh and Kesar Singh, *et al.*, (2002), "Rural Development" in *Punjab Development Report*, Planning Commission, Government of India, New Delhi, p. 175.

Table 1.22: Utilization of Funds under various Centrally Sponsored Schemes (Ninth Plan) upto February 2002

(*Rs. Lakhs*)

Sl. No.	*Scheme*	*Funds Available*	*Funds Utilized up to Feb., 2002*	*Funds Utilized as percentage of funds available*
1.	Swarnjayanti Gram Swarozgar Yojana (SGSY)	4396.00	4003.00	91.06
2.	Jawahar Gram Samridhi Yojana (JGSY)	7413.36	6605.89	89.11
3.	Indira Awas Yojana	5435.15	4550.80	83.73
4.	Pradhan Mantri Gramoday Yojana (PMGY)	610.64	455.66	74.62
	Total	17855.15	15615.35	87.46

Source: Kesar Singh *et al.,* (2002), "Rural Development" in *Punjab Development Report*, Planning Commission, Government of India, New Delhi, pp. 176-179.

the target of helping even one poor family by providing 100 days additional employment in one village per year. 22631 houses have been constructed during the five year period under both Indira Awas Yojana and Pradhan Mantri Gramoday Yojana (Kesar Singh, *et al.*, 2002). The data show that on the average less than two houses have been built for poor per village during the five year period. Thus, the employment generation and construction of houses show very poor record of performance of anti-poverty programmes in the state.

At ground level, some insight is available from study reports of IAS probationers about the operation of centrally sponsored schemes for poverty alleviation of the 15 villages studied (Gurdaspur 1, Jalandhar 2, Nawanshahar 1, Patiala 5, Sangrur 4, Ropar 2). JRY/JGSY was in operation in 10 villages. This scheme has not operated in the remaining 5 villages. So, the target of providing 100 days employment in the lean period to the rural poor is not achieved in these villages. Earlier IRDP and SGSY was in operation in 8 villages out of 15 studied. Thus nearly one-half of the villages remain uncovered. Houses for the rural poor under IAY have been constructed in 5 out of 10 villages studied. Only in one village Harditpura (Sangrur) a Self Help Group of SC women has been formed and is successfully working. The reports show that vast areas of rural Punjab remained untouched so far as poverty alleviation programmes are concerned. This puts question mark on the claim of employment generation of the Rural Development of Government of Punjab. In the operation of JRY/JGSY there is very serious problem related to the rate of wage payment. The market wage rate is higher than the wage rate permissible under this programme. Therefore, most of the rural poor are reluctant to get employed in this programme. At many places work is got done on contract by the contractors who bring their own labour mainly migrants from UP and Bihar who are willing to work on lower wages.

IRDP and host of other programmes have been merged into Swarnjayanti Gram Swarozgar Yojana for helping the rural poor. Those who are identified as the rural poor are eligible to get assistance. There is a very serious problem of identification of the rural poor in Punjab. In operation of these programmes, the Yellow Card holders are recognized as poor. But a large number of the poor don't have Yellow Cards and many of the card holders are not poor. Consequently most of the poor either do not get assistance or a large number of rural non-poor are able to manage assistance using their influence with officials and politicians. Moreover the income eligibility criterion is very low, fixed on the basis of requirements of the poor states. Most of the study reports point out that poverty alleviation programmes need to be modified in terms of requirements of the state. These programmes have been launched on the basis of all India average. It is necessary to recall an observation of Dantwala on rural employment many years back:

> "It is therefore essential for employment planning to match employment generation with the demand for work, if not for each individual, at least for each major category of unemployed.... A large majority of persons in the 'labour market' may not want new jobs, they want more stable and more remunerative employment in the existing or allied occupations" (Dantwala, 1979: 1056).

This explains massive rural unemployment and underemployment in Punjab. The work which is available including in various centrally sponsored schemes (at low wages) is not acceptable to a large number of unemployed persons. They want more stable and regular jobs at relatively higher wage rate/salary. While recognizing the importance of public works and special employment schemes, Dantwala cautions against them as main plank of employment policy. In his words:

> "They must not become the main plank of the employment programme and thus divert the attention of the planners from the task of rural development, namely, removal of all hurdles which impede the efforts of the poor and the unemployed to be self-reliant and earn livelihood through their own work and merit" (Dantwala, 1979: 1056).

Given the stage of development, the state requires employment planning which is different from what is required in other areas of the country such as east U.P., Bihar or Madhya Pradesh. The employment generation must meet the aspiration and demands of majority of job seekers. Otherwise jobs may be created which people don't accept leading to the situation of no takers for such work. This is what is happening in Punjab in case of JRY and other related programmes. The centrally sponsored programmes are not suited to the needs of the rural Punjab and are being implemented half heartedly and in patchy ways and many a times a source of misappropriation of scarce public resources. They need to be rooted in the soil and ground reality of the rural Punjab.

RURAL ECONOMIC ACTIVITIES AND AGRARIAN RELATIONS

Economic activities in the state are showing structural change over period of time. Primary sector is experiencing a decline both in its share of state domestic product (SDP) as well as the share of workforce. This sector accounted for 49.13 per cent of the share of SDP in 1980-81 which declined to 40.32 per cent in 2001-02. Correspondingly the share of secondary and tertiary sectors have increased respectively from 20.01 per cent and 30.86 per cent in 1980-81 to 21.42 per cent and 37.02 of the SDP (Table 1.23). The share of agriculture and live stock in SDP of primary sector has been more than 98.10 per cent during 1980-81 to 2001. The share of agriculture alone (cultivators and agricultural labourers) in the total workforce of the state stood at 58.01 in 1981 but declined to 39.4 per cent in 2001. Thus agriculture and livestock though experiencing a decline in their importance yet remains the single largest sector of economy of the state.

The backbone of the rural economy continues to be agriculture and allied activities (mainly livestock). Cultivators and agricultural labourers, directly dependent on agriculture, account for 53.5 per cent of the rural workforce in terms of 2001 census data (Table 1.7) and 62.7 per cent in terms of 1999-2000 NSS data (Table 1.8). Recently the share of other activities such as transport, communication, storage, construction and manufacturing has grown yet remain dependent on agriculture and allied sector. NSS data (Table 1.8) reveal that 37.3 per cent (46.5 per cent according to 2001 Census) of the workforce in the rural areas is engaged in non- agricultural activities. These include trade, hotel and restaurant (8.0 per cent), manufacturing (7.9 per cent), construction (7.4 per cent), public administration, education and communication (7.2 per cent), transport (5.3 per cent), electricity, water etc. (1.1 per cent) and financial services and business (1.1 per cent).

Table 1.23: Percentage Distribution of Net State Domestic Product at Factor Cost at Constant Prices

Sl. No.	*Sector*	*1980-81*	*1990-91*	*2000-01*
1.	Agriculture	33.76	31.17	27.33
2.	Livestock	14.44	15.19	14.14
3.	Forestry and Logging	0.88	0.53	0.16
4.	Fishing	0.03	0.08	0.40
5.	Mining and Quarrying	0.02	0.04	0.00
	Sub-total (Primary)	**49.13**	**47.01**	**42.03**
6.	Registered manufacturing	6.70	10.10	10.10
7.	Unregistered manufacturing	4.96	6.69	5.19
8.	Electricity, Gas and Water supply	2.64	3.79	0.73
9.	Construction	5.71	3.76	5.40
	Sub-total (Secondary)	**20.01**	**24.34**	**21.42**
10.	Trade, Hotels and Restaurants	13.10	10.37	14.02
11.	Transport, Storage and Communication	2.61	3.11	4.05
12.	Banking and Insurance	2.30	4.28	6.08
13.	Real Estate, Ownership of Dwellings and Business Services	4.70	3.49	3.40
14.	Public Administration	2.85	3.35	4.57
15.	Other services and Sanitary Services	5.30	4.05	4.34
	Sub-total (Tertiary)	**30.86**	**28.65**	**37.02**
	Total State Domestic Product	**100.00**	**100.00**	**100.00**

Note: Figures for 1980-81 and 1990-91 are at 1980-81 prices and for 2000-01 at 1993-94 prices.

Source: *Statistical Abstract of Punjab*, 1992 (pp. 106-107) and 2002 (pp. 134-135), Government of Punjab, Chandigarh.

Thus, agriculture is not only the most dominant activity but an activity around which other activities are woven. The performance of agriculture determines the scope and rate of development of other activities.

Cropping Pattern

Punjab had a fairly diversified cropping pattern before green revolution. The share of cereals in the total cropped area was 45.65 per cent and foodgrains 64.33 per cent as pulses accounted for 19.08 per cent of the area in 1960-61. Other important crops were cotton, oil seeds and sugarcane respectively grown on 9.45 per cent, 3.91 per cent and 2.81 per cent of the total cropped area. Though wheat was the most dominant crop, it was cultivated on 29.59 per cent of the area. The share of rice in the area was only 4.80 per cent in 1960-61. Over the years the Punjab agriculture has progressively moved towards the mono crop culture. This situation was nearly obtained by 1980-81. The area under food grains had increased to 77.77 per cent and under cereals to 66.76 per cent. The area under wheat had increased to 41.57 per cent and under rice to 17.49 per cent of the cropped area. The crop like oilseeds, sugarcane and pulses were nearly decimated with respective share of 1.39 per cent, 1.35 per cent and 1.91 per cent of the total area under cultivation. The situation has

Table 1.24: Shift in Cropping Pattern in Punjab, 1960-61 to 2000-01

(*Percentage of Gross Cropped Area*)

Year	Food-grains	Cereals	Wheat	Rice	Cotton	Oil seeds	Sugar-cane	Pulses
1960-61	64.33	45.65	29.59	4.80	9.45	3.91	2.81	19.08
1970-71	69.18	61.89	40.49	6.87	6.99	5.20	2.25	7.29
1980-81	77.77	66.76	41.57	17.49	9.60	3.52	1.05	5.04
1990-91	75.55	73.65	43.63	26.86	9.34	1.39	1.35	1.91
1995-96	74.17	72.94	41.17	28.33	9.62	3.07	1.76	1.23
1997-98	72.87	71.63	41.34	27.62	9.16	3.15	2.23	1.24
1998-99	74.60	73.55	41.94	28.94	9.20	1.77	1.60	1.05
1999-00	78.29	77.35	42.35	32.53	7.27	2.07	1.33	0.94
2000-01	79.11	78.41	42.95	32.92	5.96	1.08	1.52	0.69

Source: *Statistical Abstract of Punjab*, 2002, Government of Punjab, Chandigarh, pp. 164-165.

gone from bad to worse by 2000-01. The share of food grains in the total area has increased to 79.11 per cent of the total cropped area and that of cereals to 78.41 per cent which is nearly occupied by wheat-rice combination accounting for 75.87 per cent of the total cropped area. Along with oilseeds, sugarcane and pulses, cotton has also suffered in the decade of nineties. The share of cotton in total area has been above 9 per cent between 1960-61 to 1999-2000 has declined to 5.96 per cent in 2000-01 (Table 1.24). The share of all other (than wheat-rice) crops has been reduced to 24.13 per cent in the total cropped area. In winter it is wheat everywhere and in summer rice is cultivated in the fields of Punjab.

Stagnating Productivity

The green revolution technology raised productivity of both wheat and rice significantly. Per hectare yield of wheat increased from 2095 kg during 1967-68 to 1969-70 to 4530 kg during 1998-99 to 2000-01 and rice from 1392 kg to 3335 kg during this period. But recently productivity rise is either very slow or stagnating showing exhausting potentials of green revolution technology. The per hectare yield of rice has stagnated around 3335-3341 kg during the last one decade (1990-91 to 2000-01). The case of wheat is different. The wheat productivity

Table 1.25: Average Yield of Wheat, Rice and Cotton in Punjab

(*Kg/ha*)

Period	*Wheat*	*Rice*	*Cotton American (in lint)*
1967-68 to 1969-70	2095	1392	374
1971-72 to 1973-74	2279	2113	415
1974-75 to 1976-77	2400	2410	400
1977-78 to 1979-80	2683	2818	368
1981-82 to 1983-84	2985	3055	280
1985-86 to 1987-88	3346	3230	505
1990-91 to 1992-93	3762	3292	569
1993-94 to 1995-96	3995	3341	481
1996-97 to 1998-99	4134	3337	280
1998-99 to 2000-01	4530	3335	318

Source: *Statistical Abstract of Punjab*, 1978 (pp. 118-119), 1988 (pp. 144-145), 1995 (pp. 152-153), 2002 (pp. 176-177), Government of Punjab, Chandigarh.

(per hectare yield) is continuously growing but in case of cotton the productivity level has declined in absolute terms giving a negative growth rate (Table 1.25). The farmers have achieved 75 per cent of realizable potential yield of rice and wheat (PAU, 1998, p. 5). The irrigation potentials are fully exhausted and irrigated area as percentage of net sown area has stagnated at 95 per cent (Table 1.5). There is no scope of increasing area under cultivation. At the same time Punjab has become nearly double crop area with cropping intensity also stagnating around 186 (Table 1.26).

Table 1.26: Net Sown Area and Cropping Intensity

Year	*Net Sown Area ('000 hectare)*	*Cropping Intensity*
1960-61	3757	126
1970-71	4053	140
1980-81	4191	161
1990-91	4218	178
1996-97	4234	185
2000-01	4264	186

Source: *Statistical Abstract of Punjab*, 2002, Government of Punjab, Chandigarh, pp. 158-159.

Declining Returns and Viability of Farming

The initial years of green revolution brought sharp increase in productivity in the major crops leading to reduction in cost of production of output. The increase in use of input such as fertilizers and other chemical inputs, machinery, fuel etc. was at the slower rate than increase in productivity. From 1971-74 to 1985-88, the total cost of production per unit of output in case of wheat, rice and cotton declined at constant prices of 1971-72. But after 1985-88 to 1993-96 the total cost of production per unit of output experienced a marginal increase (Rs. 39.13 to Rs. 40.64 per quintal) in case of wheat, a bit higher rate in case of paddy (Rs. 31.74 to Rs. 35.35) and sharp rise in case of cotton (from Rs. 90.39 to Rs. 166.67). The main reason has been rise in fixed cost (due to over capitalization) both in case of wheat and rice. But in case of cotton both variable as well as fixed costs have increased during this period. With rising costs of production, the rise in MSP, at which market clearance takes place in

Punjab, have not compensated the agriculture. Leaving the case of wheat which continues to give rising rate of return per hectare, return on rice (declined from Rs. 684 in 1991-92 to Rs. 298 in 1995-96 at constant prices) and cotton (declined from Rs. 1418 in 1991-92 to Rs. 217 in 1995-96) have fallen (Sidhu and Johl, 2002: 23).

Similar findings are also reported by another study (Ghuman, 2002). It is estimated that on 5 acres (2 hectare) farm in 1995-96 with existing level of technology generate gross income of Rs. 72,370. After meeting paid out costs, a farmer is left with income of Rs. 40,740 from wheat-rice rotation. However, returns over cash costs for this farm with wheat-rice-dairy farming system increased to Rs. 42,180. This works out to be less than salary of an unskilled worker in service sector which stood at Rs. 45,134 and for skilled worker at Rs. 73,224 per annum at minimum of their pay scales. Even by raising 10-15 per cent productivity from the present 75 per cent of the realizable potential, these farmers cannot be taken out of poverty cycle (PAU, 1998: 11). The present pattern of agricultural practices has put a question mark on the viability of small and marginal farmers who constitute 45 per cent of the total cultivators (1990-91). These cultivators remain trapped in agriculture for want of jobs, though many of them want to leave agriculture.

The rising cost of production and commercialization has made Punjab agriculture high cost and risk sensitive to crop failure. The falling income along with occasional crop failure accompanied by high consumption standards (determined by peak income levels) and inflated aspirations demonstrated by ostentatious expenditure on celebrations has brought various sections of peasantry under mounting debt.

In 1997 it has been estimated that the debt burden on farmers of Punjab stood at Rs. 5700.91 crore. The share of formal credit agencies (commercial banks and co-operative institutions) stood at 46.56 per cent while the share of non-formal credit agencies (commission agents 46.32 per cent and agricultural mortgages 7.12 per cent) was 53.34 per cent (Table 1.27). The average debt on per acre cultivated land stood at Rs. 5,721 but it was highest among small (and marginal) farmers, i.e. Rs. 10,105 as compared to Rs. 4,228 (lowest) among the medium category of farmers (Table 1.28). The small and marginal farmers have greater debt burden in relation to their resource base. Moreover, it is this category of farmers who have a high mortgage debt. The

Table 1.27: Estimates of Indebtedness of Punjab Farmers in 1997

(*Rs. crore*)

Sl. No.	*Nature of Debt*	*Credit Agency*				*Total*
		Commercial Banks	*Cooperative Institutions*	*Commission Agents*	*Agricultural Mortgages*	
1.	Short Term Productive Credit (Annual Flow)	146.89	1059.86	1912.58	—	3119.33 (54.72)
2.	Long Term Productive Outstanding Loans	960.06	487.56	—	—	1447.62 (25.39)
3.	Long term Non-Productive Outstanding Loans	—	—	727.94	—	727.94 (12.77)
4.	Long term Mortgage Debt	—	—	—	406.02	406.02 (7.12)
	Total Debt	**1106.95 (19.42)**	**1547.42 (27.14)**	**2640.52 (46.32)**	**406.02 (7.12)**	**5700.91 (100.00)**

Note: Figures in parentheses are percentages.
Source: H.S. Shergill (1998), *Rural Credit and Indebtedness in Punjab*, IDC, Chandigarh, p. 63.

Table 1.28: Size Classes and Indebtedness of Punjab Farmers

Sl. No.	*Size Class*	*Total Debt (Rs. crore)*	*Debt Per Operated Acre (Rupees)*
1.	Small (up to 5 Acres)	1229.58 (21.57)	10,105
2.	Semi-medium (5-10 Acres)	1651.31 (28.97)	7,941
3.	Medium (10-15 Acres)	1694.49 (29.72)	4,228
4.	Large (Above 15 Acres)	1125.53 (19.74)	4,230
	All holdings	5700.91	5,721

Note: Figures in parentheses are percentages.
Source: H.S. Shergill (1998), *Rural Credit and Indebtedness in Punjab*, IDC, Chandigarh, p. 65.

mortgage debt make their dependence on informal sources much greater than other categories of farmers (Shergill, 1998: 65). It is well known fact that interest rate on informal debt is much higher than the formal debt. Some of the farmers from this category have resorted to suicide when pressed to pay debt or face auction of their land. The unbearable debt burden becomes deadly when there is crop failure due to floods, pest attack etc. Many of these farmers are facing crisis of viability and their existence as farmers is threatened.

Market Clearance Problems

With introduction of Targeted Public Distribution System (TPDS) in 1997, the off take of the food grains (wheat-rice) has considerably fallen compared to allocation. This has led to building up of huge stocks of food grains with the government. Against the minimum norm of 24.3 million tonnes, the actual stocks of wheat and rice had increased to 33.1 million tonnes in July 1999, 42.2 million tonnes in July 2000, 61.7 million tonnes in July 2001 and 63.0 million tonnes in July 2002 (Government of India, 2003: 92). This has put a heavy financial burden on the exchequer along with cost of management and logistic efforts for purchasing, handling, transportation and storage of these stocks. Under the new policy regime, the government agencies have been entering late in procurement of food grains at MSP, causing procurement and market crisis in Punjab. Punjab being the largest contributor (46.72 per cent in 2001-02) to central stock faces immediate crisis as and when procurement agencies show slackness in the market. This is reflected in flooding of market yards with food grains at the time of harvest and loud protests by farmers against the procurement agencies. Every year this is being faced by farmers of the state for the last many years. This has led, many times, to a situation when farmers sell their produce at a price below MSP. This has caused harm to farmers and lowered their income and added uncertainty to future procurement. A message has spread that procurement of wheat and rice is under threat.

The recommendation of Sen Committee (July 2002) for withdrawal of central agencies from procurement and replacement of state agencies in north-western states along with freezing of procurement price and policy statements by Punjab Government spokespersons suggesting cropping shift away from wheat-rice following submission of report by Chief Minister's Advisory Committee on Agriculture Policy and Restructuring (2002) contributed to the impression that wheat-rice crops are not needed in the state and future procurements and market clearance are in doubt.

The uncertainty about procurement at MSP of wheat and rice and absence of any other viable cropping pattern equally remunerative is a source of resentment and unrest among the farmers. The farmers have tried in the past with sunflower (oilseeds) vegetable and fruit cultivation in past but failed due to problems of market clearance. The livestock, the second major source of income of rural people, is facing problems with stagnating prices of milk in face of rising cost of production.

Degrading Environment and Sustainability of Agriculture

The present cropping pattern has put heavy pressure on the physical resources of the state. The resource which has been strained the most is water for irrigation. Irrigation is life line of the agriculture of the state. But the wheat-rice production system has created serious imbalance in use of water resources. The total demand for irrigation water in a year in the state is estimated at 4.377 million hectare metres with existing technology and cropping pattern, against a total supply of 3.130 million hectare metres both from surface and annual recharge of groundwater sources. This is leading to annual deficit of 1.247 million (39.84 per cent) hectare metres (Sondhi and Khepar, 1995). The over-exploitation of ground water resources through tube wells has led to falling water table at alarming rate. The proportion of area with more than 10 metres depth of water table increased from 12.7 per cent in 1973 to 29.8 per cent in 1996 and of 5-10 metres from 50.6 per cent to 56.1 per cent. There are only six blocks in Punjab which are white as well as technically exploitable (Sidhu and Johl, 2002). Most of the area in the state falls either in dark or grey blocks. This is likely to cause drinking water problems both in rural as well as urban area. With river getting polluted, canal water is increasingly becoming unfit for drinking. On the other hand, south-west Punjab is facing water logging due to greater supply of canal water as ground water is saline.

The increased cropping intensity has overexploited the soil and lowered its fertility. The chemical fertilizers are excessively used leading to greater use of basic elements of soil than what is added. The low application of organic manure has reduced the organic carbon to very low level. Consequently, the soil has become poor in nitrogen (N). The same is the case with phosphorous (P). The soil has also become deficit in such micro-nutrients as iron and manganese.

The area under forest cover is alarmingly low (5.6 per cent). Thus the declining water resources, depleting quality of soil and degrading environment has put a question mark on the present cropping pattern and system of farming. Apart from rising cost of production and falling incomes, the rural areas are likely to face new problems like drinking water scarcity and attack of old and new disease pattern, the sign of which are already visible in the state.

Agrarian Relations

A remarkable change which Punjab agriculture witnessed after the green revolution in production and productivity has made the state agriculturally most advanced among states in the country. This change has been observed at level of technology and intensive use of modern inputs. These include mechanical implement/machines, chemical fertilizers, weedicides, insecticides, pesticides etc. and seeds earlier hybrid varieties and recently genetically modified. These changes have increased cropping intensity, per acre yield and production by several folds. The changes in the field of technology and inputs have made agriculture of the state highly commercialized economic activity. Agriculture of the state is very sensitive to market conditions and signals. As mentioned in the earlier section, the risk and uncertainty influence farmers decision because agriculture is high cost and capital intensive. The changes in farm practices and orientation of agriculture towards market has significantly influenced agrarian relations.

The agriculture in the state is no longer a way of life. It has become commercial activity where various decisions are governed by profitability/rate of return. Though some sections of producers are trapped in agriculture, yet they are also substantially affected by market forces and take decisions accordingly. The agriculture of the state can be characterized by dominance of capitalism. On one side there are big farm households with operational holdings of above 10 hectares (25 acres) who cultivate 26.70 per cent of the area and constitute 6.01 per cent (in 1990-91) of the cultivators. They include most enterprising farmers like potato growers of Jalandhar/Hoshiarpur region (Brar and Gill, 2001: 214-237), horse breeders and orchard owners of Mukatsar/Bathinda region and like. Most of the rural origin politicians belong to this category. They have also interests in urban property and business particularly transport, cinema, hotel, commission agent work etc. On the other extreme are agricultural labourers who constituted 31.62 per cent of workforce in 1991 (and 22.0 per cent in 2001). They earn their living by selling their labour to cultivators and themselves don't own land and they also belong to SC and BC population. Above the agricultural labourer but quite near to them in economic status come marginal farmers each cultivating less than one hectare of land. They constituted 26.47 per cent of the farm households and cultivated 4.07 per cent of the total area in 1990-91. Above this category are small farmers cultivating land between 1-2 hectares. They account for 18.24 per cent of the farmers and cultivate 8.13 per cent of the cultivated area. The marginal and small farmers together account for 44.71 per cent of the farmers in the state and cultivate only 12.20 per cent of the land. Their proportion is expected to be around 50 per cent by 2000-01. These categories of the farmers are in serious crisis. They are fighting for their existence which is under threat. Caste-wise they belong to other categories of farmers (Jat Sikhs). They are in debt trap with income levels quite low. There is a large chunk of farmers who cultivate area between 2-4 hectares and 4-10 hectares. This size class of 2-4 hectares farmers constitutes 25.85 per cent of the total and cultivate 20.87 per cent of the area while the size class of 4-10 hectares farmers constitutes 23.40 per cent of the farmers and cultivate 40.23 per cent of the area. Both these categories are called (lower and upper) medium farmers. They are considered to be very active and backbone of the farming in the state. They are moderately under debt and falling returns from cultivation is also affecting them.

The cultivation/farming is highly mechanized and based on market both for input acquisition and output disposal. In terms of use of machinery, chemical inputs, hybrid varities of seeds, irrigation, Punjab is ranked number one in the country (Bhalla and Singh, 2001: 36-37). The cultivation in the state is organized on the basis of individually owned family farms. The organization of agriculture is based predominantly on hired labour (Sidhu and Johl, 2002: 26; Gill and Ghuman, 2001: 817-818). All categories of farmers hire labour but medium and large farmers heavily depend on hired labour. Similarly, all categories of farmers are producing marketable surplus but medium and large farmers' share is much larger. There is differentiation among the farmers in terms of economic status but unity in terms of caste composition, participation in labour hiring in and selling of marketable surplus output. The differentiation is also found in terms of educational levels of the farmers and the type of schooling their children are getting. The medium and big farmers are more educated and are increasingly sending their children to city based private English medium schools which are coming up in the rural areas also. While children of small and marginal farmers and those of agricultural labourers join government schools with miserable teaching standards. Punjab agriculture is at the threshold where the differentiation among the farmers will further result in marginalization of the small and marginal cultivators.

This process is already taking place *via* three routes. One root is *via* tenancy. In the earlier period (1950s), it was the small owners who leased in land to supplement their operational holdings and large owners unable to cultivate their land indulged in leasing out. But today it is the medium owners who lease in land and small owners lease out their land. Many marginal and small farmers with low income level are in search of jobs outside agriculture. As and when they find alterative source of employment they move out of agriculture leasing out their land. Though many studies are not available yet a major shift of rural workforce away from agriculture during the last decade is partly explained by this factor. Consequently, dominant form of tenancy generally unrecorded is leasing in land by middle and big cultivators from small and marginal owners referred to as reverse tenancy (Gill, 1989: A79-85; Singh, 1989: 86-92; Singh and Grewal, 2001: 203-14; Brar and Gill, 2001: 215-37).

The second way of shifting land away from small and marginal owners is *via* mortgage. Faced with acute financial needs when other sources of credit both formal and informal are closed. These poor farmers resort to mortgage of land, generally to medium and large cultivators (and sometimes to commission agents also). Of the total estimated mortgage loan (Rs. 406.02 crore) the share of small and marginal farmers was 60.05 per cent in 1997. This is much larger than (five times) their combined share of (12.20 per cent) of the total cultivated area by them. The share of middle farmers was 10.03 per cent while the share of large farmers was 29.92 per cent (Shergill 1998: 60). This indicates that some land *via* mortgages is getting transferred from small and marginal farmers to middle farmers.

Thirdly, some land is also getting transferred from small and marginal farmers to large cultivators through sale-purchase of land (Baldev Singh, 1982, pp. 67-68). The recent studies on this theme are not available yet this phenomenon is continuing in the rural areas. The scale of land transfers are low through mortgages and sale-purchase process. But transfers *via* tenancy are relatively high. These processes are leading to concentration of land with medium and large cultivators while small and marginal farmers are losing the battle and leaving cultivation.

The changing agrarian relations have undermined the traditional *Jijmani System* by employer-employee system in cultivation. The traditional support system for the weaker and the poor is replaced by commercial relations where the weaker and poor are losing their productive assets to the rich. The rich would like to purchase land and other resources of the weaker in crisis instead of helping him. This is the crux of agrarian relations in todays Punjab which also partly explains the phenomenon of suicides among farmers in some regions of Punjab.

MAIN ISSUES OF RURAL DEVELOPMENT AND POLICY PERSPECTIVE

The rural development in Punjab is in the state of neglect for more than two decades. One decade (1982-1992) was consumed by disturbed conditions and problems associated with them. The second decade (1992-2002) and afterwards have been a period of callous neglect on the part of shortsighted politicians and unconcerned bureaucracy due to absence of meaningful social movement of the rural people. There is no appreciation of the fact in the ruling circles that the disturbed decade was the byproduct of the socio-economic model and its consequences in the rural areas. This is the reason that even after more than a decade after political normalization in the state as yet there is no bold initiative to solve the problems of the rural people. The social movement is fragmented and dominated by leadership which lacks creativity to grasp complex reality. Thus, people are confused and helpless. They have internalized their pain and helplessness. They are harming themselves through use of a variety of drugs and intoxicants leading to slow deaths and restless among them are resorting to suicides. Some of them are also seeking, legally and illegally, greener pastures abroad. The situation is crying for early interventions to give constructive direction to the society. The intervention can be made by the government or social movement of farmers or by government sponsored NGOs or by all in their own way.

The green revolution potentials are exhausted in the state and agriculture is in crisis. This crisis is proving fatal for the poor cultivators and agriculture laboureres. There is need to make farming viable and save the poor cultivators and agricultural labour from bankruptcy. There has been a talk of second green revolution and technology based solutions called diversification of agriculture and setting up of agro based industries (Johl Committee I, 1986; and Johl Committee II, 2002). Who would accomplish the task of introduction of high value crops and value addition to existing crops through agro processing? It was believed that globalization would bring foreign capital, technology and market but it has not proved helpful. It was also believed that liberalization would bring capital for agro processing but this has not happened. The state government is in financial crisis, and this crisis has continued for more than a decade, therefore, the government has no capacity to intervene. Some measures are announced but remain ineffective due to lack of financial resources. Some appeal is made to the Union government for help but no response comes. Whatever resources are available, they are cornered by wheelers and dealers in and outside the government. Therefore, the first issue which needs attention is generation of financial capability in the state to intervene for rural development. This is not possible without disciplining tax collection machinery (to avoid tax evasion) and development machinery (responsible for pilferage of resources).

The second issue is concerned with generating capability among the people to involve themselves in development activity and make them partners in social and economic progress. This can be done through revival of rural education and health. Equal and quality education near ones place of residence is of dire need. At present there are wide gaps between rural and urban areas in education and health indicators. In these matters the task has to be performed by the government. The state has already a good physical infrastructure but utilization is very poor and the government is unnecessarily withdrawing from the scene.

The third issue is concerned with integration of agricultural production activities to marketing and processing activities. At present solutions are suggested without making the local population in the centre of the solutions. It is either suggested that the private capital both Indian and foreign would perform this task or public sector would do it. These solutions have not worked. Had these things worked rural people would have been further marginalized. There is psyche at work to exclude rural people from development process. They are thought unfit for this purpose and have been made so also. There is deskilling among them. Harnessing their collective energy is an ideological question and alien to thinking of policy makers. This needs to be reversed.

The co-operatives of new generation and different in forms need to be experimented in the state. The farmers and agricultural labourers have to be engaged in agricultural production, marketing and processing of agricultural produce to increase their income and days of employment. It is here that role of social movement and NGOs becomes very important. Punjab's rural areas have a long tradition of self help in the hours of crisis. This need to be harnessed. The involvement of corrupt bureaucrats and technocrats would worsen the situation. Therefore, this task has to be performed by organizations of the rural people. Punjab can learn from positive experiments undertaken in other states of India and even abroad. This is a gigantic task which requires big initiative of the social movement and disengagement of myopic politicians and corrupt bureaucracy. If integration of agricultural production, marketing and processing activities with people's involvement takes place, rural Punjab can usher in a new era of development. This would create a large number of jobs to provide gainful employment to the poor farmers, agricultural labourers and artisans who are experiencing redundancy and large scale joblessness (including underemployment). This would also prepare the rural society to better absorb innovations in agriculture, marketing and processing and harness the services of extension experts in the various fields. This would also arrest exodus of rural youth to urban slums or illegal emigration abroad.

The outmoded Co-operative Act needs to be repealed and new Co-operative Act which frees co-operatives from the clutches of bureaucracy need to be enacted. Model Co-operative Societies Act drafted by Planning Commission (1990) needs to be examined. It is necessary to recognize co-operative societies as democratic institutions owned, controlled and managed by members for their economic and social betterment, operating their business with mutual aid and on co-operative principles. Further, the state shall not interfere in the management and operation of co-operatives (Planning Commission, 1990). To save the rural economy, agriculture of the state need restructuring in cropping pattern and adoption of new farm practices to avoid crisis of market clearance, save precious ground water resources and avoid depletion of soil (and its fertility). This requires immediately establishment of mechanism for MSP for new/proposed crops, arrangement for procurement (on pattern of wheat and rice), storage and processing facilities. This demands a massive public (including private) investment in establishment of marketing infrastructure, cold storage, refrigerated transport and processing activities.

Besides, the poor farmers and agricultural labourers who are in debt trap need to be identified. A survey can be done for their identification to help them. Immediately, a programme need to be introduced for rehabilitation of the families falling victim to suicide by the sole earner. This must include debt redemption (both of public and private sector agencies) and material help to save families from becoming destitute. At the same time rural poor families in debt trap (with debt amount being double the value of land/productive assets) need a debt moratorium for next five years. In fact, the Finance Minister of Punjab announced one such programme in his budget speech in 2001. This needs to be given a concrete shape by working out details, passing necessary orders and making provision for financial resources in the Finance Bill.

The experience of implementing anti-poverty programmes and centrally sponsored scheme is not encouraging. These schemes do not match the ground reality of the rural Punjab. They need to be modified in terms of the specific reality of the state. This would make them effective and coverage can be made more comprehensive. The State Rural Development Department would have to work out detailed modalities in consultation with the Planning Commission. This must incorporate the issue of minimum wage rate to be paid under employment generation programmes so that it is made equal to market wage rate (above the nationally prescribed wage rate). The minimum income level prescribed for entitlement of benefit under SGSY and IAY need to be revised upward to ensure its benefit to the needy persons in the state. This is not the place to go in detail, the whole gamut of these schemes need to be reshaped in terms of requirements of the rural society of the state.

The working of village panchayats reveals that in spite of the reservation for SCs and women they are not representing aspirations of the weaker sections and women. The SC members and women are not in the position to exercise their will freely in the working of the panchayats. The entitlement of membership is not sufficient for their empowerment. They lack both ownership of productive assets as well as necessary awareness. In the long run, the membership entitlement can be converted into their empowerment through raising literacy rates and mean years of schooling among SCs and women. But immediately, some awareness about the rights and duties can be created through effective training of elected members of PRIs. The training should be for a period of effective ten days instead of two/ three days. The necessary allocation for funds need to be raised for this purpose and more institutions can be involved in training programmes. In absence of the necessary awareness if 29 subjects are transferred to the panchayats, the purpose of 73rd Amendment may be subverted. In order to increase effectiveness of these institutions, the panchayats need to be made free from party politics and also from corruption.

It has been observed that in the plan period very small proportion of financial resources are earmarked for rural development. This bias need to be corrected by making higher allocation and making resources available to panchayats as per recommendations of the State Finance Commission. The experience of Punjab State is that as yet dominant political leadership is not ready to allow the PRIs to play the role assigned to them.

The delayed empowerment of PRIs in the state is mainly due to opposition of MLAs and MPs whose importance will decline and those of Chairman of Block Samiti and Zila Parishad would increase. But those who are to gain have not raised this issue either through public mobilization or through press. This, itself is sign of low level of awareness among elected representatives of PRIs and neglect on the part of social movement in the state.

The rural development would get proper focus if the rural people assert their position. Two-third of the population of the state is living in the rural areas need to raise their voice. The quality of rural life is relatively poor compared to that in urban areas. The majority of the elected members in the state assembly are elected by the rural voters, unless the people raise the issue of rural development effectively, the issue would suffer apathy and discrimination from the power that be.

NOTES

1. Though compulsory consolidation of land holding was started in April 1948 after the East Punjab Holdings (Consideration and Fragmentation) Act, 1948 was passed yet the actual work started from 1951 onwards. Priority was given, for first two years (1949-51), for resettlement of those farmers who had migrated from West Punjab due to partition of the country. 98.85 per cent (89.37 lakh hectares) of the total area (90.41 lakh hectares) was consolidated between 1951-52 to 1965-66. The rest of the 1.15 per cent (1.04 lakh hectare) area was consolidated during 1966-85 (Singh, 1993).
2. In 1977-78 the state was divided into 12 districts and 117 development blocks. The number of districts has been increased to 17 and the development blocks to 140 (Statistical Abstract of Punjab, 2002).
3. 73rd Amendment to the Constitution was enacted in 1992 but became effective w.e.f. 24-4-1993. The 29 departments included in the Eleventh Schedule are:
   - (i) Agriculture including agricultural extension.
   - (ii) Land improvement, implementation of land reforms, land consolidation and soil conservation.
   - (iii) Minor irrigation, water management and watershed development.
   - (iv) Animal husbandry, dairying and poultry.
   - (v) Fisheries.
   - (vi) Social forestry and farm forestry.
   - (vii) Minor forest produce.
   - (viii) Small scale industries.
   - (ix) Khadi and village industries.
   - (x) Rural housing.
   - (xi) Drinking water.
   - (xii) Fuel and Fodder.
   - (xiii) Roads, culverts, bridges, ferries, waterways and other means of communication.
   - (xiv) Rural electrification, including distribution of electricity.
   - (xv) Non-conventional energy sources.
   - (xvi) Poverty alleviation programme.
   - (xvii) Education, including primary and secondary schools.
   - (xviii) Technical training and vocational education.
   - (xix) Adult and non-formal education.

(xx) Libraries.

(xxi) Cultural activities.

(xxii) Markets and fairs.

(xxiii) Health and sanitation, including hospitals, primary health centres and dispensaries.

(xxiv) Family welfare.

(xxv) Women and child development.

(xxvi) Social Welfare, including welfare of handicapped and mentally retarded.

(xxvii) Welfare of weaker sections, and in particular, of the Scheduled Castes and Scheduled Tribes.

(xxviii) Public distribution system.

(xxix) Maintenance of community assets.

4. When Akali-BJP Government was formed under Chief Ministership of S. Prakash Singh Badal in February 1997, the Chief Minister showed a lot of interest in the revival of focal point strategy for rural development in the state. Rs. 38.64 lakh was spent on getting prepared 23 block development plans for this purpose. In fact, focal point development strategy was launched in 1978 during the earlier tenure of S. Prakash Singh Badal as Chief Minister (1977-80) but was discontinued after fall of his government in 1980 and formation of Congress government with S. Darbara Singh as the Chief Minister.
5. With installation of Akali-BJP Government led by S. Prakash Singh Badal in 1997, the electricity supply to tubewells and canal water for irrigation to farmers were made free of cost. The free supply of electricity was criticized by economists and also by international financial institutions like the World Bank. This facility was withdrawn by Congress Government led by Captain Amrinder Singh in 2003.
6. Caste based literacy data pertaining to 2001 are not released as yet. Mansa district came into existence after 1991.
7. Data on religious composition of population of Punjab has not been released as yet.
8. List of the reports is given in bibliography.
9. Recently, Punjab Chief Minister has announced to transfer six of the 29 listed subjects to the panchayats from October 2, 2003.
10. This estimate is based on estimated expenditure of Rs. 1200 per Gram Panchayat member, Rs. 1500 per Block Samiti member and Rs. 2000 per Zila Parishad member. This is estimated at current prices of 2002. They would need revision for using them for future years.

11. The average utilization of tractor in Punjab is 20 per cent of its capacity. On small farms, the utilization is as low as 4 per cent and on medium farms 16 per cent. The utilization of diesel engines is only 22 per cent (Sain *et al.*).
12. In 2002 panchayat of Harkishanpur village in Bathinda district has put a sign board on road outside the village that the whole village is for sale. This sign board attracted media's attention and created some flutter in Government circles but with no consequences for the poor cultivators.

BIBLIOGRAPHY

Abhi, B.L. and Singh, Kesar (1997), *Post-Green Revolution Rural Punjab—A Profile of Scio-Cultural Change (1965-95)*, CRRID, Chandigarh.

Bhalla, G.S. and Singh Gurmail (2001), *Indian Agriculture: Three Decades of Development*, Sage Publications, New Delhi.

Brar, Jaswinder Singh and Gill, Sucha Singh (2001), "Tenancy Reversal and Operational Enclosures: A Study of Doaba Region", in Sucha Singh Gill (ed.) *Land Reforms in India Vol. 6: Intervention for Agrarian Capitalist Transformation in Punjab and Haryana*, Sage Publications, New Delhi.

Chadha, G.K. (1986), *The State and Rural Economic Transformation: The Case of Punjab (1950-85)*, Sage Publications, New Delhi.

Chenery, Holis, (1979), *Structural Change and Development Policy*, Oxford University Press, New York.

Chaudhari, D.P. (1979), *Education, Innovation and Agricultural Development*, Vikas Publishing House, New Delhi.

Dantwala, M.L. (1979), "Rural Employment: Facts and Issues", *Economic and Political Weekly*, Vol. 14, No. 25.

Gill, Sucha Singh (1989), "Changing Land Relations and Implications for Land Reforms", *Economic and Political Weekly*, Vol. 24, No. 25.

—— (2002), "Agriculture, Crop Technology and Employment Generation in Punjab", in S.S. Johl and S.K. Ray (Eds.), *Future of Punjab Agriculture*, CRRID, Chandigarh.

Gill, Sucha Singh and Ghuman, R.S. (2000), "Changing Agrarian Relation in India: Some Reflections From Recent Data", *The Indian Journal of Labour Economics*, Vol. 44, No. 4.

Ghuman, R.S. (2002), "World Trade Organization and Indian Agriculture with Special Reference to Punjab", in S.S. Johl and S.K. Ray (Eds.), *Future of Punjab Agriculture*, CRRID, Chandigarh.

Government of India (2002), *The Report of the High Level Committee on Long Term Grain Policy* (Sen Committee), New Delhi.

—— (2003), *Economic Survey 2002-03*, Ministry of Finance, New Delhi.

Government of Punjab (1978), *Integrated Rural Development, Punjab*, Development Department, Chandigarh.

—— (1986), *Report of Export Committee on Diversification of Agriculture in Punjab*, (Johl Committee I), Chandigarh.

—— (1987), *Integrated Rural Development Programme*, Publication No. 544, The Economic Adviser to Government of Punjab, Chandigarh.

—— (1995), *Report of the First Finance Commission*, Department of Finance, Chandigarh.

—— (2002), *Report of the Second Finance Commission*, Department of Finance, Chandigarh.

—— (2002), *Agricultural Production Pattern Adjustment Programme in Punjab for Productivity Growth*, Chief Minister's Advisory Committee on Agriculture (Johl Committee II), Chandigarh.

Hendrix, W.E. (1981), "Availability of Capital and Production Innovation on Low Income Farms", *Journal of Farm Economics*, January.

Isaac, Thomas with Frank, Richard (2000), *Local Democracy and Development: People's Campaign for Decentralized Planning in Kerala, Left Word*, New Delhi.

Jodhka, Surinder S. and Luis, Prakash (2003), "Caste Tensions in Punjab: Talhan and Beyond", *Economic and Political Weekly*, Vol. 38, No. 26.

Kaur, Varinder (2004), *Changing Consumption Pattern in Punjab*, unpublished, Ph.D. Thesis, Punjabi University, Patiala.

Kuznets, Simon (1956), *Modern Economic Growth: Rate Structure and Spread*, Yale University Press, New Haven.

Planning Commission (1990), *Model Co-operative Societies Act*, Government of India, New Delhi.

——, (1993), *Report of the Expert Group on Estimation of Proportion and Number of Poor*, Government of India, New Delhi.

Punjab Agricultural University (1998), *Proceedings of Brainstorming Meeting on Farmers and Farming in Punjab*, Ludhiana.

Raul, C. (2001), *From Bitter to Better Harvest: Post-Green Revolution Agricultural and Marketing Strategy in India,* Northern Book Centre, New Delhi.

Sain, Inder; Joshi, A.S.; Singh, Amarjit and Sharma, V.K. (1999), *A Study into the Economics of Farming and the Pattern of Income and*

Expenditure Distribution in Punjab Agriculture: A Project Report, Department of Economics and Sociology, PAU, Ludhiana.

Shergill, H.S. (1998), *Rural Credit and Indebtedness in Punjab*, IDC, Chandigarh.

Sidhu, R.S. and Johl, S.S. (2002), "Three Decades of Intensive Agriculture with Special Reference to Punjab: Crisis and Challenges", in S.S. Johl and S.K. Ray (eds.), *Future of Punjab Agriculture*, CRRID, Chandigarh.

Shultz, T.W. (1964), *Transforming Traditional Agriculture*, Yale University Press, New Haven.

Singh, Baldev (1982), *Land Market: Theory and Practice in India*, Agricole, New Delhi.

Singh, Brijpal (1993), "Consolidation of Land Holding in Punjab: Lessons for Bihar" in B.N. Yugandhar and K. Gopal Iyer (eds.), *Land Reforms in India Vol. I: Bihar Institutional Constraints*, Sage Publications, New Delhi.

Singh, Iqbal (1989), "Reverse Tenancy in Punjab Agriculture: Impact of Technological Change", *Economic and Political Weekly*, Vol. 24, No. 25.

Singh, Kesar *et al.* (2002), "Rural Development", in *Punjab Development Report*, Planning Commission, Government of India, New Delhi.

Singh, R.P. and Grewal S.S. (2001), "Tenancy Pattern in Post Green Revolution Punjab" in Sucha Singh Gill (ed.), *Land Reforms in India, Vol. 6: Intervention for Agrarian Capitalist Transformation in Punjab and Haryana*, Sage Publication, New Delhi.

Sondhi, S.K. and Khepar, S.D. (1995), Water Resources Development and Management for Sustainable Agriculture Production", in *Proceedings of Water Management Symposium*, PAU, Ludhiana.

Todaro, Micheal P. and Stephen C. Smith (2003), *Economic Development in the Third World*, Longman, New York.

Unpublished Socio-Economic Reports of IAS Probationers, submitted to CRS, LBSNAA, Mussoorie

Avhad, Nilkanth (2001), *Socio-Economic Study of Village Bhamabadi* (Sangrur District).

Bhandari, Rahul (1999), *Case Study of Village Jogipur* (Patiala District).

Bhandari, Rakhee Gupta (1999), *Case Study of a Village Akbarpura* (Patiala District).

Garg, Bhawna (2001), *Village Study Assignment* (Malian, District Jalandhar).

Garg, Vikas (2000), *Village Study Assignment*, (Dhapai, Gurdaspur District).

Gurjar, Sumer Singh (2000), Socio-Economic Survey of Village Akol (District Sangrur).

Kaur, Dilraj (2002), *A Study of Socio-Economic Survey* (Abhipur, Ropar District).

Lal, Hussan (1997), *Socio-Economic Survey* (Alipur Jattan, Patiala District).

Meena, V.K. (1999), *Socio-Economic Study of Ghabdan Village* (Sangrur District).

Partap, Vikas (1996), *Socio-Economic Study of Village Laloda, Block Nabha* (District Patiala).

Sharma, Ajay (2001), *Village Study Assignment* (Kahlwan, Jalandhar District).

Singh, Vivek Pratap (1998), *Socio-Economic Survey* (Makauri, Rupnagar District).

Sinha, Ajay Kumar, *Socio-Economic Survey Report* (Village Auza, Patiala District).

Tewari, Rahul (2003), *Socio-Economic Report of Village Harditpura* (Sangrur District).

Tiwari, D.K. (1996), *Socio-Economic Study of Village Langroya Block Nawanshahar* (Jalandhar/Now Nawanshahar District).

2

Haryana

PADAMVIR SINGH

Aims and Methodology

The aim of this chapter is to introduce the reader to Haryana, to its districts and to its villages. In doing so, the study has been limited to Agriculture and Animal Husbandry on the one hand, they being the principal income generating sectors of the economy of Haryana, and to Education and Health, the principal social sectors. The chapter closes with the Poverty Alleviation Programmes, the principal safety net sector.

While the overview of the state and of the districts is largely based on secondary data derived from standard state publications of Haryana and the Census of India, the village level picture is based wholly on the Socio-economic studies conducted by I.A.S. probationers between 1994 and 2002 as part of their training assignments during their district training. While the state data provides the overview, the real content of the paper is based and made up of the village level observations of the probationers. To preserve the freshness of the observations of the probationers as well as to acknowledge the quality of their individual findings, unedited excerpts from their studies have been interspersed throughout the paper. Although the skeleton of the chapter is built up from secondary data, the flesh and blood of the chapter is made up of these unadulterated findings of the probationers.

While selecting the excerpts, I have been guided principally by the quality of the observations and by their complementary nature. I have tried to pick up pieces of the story from the different studies to give a feel of what different observers at different places, at different points of time, have had to say about village realities in Haryana. Many of the pieces sometimes stand alone and do not fully and successfully knit into the general narrative. That is a shortcoming of the general structure of the chapter. At the end of each excerpt, the surname of the probationer, the year in which the study was completed, the village studied and the name of the district are mentioned, [e.g. Khandelwal, 87: Village Nahla (Hisar)]. A list of the studies is available at Annexure 1.

The total number of village studies available for the period were 9. These studies have been conducted in different villages of different districts of Haryana. The limitations of the studies are:

1. The samples are much too small for the purpose of generalisations. As compared to the earlier study which was based on 49 surveys in 49 villages, this study is based on only 9 surveyed villages.
2. Since all the studies deal with different villages and a different set of households, inter-temporal study of development and the impact of Government intervention becomes very difficult.
3. Data collected by the probationers at the village level is inadequate and sketchy. Quantitative analysis of the data is very difficult.

Box 2.1
Objectives of the Study

1. To understand the social, economic, cultural and geographical features of the village, which affect the quality of life of the rural people.
2. Sensitisation towards the problems faced by the people by recording qualitative information about the people, their felt needs and immediate concerns, their own thinking on the problems faced by them and on the ways of dealing with those problems, the extent of local interest and resources and ways of people's participation in the development programmes.
3. To make an appraisal of the implementation of the poverty alleviation programmes in the village.
4. To make an appraisal of the implementation of the Land Reforms measures in the village.

(*Contd.*)

Box 2.1 (Contd.)

5. To study the prevalence of all sorts of untouchability towards the Scheduled Castes and other weaker sections in the village.
6. To facilitate the understanding of factors which cast crucial influence upon administrative planning and decision making.
7. To further use the study as an input for the policy framing as well as micro-planning at the village level. [Tayal, 2000: Ransika (Gurgaon)]

Box 2.2
Methodology of the Field Study

The village study report is meant to be a representative study for the district as a whole and so it is important to have a random choice of the village to be selected for the study. Selection of the village was done scrupulously in accordance with the guidelines for random sampling. A list of all census villages in Pataudi block was prepared along with their respective population. The names of villages with population less than 300 and more than 3000 were removed as required in the guidelines. A random sample was chosen from the table of random numbers provided. The sample number being greater than the number of villages, it was divided by the number of villages and the remainder taken as the serial number of the village to be studied. This corresponded to our survey village of Ransika.

The same random sampling method was followed in the selection of households for the household survey. A list of all the households was drawn up habitation-wise and proportionate random sampling was done for each of the habitations.

For the Focus Group Discussion Schedule, discussions were held in each of the habitations. These discussions were mainly held in the evenings after the villagers returned from the fields. PRA techniques were used in the Focus Group Discussions with emphasis on qualitative data for better communication. Mapping of the village was done with the help of the people to build up enthusiasm and a degree of rapport. A transact walk was done accompanied by some of the people involved in making the map. Individual interviews for household survey were taken up only after a series of Focus Group Discussions.

In doing the Case Studies, apart from the interviews, time was spent with the subjects while they were engaged in their occupations. This was done however only after a certain degree of rapport was built up with the subject. [Tayal, 2000: Ransika (Gurgaon)]

OVERVIEW OF HARYANA

The state of Haryana came into being on November 1, 1966, when the plains of former Punjab state were bifurcated to form the states of Haryana and the present Punjab. With just 1.37 per cent of the total geographical area and about 2 per cent of India's population, Haryana has carved a place of distinction for itself during the past three decades.

Administratively the state is made up of 4 divisions and 19 districts. The districts are further subdivided into 47 sub-divisions, 67 tehsils, 45 sub-tehsils and 116 blocks. The state has 6759 villages and 106 cities and towns. The administrative units were reorganised in 1989 when four new districts, Panipat, Rewari, Yamunanagar and Kaithal were carved out of the 12 districts that existed previously. Later 3 more districts were added.

While presenting the following overview of the state, data has been drawn from the Census of India and from state publications. One may find that all the figures do not match. That would occur because of the different sources and the different points of time that the figures refer to. Data has been picked up looking to its relevance rather than its consistency with other data.

Physical Features

Haryana has an area of 44,212 sq. kms. and after Delhi, Nagaland and Kerala, is the smallest state in the Indian Union. Situated in the northern region of the Indian Union, the state is bounded by the plains of Punjab in the north-west, sharply rising hills in the north-east, Uttar Pradesh separated by the river Yamuna and the state of Delhi in the east and the sandy tract of Rajasthan in the south and the south-west. The state is bounded by river Ghaggar in the west. Topographically, the state possesses large tracts of level or near level land well suited to arable farming and the use of farm machinery. The average height of topography ranges from 700 to 900 feet above sea level. Physically, Haryana falls into two broad natural divisions, the sub-Himalayan and the Indo-Gangetic Plain which run into a south-eastern direction, almost parallel to each other.

Soil

A major part of the soil in Haryana is alluvial loam (central Haryana), the rest being silty loam, coarse loam, sandy loam or sandy. The soils are largely fertile and responsive to irrigation. Rocky and '*pahari*' areas are almost insignificant.

Climate

The climate is very hot in summer and markedly cold in winter. The maximum temperature, recorded during May and June goes as high as 49 degrees Celsius; on the other hand it drops to as low as 2 to 3 degrees Celsius in January.

Except in a few areas the rainfall in the region is low and erratic obviating the need for irrigation. The maximum rainfall is about 216 cm. occurring mainly in the foothills. The minimum rainfall is 25 to 38 cm. in the southern part of the state. About 80 per cent of the overall rainfall occurs between July and September, often resulting in local floods.

Agro-Climatic Zones

North Eastern Zone

(Karnal-Kurukshetra-Ambala)

The zone has very hot summers with temperatures going as high as 45°C in May, June and July and cold winters with temperatures as low as 2°C in December and January. The average total rainfall during the year is about 110 cm. and is received mainly in July-September. The rivers Yamuna, Ghaggar, Markanda, Tangra, Saraswati etc. carry heavy discharge during the monsoon and often cause floods. The soil is mainly loamy.

Central Zone

(Rohtak-Sonipat-Jind)

Very similar to the above zone with respect to climate, this zone has sandy loam soil and an average annual rainfall of about 71 cm. On account of its topography this region is also frequented by floods during the monsoon.

South Western Semi-arid Zone

A. *(Hissar-Bhiwani-Sirsa)*

Bordering the Rajasthan desert the area is arid. The average annual rainfall is only 48 cm. Hot and dry winds and duststorms are common during the summer.

B. (Gurgaon-Faridabad-Mahendragarh)

This zone is also arid and dry. The rainfall is scanty and unevenly distributed averaging about 59 cm. annually. The soil texture of Mahendragarh bordering Rajasthan is sandy and hard calcareous whereas that of Gurgaon and Faridabad is sandy-to-sandy loam.

Demography

The total population of Haryana is 21.08 million (2001 census) constituting 2.05 per cent of the total population of India with a proportionate area of 1.3 per cent. The density of population was 476 per sq. km in 2001 and 372 per sq. km in 1991 as against 318 per sq. km for India as a whole in 2001 and 267 per sq. km in 1991.

The increase in population during 1991-2001 was 28.06 per cent as against 27.4 per cent in 1981-1991, 28 per cent in 1971-81 and 32 per cent in 1961-1971. The corresponding figures for the Indian Union are 21.34 per cent (1991-2001), 23.5 per cent (1981-1991), 25 per cent (1971-1981) and 24.8 per cent (1961-71). The achievements of population control in the state during the period 1971-1981 could not be sustained during the subsequent decades. The rural population as a percentage of the total population declined from 82.3 per cent in 1971 to 78.1 per cent in 1981 and then to 75.4 per cent in 1991, indicating an accelerated pace of urbanisation. The corresponding figures for the Indian Union are 80.1 per cent (1971), 76.7 per cent (1981) and 74.3 per cent (1991). Cultivators as percentage of total workers in Haryana are 38.77 per cent (1991) as against 38.75 per cent (1991) for the Indian Union. However, agricultural labourers as percentage of total workers for Haryana is only 19 per cent (1991) compared to 26.15 per cent for India as a whole. This indicates the predominance of the owner-cultivator in Haryana. The Scheduled Caste population as percentage of total population in Haryana, is 19.75 per cent as compared to 15.8 per cent for the Indian Union. However, in general demographic terms, Haryana appears to be a good representative sample of the Indian Union. (See Table 2.1)

Table 2.1: Demographic Indicators of Haryana

	Haryana	*All India*
Population	16,463,648	846,302,688
Population of Haryana as per cent of total population of India	1.95	
Rural population as per cent of total population	75.37	74.29
Scheduled Caste population as per cent of total population	19.75	15.80
Density	372 per sq. km	257 per sq. km
Decennial Growth rate of Population	27.40	23.51
Sex ratio	865	929
Cultivators	1,829,530	110,588,822
Cultivators as per cent of total workers	38.77	38.75
Agricultural labourers	8,96,782	74,649,217
Agricultural labourers as per cent of total workers	19.00	26.15
Household industry workers	72,195	10,373,099
Household industry workers as per cent of total workers	1.53	3.63
Other categories of workers	1,920,219	89,811,775
Other category workers as per cent of total workers	40.70	31.47

Source: Derived from *Statistical Abstract of Haryana (1991-1992)*, Government of Haryana.

The sex ratio of Haryana is however much lower than the Indian Union: 861 (2001) and 865 (1991) compared to 933 (2001) and 929 (1991) for the Indian Union. The Literacy rate in Haryana is 57.98 per cent (2001) as compared to 55.17 per cent (2001) for the Indian Union.

Agriculture and Land Utilisation

The total area of Haryana is only 1.3 per cent of the total area of India. However, the net area sown is 2.5 per cent of the net sown area of India; and the total cropped area is 3.3 per cent of the total cropped area of India, indicating an intensity of agriculture around double that of India as a whole.

The area under rice in Haryana is only 1.5 per cent of the area under rice in India. However, the production is 2.5 per cent of the total rice production in India. The area under Bajra is 6.4 per cent with a corresponding production of 7.6 per cent of the total production in India. The area under wheat in Haryana is 7.7 per cent of the total area under wheat in India; the corresponding production figure is 13 per cent. The total area under cereals in Haryana is 3.3 per cent of the total area under cereals in India; the corresponding production figure is 5.6 per cent. The area under gram is 10.1 per cent with production at 9 per cent. The area under Pulses is 3.0 per cent with Haryana producing 3.8 per cent of the total production of pulses in India. The total area under foodgrains is 3.3 per cent of the total area under foodgrains in India. Area under sugar cane is 4.3 per cent and under cotton 6.7 per cent. (see Table 2.2 and Table 2.3)

The above data clearly demonstrates the increases in agricultural productivity which Haryana has been able to achieve, especially in foodgrains production. On the basis of 1990-91 agricultural data, the yield of rice per hectare in Haryana was 2775 kg compared to 1751 kg for India. In the case of wheat, the yield per hectare in Haryana was 3479 kg compared to 2274 kg for India. Similarly, in the case of Bajra, the yield per hectare in Haryana was 864 kg compared to 661 kg for India.

The average consumption of fertilizers per hectare rose from 3 kg. in 1966-67 to 115.15 kg. in 1994-95. Similarly, the consumption of certified seeds rose from 17,000 tonnes in 1966-67 to 2,89,000 tonnes in 1993-94. The number of tractors in Haryana during the same period rose from 4,800 to 1,65,000. In 1989-90 the per hectare consumption of plant nutrients for Haryana was 90 kg compared to 62.4 kg for India.[1]

Table 2.2: Land Use and Area under Major Crops (1990-91)

(in hectares)

	Haryana	*All India*
Total area	4,378,000	328,726,300
Culturable area	3,792,000	
Net area sown	3,575,000	1,41,700,000
Area sown more than once	2,344,000	
Total cropped area	5,919,000	1,80,100,000
Area under Rice	661,200	42,600,000
Area under Rice as per cent of total cropped area	11.16	23.60
Area under Bajra	608,600	10,500,000
Area under Bajra as per cent of total cropped area	10.30	5.80
Area under Wheat	1,850,100	24,000,000
Area under Wheat as per cent of total cropped area	31.00	13.30
Area under other cereals	217,000	26,000,000
Area under other cereals as per cent of total cropped area	3.70	13.60

(Contd.)

(Contd.)

(in hectares)

	Haryana	*All India*
Area under cereals	3,337,300	103,100,000
Area under cereals as per cent of total cropped area	56.40	57.20
Area under Gram	649,300	7,400,000
Area under Gram as per cent of total cropped area	11.00	4.10
Area under other pulses	92,700	13,400,000
Area under other pulses as per cent of total cropped area	1.60	7.40
Area under pulses	742,000	24,400,000
Area under pulses as per cent of total cropped area	12.50	13.50
Area under foodgrains	4,079,300	127,500,000
Area under foodgrains as per cent of total cropped area	68.90	70.80
Area under oilseeds	488,500	24,000,000
Area under oilseeds as per cent of total cropped area	8.25	13.30
Area under Sugar Cane	147,800	3,682,000
Area under Sugar Cane as per cent of total cropped area	2.50	2.00
Area under Cotton	490,600	7,780,000
Area under Cotton as per cent of total cropped area	8.30	4.30

Source: Derived from *Statistical Abstract of Haryana* (1991-1992), Government of Haryana and Statistical Pocket Book of India (1992), Government of India.

Table 2.3: Area, Agricultural Production and Yields

	Proportionate area in Haryana compared to the Indian Union	*Proportionate production in Haryana compared to the Indian Union*	*Total Production Haryana 1990-91 (in '000 tonnes)*	*Total Production India 1990-91 (in '000 tonnes)*	*Yield Haryana (in kg. per hectare) 1990-91*	*Yield India (in kg. per hectare) 1990-91*
Rice	1.5	2.5	1834	74600	2775	1751
Bajra	6.4	7.6	526	6900	864	661
Wheat	7.7	13.0	7083	54500	3479	2274
Cereals	3.3	5.6	9017	162200		
Gram	10.1	9.0	469	5200	722	701
Other pulses	0.7	1.1	73	6400		

(Contd.)

(Contd.)

	Proportionate area in Haryana compared to the Indian Union	Proportionate production in Haryana compared to the Indian Union	Total Production Haryana 1990-91 (in '000 tonnes)	Total Production India 1990-91 (in '000 tonnes)	Yield Haryana (in kg. per hectare) 1990-91	Yield India (in kg. per hectare) 1990-91
Pulses	3.0	3.8	542	14100		
Oilseeds	2.0	3.4	638	18500		
Cotton	6.3	12.0	1155*	9579*		

* in '000 bales of 170 kg. each

Source: Derived from *Statistical Abstract of Haryana (1991-1992)*, Government of Haryana and *Statistical Pocket Book of India (1992)*, Government of India.

Land Distribution

The distribution of agricultural holdings are far more progressive than the national averages. Whereas 75 per cent of agricultural land holdings at the all India level are small or marginal, i.e. having less than 2 hectares of land, only 57 per cent of the holdings in Haryana are small or marginal. On the other hand, whereas only 23 per cent of the all India holdings are semi-medium/medium, i.e. having 2-10 hectares of land, in Haryana, 38.5 per cent of the holdings belong to this category. The average size of operational holdings in Haryana is also considerably higher than the national average. The distribution pattern of operational holdings in Haryana seems to have had a

Table 2.4: Operational Holdings—Haryana (1985-86)

	Haryana
% of Operational holdings of size 0-0.5 ha.	22.18
% of Operational holdings of size 0.5-1.0 ha.	15.09
% of Operational holdings of size 1-2 ha.	19.65
% of Operational holdings of size 2-3 ha.	12.37
% of Operational holdings of size 3-4 ha.	8.51
% of Operational holdings of size 4-5 ha.	6.08
% of Operational holdings of size 5-10 ha.	11.66
% of Operational holdings of size 10-20 ha.	3.81
% of Operational holdings of size 20 ha. and above	0.65

Source: *Statistical Abstract of Haryana (1991-1992)*, Government of Haryana.

positive impact on productivity levels in agriculture. However, it is a matter of concern that the average size of holdings in Haryana has been contracting at a very rapid rate. (Table 2.4 and Table 2.5)

Table 2.5: Operational Holdings—Haryana and India (1985-86)

		Haryana	*All India*
% of Operational holdings of size 0-1.0 ha.	Marginal	37.27	57
% of Operational holdings of size 1-2 ha.	Small	19.65	18
% of Operational holdings of size 2-4 ha.	Semi-medium	20.89	14
% of Operational holdings of size 4-10 ha.	Medium	17.74	9
% of Operational holdings of size 10 ha. and above	Large	4.46	2

Source: Derived from *Statistical Abstracts of Haryana*, Government of Haryana and *Agricultural Census 1985-86*, Government of India.

Animal Husbandry

Haryana is rich in productive livestock. In numbers too, Haryana has a relatively greater proportion of cattle and buffalo population as compared to the area of the state. The state has only 1.3 per cent of the area but possesses about 2.2 per cent of the cattle and buffalo population.[2] It has the second highest population of buffaloes per household in the country. Whereas Punjab had 226 buffaloes per hundred rural households in 1982, Haryana had 204 buffaloes. Haryana is well known for its famous breeds of Haryana cows and Murrah buffaloes. The average milk yield for cows and buffaloes in the state has been estimated at 550 and 1300 kg. per lactation period. This is much higher than the all India average of 173 and 491 kg respectively.[3]

Per Capita Income and Poverty

The overall progress that Haryana has been able to achieve is reflected in the rise in per capita income and the reduction in poverty especially in rural areas. Planning Commission statistics of 1987-88 show only 11.7 per cent of the rural population in Haryana living below the poverty line, compared to 33.4 per cent for India as a whole. Even with respect to the urban population, in Haryana the population living below the poverty line was 11.7 per cent compared to 20.1 per cent for India as a whole. Similarly, the per capita Net State Domestic Product during 1990-91 (at current prices) for Haryana was Rs. 6936 whereas the per capita national income for the country for the same period was only Rs. 4974.[4]

Table 2.6 further demonstrates the accelerating growth rate of the Haryana economy. In 1991-92, the growth rate of the Net State Domestic Product (NSDP) and the per capita NSDP had overtaken that of Punjab. Whereas during this period, the NSDP of Punjab grew by 6.17 per cent, that of Haryana grew by 7.38 per cent. Similarly, the growth in the per capita NSDP registered an increase of 4.9 per cent compared to 4.3 per cent for Punjab. The table also demonstrates the dramatic increase in the share of the Tertiary and the Secondary sectors in the NSDP. The share of the Secondary sector rose from 11.7 per cent in 1971-72 to 21.5 per cent in 1991-92 and that of the Tertiary Sector from 9.8 per cent to 31.9 per cent. Thus, whereas the share of the Primary sector fell by only 13 per cent in Punjab during the period 1971-72 to 1991-92, Haryana registered a 32 per cent decline in the share of the Primary sector during this period. These changes can partly be explained by the proximity of Haryana to Delhi, but the fact remains that the pace of change in Haryana appears to be outstripping that in the most prosperous state of Punjab. Although in agricultural

Table 2.6: Net State Domestic Product (NSDP), growth rate, per capita (at 1970-71 prices) and sectoral contribution (per cent share) in Punjab and Haryana

Period	*NSDP (Rs. crores)*		*Per capita NSDP (Rs.)*		*Primary Sector*		*Secondary Sector*		*Tertiary Sector*	
	Punjab	*Haryana*	*Punjab*	*Haryana*	*Punjab*	*Haryana*	*Punjab*	*Haryana*	*Punjab*	*Haryana*
1971-72	1399.4	893.6	1022.7	878.8	59.6	78.5	13.6	11.7	26.8	9.8
1981-82	1843.8 [3.34]	1211.6 [3.11]	1084.6 [0.6]	924.6 [0.5]	44.1	53.5	21.3	20.7	34.6	25.8
1991-92	3356.6 [6.17]	2469.8 [7.38]	1649.7 [4.3]	1486.6 [4.9]	46.6	46.6	21.4	21.5	32.0	31.9

Note: Figures in brackets show the compound growth rates in the respective years.

Source: 1. *Statistical Abstract of Punjab* (for various years), Government of India.

2. *Statistical Abstract of Haryana* (for various years), Government of Haryana.

productivity Haryana is still lagging behind Punjab as may be seen from Table 2.7, the increasing role of the tertiary and secondary sectors may well compensate for this handicap.

Table 2.7: Yield of Major Crops in Punjab and Haryana

(kgs. per hectare)

Period	Rice			Wheat			American Cotton		
	Punjab	Haryana	All India	Punjab	Haryana	All India	Punjab	Haryana	All India
1971-72	2045	1843	1141	2406	2041	1380	407	354	151
1981-82	2955	2475	1308	2932	2357	1691	334	387	166
1991-92 (P)	3257	2831	1751	3803	3597	2394	636	464	216

Source: 1. *Statistical Abstract of Punjab* (for various years), Government of India.
2. *Statistical Abstract of Haryana* (for various years), Government of Haryana.
3. Area and Production of Principal Crops in India 1986-88, Ministry of Agriculture, Government of India.
4. Agricultural Statistics at a Glance, Ministry of Agriculture, Government of India.

Infrastructure

The development of infrastructure has also kept pace with the overall economic growth. Hundred per cent of the villages in Haryana have been electrified compared to 79 per cent for the country as a whole. The length of surfaced and unsurfaced roads per 100 sq. km. for Haryana in 1988 was 58.7 km. compared to 56.1 km. for the country as a whole. The percentage of net area irrigated to net area sown for Haryana is 72.7 per cent (1990-91) compared to 31.9 per cent for India.

In social sectors the performance of Haryana has not kept pace with its economic development. The literacy percentage is only a little higher than the all India figure. Haryana's literacy is 57.98 per cent compared to 55.17 per cent for India. The number of beds in hospitals is 64 per lakh population compared to 92 per lakh population for India as a whole. The position of the state is third from the bottom, with only Uttar Pradesh and Orissa faring worse.

Table 2.8: Tractors, Tube wells, Electrification, Literacy, Roads, Hospital Beds, Population Below Poverty Line and Per Capita NSDP in Haryana and India

	Haryana	*All India*
Tractors	1,65,648	
Tube wells	5,11,059	
Villages Electrified (Central Electricity Authority, Ministry of Energy, GOI, 1990)	100%	79%
Literacy	55.85	52.11
Length of Surfaced and Unsurfaced roads (per 100 sq. km.) (Ministry of Surface Transport, GOI, 1988)	58.7	56.1
No. of Beds in Hospitals (per lakh population) (DGHS, Ministry of Health and Family Welfare, GOI, 1991)	64	92
Population below poverty line, Rural India (as per cent of total rural population) (Planning Commission, GOI, 1987-88)	11.7	33.4
Population below poverty line, Urban India	11.7	20.1
Per capita Net State Domestic Product (at current prices, 1989-90) (Directorate of Economics and Statistics)	6248	4252 per capita national income

Source: *Statistical Handbook of Haryana* (*1991-92*), Government of Haryana and *Statistical Pocket Book of India* (*1992*), Government of India along with the sources mentioned in parenthesis against each item.

The Presentation

The macro-picture of development in the state which is largely based on state level quantitative information, while providing important indicators of development, fails to give a feel of the real life in the villages or even in the districts. Figures are useful abstractions for the purpose of analysis but fail altogether in putting life and blood into a description of reality. Thus the main narrative of the chapters that follow, which is made up of generalisations on the basis of quantitative analysis of state and district level data, is enriched by village level observations contained in the boxes, which either follow the narrative or are interspersed with the narrative.

DEMOGRAPHIC PROFILE OF THE DISTRICTS

Haryana has been carved into 19 districts. The state has 6988 villages of which 6759 are inhabited. Against an average number of 437 villages to a district, Ambala, Gurgaon, Yamunanagar, Hisar, Rohtak, Bhiwani and Faridabad have more than the average number for the state, with Ambala having the largest number of 738 villages. Panipat has the lowest number with only 232 villages. So far as urban habitats are concerned, the state has 106 towns (Census, 2001). The largest number of towns are in Gurgaon district with 11 towns, and the smallest number of towns are in Rewari, Panipat and Sonipat, with 3 towns in each of the districts (Table 2.9).

Table 2.9: Districts of Haryana

District	*Date of formation*	*Area (sq. km)*	*Population*	*District HQ*
Ambala	1 November 1966	1,569	1106000	Ambala
Kurukshetra	23 January, 1973	1,217	641000	Kurukshetra
Karnal	1 November, 1966	1,967	885000	Karnal
Jind	1 November, 1966	2,736	963000	Jind
Sonipat	22 December, 1972	2,260	1064000	Sonipat
Panipat	1 January, 1992	1,754	833000	Panipat
Rohtak	1 November, 1966	1,708	779000	Rohtak
Faridabad	2 August, 1979	2,760	1477000	Faridabad
Gurgaon	1 November, 1966	2,105	1146000	Gurgaon
Mahendragarh	1 November, 1966	1,683	681000	Narnaul
Bhiwani	22 December, 1972	5,140	1139000	Bhiwani
Hisar	1 November, 1966	4,191	1230000	Hisar
Sirsa	26 August, 1975	4,276	903000	Sirsa
Rewari	1 November, 1989	1,559	623000	Rewari
Kaithal	1 November, 1989	2,799	820000	Kaithal
Yamunanagar	1 November, 1989	1,756	821000	Yamunanagar
Panchkula	15 August, 1995	816	319000	Panchkula
Fatehabad	15 July, 1997	2415	615000	Fatehabad
Jhajjar	15 July, 1997	1890	709000	Jhajjar

Source: Haryana-online.com 2001-2003.

Demography

Panchkula has the smallest area of 816 sq. km. Bhiwani has the largest area of 5140 sq. km. In terms of population, Panchkula has the smallest population of 3.19 lakh. Faridabad has the largest population of 14.77 lakh. All the districts around Delhi, especially those located on the Grand Trunk Road going to Chandigarh, have a relatively higher density

Table 2.10: Number of Villages and Towns in Haryana

District	*Total number of villages*	*Number of inhabited villages*	*Number of towns*
Ambala	738	711	9
Gurgaon	730	688	11
Yamunanagar	654	627	10
Hisar	510	504	9
Rohtak	492	473	8
Bhiwani	439	433	6
Faridabad	439	414	5
Rewari	417	402	3
Kurukshetra	396	389	4
Karnal	394	377	6
Mahendragarh	371	366	4
Sirsa	323	319	4
Jind	305	301	5
Kaithal	288	287	4
Sonipat	260	248	3
Panipat	232	220	3
Total	6988	6759	94
Average	437	422	6

Source: *Statistical Handbook of Haryana (1991-92)*, Government of Haryana.

of population. After Faridabad, the next most densely populated districts of Haryana are Sonipat, Kurukshetra, Panipat and Ambala, all located between Delhi and Chandigarh. The low density districts are mainly those located in the western semi-arid zone and include Sirsa, Bhiwani, Kaithal, Hisar, Jind, Rewari and Mahendragarh. The decadel growth in population between 1981 and 1991 has been highest in Faridabad (49.80%), followed by Panipat (33.49%) and Gurgaon (32.66%). Again this increase corresponds with the proximity of these districts to Delhi and the rapid explosion of population in and around Delhi. The districts registering the lowest decadel growth rate have been Rohtak, Kaithal, Bhiwani and Jind in that order, with Rohtak registering a decadel growth rate of 19.28 per cent and Jind of 23.10 per cent. We thus notice that districts around Delhi have been growing almost twice as fast as some of the other districts. Regional variations in even a small state like Haryana are prominent. The sex ratio measured in terms of females per 1000 population is highest in Rewari (927) and Mahendragarh (910); and lowest in Faridabad (828) and Jind (838). It is significant that even Rewari with the most favourable ratio of 927 is lower than the national average of 929. Rural population as percentage of total population is lowest in Faridabad (51.43%), Ambala (64.46%) and Yamunanagar (66.31%) and highest in Mahendragarh (87.59%), Kaithal (85.30%) and Rewari (84.73%). Scheduled Caste population as percentage of total population is highest in Sirsa (26.65%), Yamunanagar (24.96%) and Hisar (23.21%); and lowest in Gurgaon (13.59%), Mahendragarh (15.46%) and Faridabad (16.06%) [refer Table 2.10].

Table 2.11: District-wise Area, Population, Density of Population, Decadel Variation in Population, Sex Ratio, Rural Population and Scheduled Caste Population as Percentage of Total Population

District	*Density of Population per sq. km.*	*% decadel variation in population 1981-91*	*Sex Ratio*	*Rural population as % of total population*	*Scheduled Castes as % of total population*
Sirsa	211	27.90	883	78.84	26.65
Yamunanagar	468	27.27	841	66.31	24.96
Hisar	294	23.83	861	78.88	23.21
Ambala	468	30.42	885	64.46	22.99
Kaithal	293	20.78	852	85.30	21.44
Karnal	450	26.54	865	72.54	20.02
Kurukshetra	527	23.41	879	75.99	19.77
Jind	352	23.10	838	82.81	19.56
Rewari	400	25.45	927	84.73	19.30
Bhiwani	222	22.90	880	82.75	18.97
Rohtak	410	19.28	851	78.69	18.40
Panipat	475	33.49	854	72.84	17.89
Sonipat	545	27.15	865	76.42	17.84
Faridabad	702	49.80	828	51.43	16.06
Mahendragarh	405	27.91	910	87.59	15.46
Gurgaon	415	32.66	871	79.70	13.59
Haryana	372	27.40	865	75.37	19.75
India	257	23.51	929	74.29	

Source: *Statistical Handbook of Haryana (1991-92)*, Government of Haryana.

Working Population

The percentage of cultivators to total workers is highest in Bhiwani (54.79%), Jind (50.01%) and Mahendragarh (49.10%) and lowest in Ambala (21.44%), Yamunanagar (25.60%) and Faridabad (26.32%).

The percentage of agricultural labourers is highest in Karnal (28.68%), Yamunanagar (28.32%) and Sirsa (27.69%); and lowest in Mahendragarh (10.36%), Faridabad (11.63%) and Rewari (12.40%). The percentage of other categories of workers to total workers is highest in Faridabad (61.15%), Ambala (60.28%) and Sonipat (48.94%); and lowest in Kaithal (25.94%), Jind (28.17%) and Sirsa (28.49%). The data shows how the western districts of Bhiwani, Jind, Mahendragarh, Kaithal and Sirsa continue to remain predominantly agriculture based, whereas Ambala, Yamunanagar, Faridabad and Sonipat have gradually shifted from the primary to the secondary and tertiary sectors. In fact, Haryana as a whole has made a definite shift from the primary to the secondary and tertiary sectors. Of the Net State Domestic Product by Broad sectors (at current prices) in 1980-81, 54 per cent of the NSDP came from the Primary sector, 19 per cent from the Secondary sector and 26.4 per cent from the Tertiary sector. A decade later in 1990-91, the share of the Primary sector had dropped from 54.6 per cent to 44.5 per cent, the share of the Secondary sector had gone up from 19 per cent to 24 per cent and that of the Tertiary sector from 26.4 per cent to 31.5 per cent. (Table 2.12)

Table 2.12: Percentage of Cultivators, Agricultural Labourers and Other Categories of Workers to Total Workers (1991)

District	*Population (1991 census)*	*% of cultivators to total workers*	*% of agricultural labourers to total workers*	*% of other categories to total workers*
Bhiwani	1139718	54.79	12.92	30.73
Jind	963104	50.01	20.15	28.17
Mahendragarh	681869	49.10	10.36	38.98
Kaithal	820685	47.61	24.95	25.94
Hisar	1844634	46.25	22.84	29.70
Sirsa	903536	42.64	27.69	28.49
Rohtak	1808606	42.54	15.95	40.53
Rewari	623301	42.26	12.40	43.18
Gurgaon	1146090	40.15	13.72	44.73
Panipat	833501	32.92	21.29	43.10
Kurukshetra	641943	32.66	27.68	38.54
Sonipat	754866	31.63	17.97	48.94
Karnal	885797	28.81	28.68	40.49
Faridabad	1477240	26.32	11.63	61.15
Yamunanagar	821880	25.60	28.32	43.59
Ambala	1116878	21.44	16.10	60.28

Source: Census of India, 1991.

Box 2.3
Gurgaon

Gurgaon is situated at 32° 22' N latitude 76° 64' E longitude and at an elevation of 140 metres above mean sea level. It is a part of the Gurgaon division of Haryana and it lies in the south eastern corner of the state. It is bounded by Delhi in the north, Alwar district of Rajasthan to the south-east, Rewari district of Haryana to the west and Jhajjar district of Haryana to the north-west. The headquarters of the district administration is connected both by rail and road with the rest of the state. Spread over an area of 2800 sq. km, Gurgaon district had a total population of 16,60,559 in 1991. The population of the district is mainly rural, living in 742 villages, though the general impression about Gurgaon is that of a highly urbanised district. Which is not altogether unfounded because of the manner in which new Gurgaon has come up with its main focus on modern urbanisation and close proximity to Delhi and the influx of urban population from there. And it is this picture of Gurgaon which people generally have, ignoring the vast region of Mewat, which is totally rural and perhaps among the most backward regions in the entire county, educationally and socially. All the villages of the district are connected by road.

Block Sohna

Sohna, the headquarter of the Sohna block, is situated at a distance of 26 km. from the district and subdivision headquarter, Gurgaon. Sohna is a municipality town and a Tehsil as well. The area has become famous because of the preponderance of the farm houses which have cropped in the last couple of decades because of the tremendous inflow of the rich and famous of Delhi to Gurgaon and nearby areas.

The block is constituted of 53 village panchayats which have been divided into 6 Panchayat Samitis. The elections to all the panchayats and the panchayat samitis were held in March 2000. Interestingly, out of 53 as many as 14 panchayats were elected unanimously [Singh, 1999: Kherki Daula (Gurgaon)].

Box 2.4
Hisar

Hisar is one of the 19 districts of Haryana situated on the National Highway No.10, connecting Fazilka with Delhi. It is bounded in the

(Contd.)

Box 2.4 (Contd.)

north and west by Fatehabad, district, in east by Jind and Rohtak districts and in the south by Bhiwani and Churu districts of Rajasthan. Part of Hisar district is alluvial or Ghaggar-Yamuna plain and its southern and western portions make a gradual transition to desert like soil and topography. The topography of the district owes its existence to geomorphic process having closer affinity with climatic aridity both of recent and past geological periods.

The plain locally known as Hariana is the largest topographic unit. It is the most important area of the district covering almost both the subdivisions of Hisar and Hansi. The entire district is drained by a single river, i.e. Ghaggar. The river Chautang, which used to flow in the district, is almost extinct now. The quality of underground water varies from place to place and from well to well and in many areas it is brackish making it very difficult to drink.

The climate is characterised by its dryness and extremes of temperature along with scanty rainfall. The cold season here is from November to March where as summer is from April to June.

The district of Hisar derives its name from its headquarter town Hisar, which was founded by Ferozeshah Tuqhlaq in the 14th Century. He named it as Hisar Feroze, which means "the fort of Feroze". The name subsequently became Hisar. It comprises two subdivisions, namely Hisar and Hansi and 9-development block.

Name of Subdivision	*Blocks*
Hisar	Hisar-I Hisar-II Agroha Barwala Uklana Adampur
Hansi	Hansi-I Hansi-II Narnaul

The principal food grain crops of the district are wheat, gram and *bajra* and the important cash crops are cotton and oil seeds. Hisar district has large and medium scale industries manufacturing steel pipes, cotton / synthetic yarn, gum-guar etc. It is also famous for Jindal Steels and other manufacturing units of Jindal group of industries. There are a lot of small scale industrial units in the district manufacturing agricultural implements, pipes, pipe fittings, aluminium

(Contd.)

Box 2.4 (Contd.)

and steel furniture, air guns, surgical cotton, cycle tubes, nuts and bolts, cotton ginning and processing, forging etc. The district can also boast of having a few second line of industrialists from here.

Hisar has also earned a name in the country for its Haryana breed of cattle. The buffalo of this breed gives milk in larger quantity. Haryana has a livestock farm, the biggest of its kind, at Hisar. It also has a research centre on Equines and buffaloes. The district can also take pride in educational institutes as it has two universities at the district headquarter. One is the state agriculture university named as Chaudhary Charan Singh Haryana Agricultural University and the other is a technical university known as Guru Jambeshwar University. The district has a tourist place called Agroha Dham, the birth place of Maharaja Agarsen. It has two Haryana Tourism Complexes, namely Blue Bird and Flamingo.

Hisar district is also a rural district with 1/3rd of its population living in 307 villages. The district has an area of 3787.90 sq. km according to the 1991 Census. Hisar district has a population of 15,36,417 with sex ratio of 852 and population of density of 386 (Census, 2001) against the state's sex ratio of 861 and population density of 477. The literacy rate of the district is 65.85 against the state average of 76.54 [Agarwal 2001: Sikarpur (Hisar)].

Box 2.5
Karnal

Demographic Profile of the district is:

Population: General Details (as per Census 1991)

Sl. No.	*Particulars*	*Number*	*%age to Total Population*
1.	Rural Population	780218	75.35
2.	Urban Population	255172	24.65
3.	Total Population	1035390	100.00
4.	Male	555322	53.63
5.	Female	480068	46.37
6.	SC	211941	20.47
7.	Literate	457319	54.33

(Contd.)

Box 2.5 (Contd.)

Demography of the District in brief is as follows:

Sl. No.	*Block*	*No of Villages*	*Area in Hectares*	*House-holds*	*Population*
1.	Karnal	85	38394.57	24653	145111
2.	Nilokheri	80	39022.06	18855	124411
3.	Indri	108	35207.96	15575	108119
4.	Gharaunda	65	37736.66	18445	132551
5.	Nissing	49	41031.97	20213	127842
6.	Assandh	47	49785.99	22328	142184
	Total	**434**	**241179.21**	**120069**	**780218**

[*Yadav, 2002: Bibipur (Karnal)*]

VILLAGE PROFILES

Haryana villages are electrified, connected by all weather roads and have most of the essential facilites like schools, telephones, dispensaries, banks, shops within a radius of about 5 kms. Most of the land is cultivable, fertile and irrigated by canals or tubewells. Agriculture seems to be prospering. However, the outlook of the villagers continues to be traditional and orthodox. The position of women and weaker sections of society is improving but old ways continue to have a resistance to change. Illiteracy is high especially among women. The power structures based on caste and landholdings continue to dominate the social landscape. Panchayati raj as an institution has emerged but has contributed to divisions. Development programmes of the government are being undertaken but without making any significant and visible dent in village life. The following account of the probationers bring out these generalities in terms of specific observations.

Kakani Bhadri (Sonipat)

Village Kakana Bhadri is part of Gohana tehsil. It is located around 13 km from Gohana, which is the subdivisional headquarters. All villages in Haryana are connected to each other with all weather, fully metalled roads.

The nearest market for the village is that of Gohana town. It is also the block and tehsil headquarters for Kakana Bhadri. The bus stand is around 1800 metres from the village. The nearest post office is 2 km away from the village. There are no facilities of bank, high school, primary health centre, primary health sub-centre, PDS shop, *haat*, adult literacy centre, public telephone service, ICDS centre, Kisan Sewa Kendra in the village. There is a primary school, a private primary school and a middle school in the village.

There is a water works scheme for the village which ensures regular drinking water supply. There is also a private doctor working in the village.

The nearest market (grain market) exists in Gohana although a village "*haat*" is organised on a fortnightly basis. There are two Government made *Chaupals* (*Dharamshalas*) for the use of the village folk. There is a canal for the village and as such there is no problem as regards irrigation. Assured canal irrigation is available for all seasons.

As per the 1991 census the total population of the village was 1128 out of which 600 were male and 528 females. At present, the population is 1465 out of which 773 are male and 692 are females. The sex ratio is 895 females for every 1000 males. This is much lower than the national average but more than the State average of 874. The dominant caste is Jat with almost 36 per cent of the population being Jat. The Scheduled Castes constitute 20.54 per cent. There are also Brahmins, Rajputs, Kumhars, Harijans and a few Baniyas, Khatis and Naiks in the village.

Within the village, a caste-wise pattern of habitation is clearly discernible. While Jats are settled almost in the centre of the village, the *dalits* are located in the periphery. Most of the Brahmin and Rajput households are also located in the centre of the village. The Kumhar and Harijan households are interspersed but are mostly towards the periphery of the village.

As per 1991 census, the population of workers is as follows:

	Male	*Female*
Total main workers	312	263
Cultivators	157	170
Agricultural labourers	111	90
Household industry	4	2
Construction	1	0
Trade and Commerce	1	0
Transport and Storage	4	0
Other services	34	1
Marginal workers	—	—
Non-workers	288	265

My visit to Kakana Bhadri village was not merely a data collecting exercise. It was more about learning about the people, their psyche, their culture and traditions. Overall this "survey of rural India" gave me an insight into the thinking pattern of the villages. During my first visit to the village, the villagers were very surprised and they gave a lot of information thinking that I was there to survey for BPL list. Once they realized that nothing of that sort was being done and no sops were forthcoming for them, many people left the scene. The dependence syndrome of the people was very much evident. One peculiar feature of the people from the "heart of Haryana" is that they are always complaining. They will always have a lot of grievances against the administration. They are very shrewd and they know how to take advantages from the officers/administration.

The village is located around 13 kms. from the Subdivisional headquarters. All the facilities are either available in the village or in the adjoining village.

One of the disturbing aspect about the village is as regards levels of literacy. The villagers do not consider it very important. No adult literacy programme is being run presently. The teachers and students normally attend the school. The infrastructure is available. The only problem is the attitude.

The land of the village is very fertile and irrigation is no problem. In my opinion, the farmers are very orthodox in the farming practices they have adopted. They do not want to adopt newer methods of agriculture. They keep on using more and more water which is not at all desirable and is proving harmful to the land in the long run.

As regards the various developmental programmes being undertaken by the government, the villagers have a negative approach towards the assistance provided by the government. At times, the amount provided under IAY is misdirected and the false beneficiary uses the house constructed for storage of fodder. Not much attention is paid to the maintenance of assets provided in the village under the various schemes by the Panchayat and the villagers.

In a nutshell, there are certain areas in which an all out effort has to be made by the administration in close association with the villages. Particularly the social parameters have to be taken care of. No doubt the village has achieved a certain level of growth but the real 'development' is not visible [Gupta, 1999: Kakana Bhadri (Sonipat)].

Ransika (Gurgaon)

Distance of the village (in km) from:

District headquarters	40
Block headquarters	5
Nearest bus stop	1
Nearest railway station	6
Nearest town	5
Nearest market	5
Nearest branch of bank	5
Nearest post office	0
Nearest PHC	0
Nearest grain storage facility	5

Basic Amenities in the Village

Electrification

All weather approach road

Bus stop

Post office

Primary school

Primary health centre

Public Distribution Shop

Community based safe drinking water source

Public telephone services

Integrated Child Development Scheme (ICDS) centre

Basic Amenities not Available

Bank

Middle school

High school

Veterinary dispensary

Haat

Adult literacy centre

Community latrine
Panchayat bhavan
Street light

Ransika village of Pataudi block is a small village of 98 families. Most of the people are caste Hindus and the rest are SCs. Both from the household survey and from the census data we can easily see that the sex ratio is very poor in the village at just about 92 women for every 100 men. With growing awareness and success of women's Self Help Groups coupled with the Adult Literacy Programme the sex discrimination is definitely on the decline and hopefully the situation will change for the better.

Wood continues to be the major source of fuel in the kitchens. LPG connections are the second most popular option. Kerosene oil is a poor third. Almost all the houses in the village are electrified. Kerosene finds use only in kerosene lamps during power cuts. Electricity is also used for community purposes such as the pump for the Rural Drinking Water Tank.

The only source of irrigation in the area is tubewells.

About the household-wise ownership of land, we find that most of the farmers with larger holdings are from the General category. The SCs in the village are both mainly small and marginal farmers [Tayal, 2000: Ransika (Gurgaon)].

Kherki Daula (Gurgaon)

Village Kherki Daula falls in Badshahpur panchayat samiti, which consists of 5 village panchayats. As per 1991 census, the total population of the village is 3000, which includes 1598 males and 1402 females. Schedule Castes constitute 21 per cent of the total village population. At present the population is about 2750 consisting of 1600 males and 1150 females. The population of the village has decreased by 8.5 per cent over the last decade. The village is divided into 4 hamlets. The people of the village speak Hindi or the Haryanvi dialect. The village is dominated by the Ahir community which is not only numerically predominant but politically and economically powerful. Though the sarpanch is a Balmiki, he has virtually no say in the matters of Panchayat which are decided essentially by the people of the dominant caste, i.e. the Ahirs. There is also a little sprinkling of Muslim/Meo population in the village.

The village is about 9 kms. from the district headquarters and 16 kms. from the block headquarters. The village has a post office, but does not have a primary health sub-centre. The approach road to the village from the block headquarters is an all weather road and there is regular bus service to the village. In fact, the village is just a kilometre and a half away from the National Highway No. 8 which goes to Jaipur and beyond. There is a primary school, a middle school and a high school as well. The Public Distribution System shop is run by a person called Bhag Singh, who is a relative of the local MLA. The village, like all the villages of Haryana, is electrified and public telephone service also exists. The nearest markets are at Badshahpur and Gurgaon. There is a nationalised bank in the village—the Bank of Hyderabad.

The total area of the village is approximately 519 hectares, out of which 454 hectares is cultivated. Mainly wheat and paddy are grown in this area. Around 26 hectares of land is the common land or panchayat land and another 12 hectares is covered by the adjoining mountain range—the Aravallis. There is no forest cover. Even the nearby hills have been grazed thoroughly and there are hardly any trees or vegetation on these hills. There are no government irrigation projects in the village and irrigation is done by private tubewells. It may be mentioned that the nearest canal passes some 22 kilometres away from this village. The village receives 300 mm of rainfall annually. Last year, it received 301 mm of rainfall. Out of 519 hectares of land, 454 hectares, is cultivated solely by the ownership cultivators and there are hardly any tenants. This is primarily due to the fact that the holdings of land are very small and any kind of tenancy would make agriculture economically unviable. There are no households, which own more than 20 acres of land. The only so called 'landlord' of the village is a factory which has come upon the village which covers an area of almost 56 acres. Otherwise almost all the households barring 4-5 own land which is less than 5 acres.

It is estimated that about 200-220 people from the village are employed in the factory, which has come up on the village land. However, all these employees from the village are of the unskilled variety and at best a couple of them could be termed as semi-skilled. Around 90-110 more people find employment in the various industries, which have come up in and around Gurgaon. [Singh, 1999: Kherki Daula (Gurgaon)]

Sikarpur (Hisar)

The selected village Sikarpur is situated at a distance of 13 km from the district headquarter Hisar. It is situated in the northeast of Hisar, near Sirsa by pass. The village is well connected with the district headquarter and other villages through a network of all weather roads except for a stretch of 1-2 km which is not an all weather road. There are 10 hamlets in the village known as Wards. There are 10 members of Gram Panchayat and one Sarpanch duly elected by the Gram Sabha. The nearest branch of a bank is the Hisar Sirsa Kshetriya Gramin Bank at a distance of 7 km from the village.

The total population of village Sikarpur was 2825 according to 1991 Census, out of which Schedule Caste population was 325, i.e. 10.5 per cent of the total population. Hindi and Haryanavi is the spoken language of the village. There are community centres for General Caste, backward castes and Harijans in the village. If we look at the constitution of village Panchayat, it has 3 women members out of 10 panchayat members. Out of these, only one woman was owner of more than 5 acres of land and 5 members were landless. It shows the effectiveness of democratic decentralization at the village level. The total land available for cultivation was 2843 acres out of a total of 3582 acres of land, i.e. nearly 79 per cent of land is cultivable. Out of 2843 acres of cultivable land 2474 acres of land is under irrigation.

Infrastructure

The village is electrified and nearly 70 per cent of the houses have electricity connection. It has all weather approach road from the district headquarters. The village is having a primary and middle school. It is also having a sub-centre of health department having a male and a female worker. It also have a veterinary dispensary, community based safe drinking water sources, ponds called *Johad* in the local parlance, brick-paved streets and separate *chaupals* for General and Harijan population. There are two Anganwadi Centres to take care of and propagate different activities under the ICDS in the village. Almost 90 per cent of total cultivable land of the village is having assured irrigation through canals and tube wells. The village does have 3-4 shops for general provisions but for bigger items the villagers have to access markets of district headquarter at a distance of 12 km. The village is also having public telephone services. The village in itself is self-contained and more or less the villagers were found to be a happy lot. [Agarwal, 2001: Sikarpur (Hisar)]

Bibipur (Karnal)

The village Bibipur is located about 25 km from the District Headquarters of Karnal and 11 km from block headquarters. Though a remote village, it has an all weather road connecting it to the block headquarters. It has a regular bus service twice a day with the bus stand about 2 km from the centre of the village. The Railway network in Haryana *per se* is not the primary mode of travelling except in the long routes of Chandigarh to Delhi and from Rewari to Delhi. Hence the Railway station, that is in Karnal is used when people want to travel to far off places like Kolkata for selling their goods. The nearest town is that of Ghadi Birbal which is about 5 km away. According to provisional figures of the 2001 Census the village has a population of 2881. Sikligars who are primarily SC Sikhs form the major part. The languages that are commonly spoken and used are Hindi and Punjabi.

Demographic Profile of the Village

It is considered one of the most backward of villages in the district because of it being remote and also as the panchayat lacks the funds for developmental works. The village is on the banks of the Yamuna river and hence is very flood prone. The panchayat of the village is that of Bibipur and it consists of the Bibipur village and the Sikligar Dera.

The peculiar characteristic of the village is that it has a hamlet of Sikhs located in its land, which is called the Dera Sikligar. These Sikh artisans migrate from place to place to sell their products and come back to the village during off season to work as casual labourers in the village. The Castes that are present in the village are Rajputs, Brahmins, Jeemars (SC) etc. and Sikhs who had come from Pakistan after migration. Most of them had sold the lands which were allotted to them by the government after resettlement.

Table 2.13: Demographic Profile of Village

Year of Survey	*Total Population*	*Male Population*	*Female Population*	*Scheduled Caste (Male)*	*SC (Female)*	*Literacy (Male)*	*Literacy (Female)*	*Change (%)*
1981	515	230	285	60	41	52	6	—
1991	1488	781	707	482	458	201	67	189
2001	2881	1485	1396	801	782	—	—	94

The different hamlets that are identifiable in the village are distinguishable broadly by castes (Figures according to 1991 census). They are:

Hamlet (according to main caste)	*Number of household*	*% of households*
Brahmin	35	14.7
Baraygi	13	5.5
Gadhariya	9	3.8
Badi	3	1.3
Jeemar	14	5.9
Jogi	3	1.2
Surav	2	0.8
Sikligar	141	59.5
Harijdri	17	7.2
Total	237	100.0

Infrastructure

Haryana had reached the status of full electrification and connectivity through roads way back in 1971. This village also has electricity facility with street lighting in the village. A metalled road passes through it. There is an STD / ISD booth in the village. Some of the residents of the village also have personal phone connections. Thus there is little problem of connectivity and communication. Financial institutions like banks are absent because of the service area approach in which there is a prescribed population for which a bank would open its branch. Thus the nearest branch is in the town, about 5 km away in Garhi Birbal. There are two primary schools in the village—one in proper Bibipur and another in Dera Sikligar. Also there is an Adult literacy centre in the village as part of the PLP, which is a follow-up to the NLM. The Health infrastructure of a Primary Sub-centre is functional partially but people prefer going to private practitioners. There are two Anganwadis working in the area, one for Bibipur and another in the Sikligar Dera.

Flood-embankments and marginal bunds are constructed to confine the river and prevent it from flooding the adjoining area. As per agreement with the Government of Uttar Pradesh, no major flood-embankment can be constructed on the Yamuna unless approved by the Yamuna Committee. Flood-embankment and marginal bunds have, however, been constructed on the Ghaggar, the Tangri and the Markanda.

Right Marginal Bund, Markanda—This bund is constructed on the right side of the Markanda from Jhansa. Its length is about 8,900 metres and the whole of it lies in Karnal District. The bund has been constructed to check the overflow of river Markanda. It protects the irrigation channel [Yadav, 2002: Bibipur (Karnal)].

Guskani (Rohtak)

The total population of the village is around 2500, 60 per cent of which are males and the rest females. Hindi and its dialect Haryanvi are predominantly spoken. It is situated 13 km south of Rohtak district and has five hamlets within it.

Economically the village appears to be in a good position. Extreme poverty is quite rare. However, there is no social equality between different castes in the village. Percentage of poverty is around 15 per cent, i.e. 40 families. The situation is thus much better than the average village of India.

Basic facilities such as availability of market, post office, Primary Health Centre, railway station and bank are within a vicinity of 2 km. The village is 100 per cent electrified but availability of power is erratic. Facilities like primary school, middle school, veterinary dispensary, public telephone, ICDS centre are all within a range of 1.5 km. The village is 100 per cent flood prone. A proposal for shifting the entire village has been mooted and is under final stages of consideration and approval [Suresh, 1997: Guskani (Rohtak)].

SOCIAL AND CULTURAL PRACTICES

The language in Haryana is Hindi, Haryanvi and Punjabi. Although there are areas with concentration of Muslims and Sikhs, most areas follow traditional Hindu beliefs. *Purdah* or "*ghoonghat*" is still prevalent among women. Traditional marriage systems remain along with the system of dowry. However, the joint family system is gradually getting eroded. Education and literacy among women is low. At the time of distribution of ancestral property women do not get any share. Consequently, women are not economically self-supporting despite the fact that most of the work is done by them. The caste system remains, but its influence is diminishing. Outward symbols of respect and subservience remain although there is no segregation on grounds of caste. A member of the SC still cannot sit in the company of the people of other castes and share the *hookah* with him. Utensils are not shared and they do not eat together. In the village temple, however, there is no restriction placed on anybody. Equality with the higher castes is still a dream, but the lower castes dream of it more often! With reservation, the representation of women and members of the weaker sections in village panchayats is also becoming a vehicle of change. The nature of tenancy in agriculture has undergone a radical change. The element of social inter-caste relationship has given way to a more business oriented outlook towards tenancy. The process of social empowerment is on through greater awareness, political empowerment, education and economic opportunities. Out-migration is becoming a common feature. A large number of villagers are in the Army and visit the village only once in a year. Others take on regular and casual jobs in towns and cities. There is also out-migration because of the soaring prices of agricultural land in the area. Many people have ventured out to other areas in or outside the state in search of cheaper agricultural lands.

Box 2.6
Village Kakana Bhadri

The village falls in the region of Bangru dialect. Bangru represents the western group of dialects of Hindi. To an outsider the villagers will appear to speak in pure or *theth* '*Haryanvi*'.

(*Contd.*)

Box 2.6 (Contd.)

There are only two Muslim households in the village. The entire Gohana tehsil does not have more than 2000 Muslims. The villagers follow traditional Hindu beliefs and are generally orthodox in their religious practices. They worship Shiva, Rama, Hanumana, Krishna and other minor dieties. On the occasion of *greh pravesh*, child brith, marrige etc. the priest is invited for performing ritual worship. The masses generally cling to many traditional superstitions in the ordinary acts of daily life.

The caste system with all its ramifications is observed among the Hindus but its social influence is diminishing. The joint family system which has been an important feature of the society since time immemorial, is breaking up, under the stress of the changed economic and social conditions. The bond of joint family system is weakening. The average holding is too small to support a joint family which continues growing in size. It is inevitable that some members of the family move out in search of service to the town or else there is no available means to supplement the family income. Family life is becoming more and more individualistic.

The dowry system is very much prevalent among all the communities of the district. The amount spent on dowry generally varies with the economic and social status of the person concerned. In case the father of the girl fails to give sufficient dowry, it may result in quarrels and even ill-treatment of the bride by her husband as well as the in-laws.

Place of Women in Society

The vast majority of women in the village are not economically self-supporting, but they do majority of the work. They bring water cook morning and evening meals and even carry food to men at work in the fields. In addition to numerous household jobs, they participate in nearly all agricultural operations like hoeing, weeding and harvesting except ploughing. The male folk spend most of their time discussing national/state politics or by attending courts (*Kachahri*).

In the village, the *purdah* system is still in vogue. The maidens cover their heads while the daughters-in-law cover their faces when moving among the elderly persons in the house or in the village.

Community Life

In earlier times, community life was effectively organised in the village. Folk songs were sung at the time of marriages and festivals. Women used to perform folk dances and sing folk songs. But now the things are changing. Most of the villagers are self-centred. Only the old people spend their time together during day time [Gupta, 1999: Kakana Bhadri (Sonipat)].

Box 2.7

Village Ransika

During the focus group discussion, most *Dalits* felt that over the years, their position in the societal structure has undergone a considerable change. There has been a definite though gradual transition from the old agrarian relationships between the owners of the land and other inhabitants of the village. The nature of tenancy in agriculture has undergone a radical change. The element of social inter-caste relationship has given way to a more business oriented outlook towards tenancy. This has had its ramification in the caste equations. Tenancy has become a kind of unwritten contractual understanding between the owner of land and the tenant, the consideration for which is pure money or its equivalent in terms of produce rather than some obligation continuing in perpetuity. With this the notion of "benefactors" of the village has disappeared and with it has been diluted the rigid social hierarchy that sprang from it. Direct wages also meant an increase in the economic options available to the labourer, which widened mobility, freedom and empowerment.

Outward symbols of respect and subservience remain. The lower classes still do not take their seats by the side of the upper castes though they may be landless and in penury. They either stand or sit on the ground before the upper castes. Utensils are not shared and they do not eat together.

The position of women in the family has traditionally been better in the Dalits than in the lower middle classes. With the promotion of the concept of women's SHG on a large scale, almost every village has at least a couple of such groups. The group approach, besides being more sustainable and effective for delivering poverty alleviation programmes also proves to be a very important means for social empowerment. Women now have the confidence to negotiate with

(Contd.)

Box 2.7 (Contd.)

government employees, bank staff and local level functionaries. Constant exposure, the habit of thrift and credit management has taught them the art of bargaining and entrepreneurial skills. Women have taken land on lease and carrying out cultivation on it on their own. Most of the village level committees such as the Gram Panchayat have women as members. With time, there has come responsibility, motivation and aspiration in women. "Self-Help" women's groups have become vehicles through which the government can now send messages to the masses. In fact, the success of the Adult Literacy Programme and Family Planning and Welfare in the district owes a great deal to the women's groups. In Poverty Alleviation Programmes, the SHG spirit has really caught on in a big way. The administration has also taken up a proactive approach apropos the SHGs. The success of women's groups coupled with several incentive schemes have seen people move away from the individual beneficiary mentality to the group approach. Schemes that have purely the group approach at their core have been launched and have been received very well by the people. There is now a stirring in the villages and women in groups no longer aim primarily for the revolving fund. They now look for a direct bank linkage. There seems to be a healthy move away from the subsidy and dole culture towards self-help and credit. It is a testimony to the kind of confidence that has been created in people by this approach [Tayal, 2000: Ransika (Gurgaon)].

Box 2.8
Practice of Untouchability

In Kherki Daula village of Gurgaon, it was observed that like most of the other parts of Haryana untouchability is not practiced in general. This is, however, not to say that the evils of the caste system do not exist. It is still a common sight to find the SC population of the village without any land despite the government having distributed the 'surplus land' among the SCs. The numerically largest caste and socio-economically dominant caste in the village is Ahir (Yadavs). Though in the Central Government the Ahirs of this region are included in the OBCs list. During the survey it was revealed that there is no bar for the people of SC community to move on any public road, in attending schools, or availing the other public facilities like Post Office and the

(Contd.)

Box 2.8 (Contd.)

Bank, etc. which are located in the village itself. Similarly, there is no problem in delivery of letters by the post person. It was found that even during the assembly or the panchayat elections there was no forcible casting of the votes of the weaker sections. In primary middle and high schools all students sit together and there is no segregation on grounds of caste. There is only one source of water in the schools and SC students also take water from the same source. Untouchability is not practiced between teachers and students or among the teachers or among the students. In the PDS shop there is no discrimination for SC and in other shops also they buy goods freely. In agriculture also there is no discrimination between SC and non-SC labour and they are paid equal wages.

However, this does not mean that disability of the SCs does not exist; to assume that untouchability does not exist totally would be closing one's eyes to the reality. This segregation is manifest in the fact that the SC have their own well in the village from which they draw their drinking water. They do not go to the Ahir's well to draw water. Even if they tried it is quite likely that it would invite repercussions. However, the most distinctive form of divide is visible in case of the smoking of the "*hookah*" or the smoke pipe. A member of the SC simply cannot sit in the company of the people of other castes and share the *hookah* with him. *Hookah* is considered to be caste specific and members of a community or caste sit around their own *hookah* thus displaying brotherhood and oneness of their caste. In the village temple, however, there is no restriction placed on anybody. The social interaction is something which is still restricted and the lower castes are generally made aware of their 'place' in the hierarchy through such devices as mentioned above.

Hence it can be concluded that untouchability is not practiced in the village especially at public places. But socially they do not mix with each other like going to each other's place and eating etc. Though invitation cards are sent to all in marriages etc. and these functions are also attended by all persons in the village.

Lastly, a very interesting fact that needs special mention—the Ahirs of this region do not use the suffix Yadav and take offence if someone addresses them as such! They would rather be called Rao. [Singh, 1999: Kherki Daula (Gurgaon)]

Box 2.9
Kherki Daula

Social Structure, Culture, Dalits and Women

The village is dominated by the Ahirs which are in majority. Most of the land in the village is owned by them. The majority of landless people belong to Scheduled Castes. But over the years, the society has undergone a massive transformation. Democracy is proving to be a great teacher and also a tremendous leveller. Now, people are aware of their rights and particularly their voting rights. Elections are a festive occasion here and no longer can any caste or community hope to rig an election. The oppressed speak against any exploitation and raise their demands. The SCs are no longer the weaker sections emotionally. Although most of them are poor economically and educationally but with the devolution of the powers in the new Panchayati Raj system, they have come to understand their powers. Now the Sarpanch also belongs to an SC, which has given them further confidence though they still maintain that equality with the higher castes is still a dream, but they now dream of it more often!

Women belonging to the Ahir community and those among the Muslims generally work in their houses, but most women belonging to Scheduled Caste families work in fields and as domestic servants in the houses of big landlords. Women belonging to the SC and the Muslims are more or less illiterate. The literacy rate is very low for girls, though Ahir women are generally much better placed educationally. But the trends of the recent years show that the literacy levels have been rising in this area steadily over the last 8-10 years. At the village level politics the women representatives are actively involved and they are not just filling the seats reserved for women. Thus, the fear that women are mere rubber stamps for their husbands is given a lie to a large extent. But that is not to say that all women work with such independence in the panchayat. But some of them definitely do! Veil system is prevalent among the Ahirs and the Muslims, but not among the other castes and women go out to bazars and to the public functions. The crime rate in the village is in general low but women related crimes are hardly recorded. There is dowry system in all the communities except the Muslims where bride price is the norm. At the time of distribution of ancestral property women do not get any share. Instead money is spent on their marriages in the

(Contd.)

Box 2.9 (Contd.)

form of gifts for the rest of their life. Offences like domestic violence and wife beating occur in the village. Marriages are generally arranged and women are not given opportunity to marry a boy of their choice. The schools in the village have co-education. [Singh, 1999: Kherki Daula (Gurgaon)]

Sports is commonest pastime in the village especially among the youth. In fact, the village is famous for the *Kabaddi* tournament that it hosts every year. It is generally a state-level tournament in which invariably some teams from Punjab are also invited. The estimated budget on this function's organisation is Rs. 2-3 lakhs apart from the prize money. [Singh, 1999: Kherki Daula (Gurgaon)]

Box 2.10
Gender Issues in Guskani

The total population of village Guskani is about 2500. Out of this the female population is only about 40 per cent. The birth of a girl child is still not accepted with the joy and festivity as associated with the birth of a boy. The position of women is still very much suppressed and in that sense Guskani represents the typical Haryana scenario. The participation of the women in the panchayat is practically non-existent. In the village there are about 100 persons who have studied upto class ten. Out of these only 25 are women. There are 5 graduates in the village. All are male. The women however are found to be more hard working than men who prefer to idle away their time in gossip and party politics.

NGOs

There is only one NGO working in Guskani village. It is called the Matana Youth Club. It is involved in creating awareness and motivating villagers in promoting prohibition, health and sanitation, providing assistance in developing programmes and in aiding in the marriages of the poor. It has 11 members and the villagers are satisfied with their work. The villagers however feel that it is not able to be very active because of paucity of funds. [Suresh, 1997: Guskani (Rohtak)]

Box 2.11
Migration

...the son of a farmer does not want to do farming. He feels ashamed of doing this. The youth today is attracted towards the towns. Many a youth have permanently shifted to Gohana, Sonepat and even Delhi. A large number of villagers are in the Army and visit the village only once in a year. The ex-servicemen of the village do not prefer to stay in the village. They sell off their share in the land to their brothers/ cousins. During the survey, the elders pointed out the following reasons for migration out of the village:

(a) Lack of employment
(b) Abundance of labour
(c) Attraction of towns

[*Gupta 1999: Kakana Bhadri (Sonepat)*]

Box 2.12
Landless People and Migration

Most of the Scheduled Caste families are landless. So, most of them work as casual labourers in the fields of other landowners. Some of them also work as industrial labourers in the factory and also in Gurgaon. They are able to earn about Rs. 2000-2500 per month. If they work in the village, they are able to earn on an average about Rs. 1500 per month.

Out-migration from this village to the areas in Mahendragarh and Rewari districts of Haryana has been noticeable. That is why there is a suspected reduction in the village population. This out-migration resulted because of the soaring prices of agricultural land in this area. People sold off their farm lands at very high prices to the rich people from Delhi and then with that money bought larger pieces of land in the neighbouring districts. [Singh, 1999: Kherki Daula (Gurgaon)]

Box 2.13
Occupational and Migration Pattern

Majority of the villagers are engaged in agriculture or are the Sikligars whose primary occupation is of carpenters and utensil makers. Many villagers who do not have land go for tenancy and other trades. Landless labour gets employment as daily wagers during harvesting

(*Contd.*)

Box 2.13 (Contd.)

and sowing season in the fields and otherwise in villages also. Many times they go to the district headquarter for working as labour. The labourers were quite satisfied with the wage structure and they did not have any complaint regarding it.

Dairying is also an informal activity. People use the cattle's milk for their household consumption and only in case of surplus sell it to the households in the district headquarters.

At the state level the percentage of workers in primary sector (agriculture, animal husbandry etc.) has gone down from 61.7 per cent in 1981 to 58.72 per cent in 1991. In case of cultivators the percentage has gone down from 44.67 per cent in 1981 to 38.77 per cent in 1991. But the percentage of agricultural labour has gone from 16.11 per cent to 19.0 per cent. From this data it appears that over the years small peasants and tenants have been reduced to the level of agricultural labour.

Migration is also a common feature of the village among the Sikligars who form the main caste of the village. They migrate to places in Haryana and outside, some as far as Calcutta where they have relatives who have setup markets to sell their products, which are usually, products made of iron. About 60-70 families migrate regularly in a year and that has its effect on the education of their children. [Yadav, 2002: Bibipur (Karnal)]

LAND USE, LAND DISTRIBUTION AND TENANCY

The peasant cultivator mode of production prevalent in Haryana has led to a distribution of agricultural holdings which are far more progressive than the national averages. Whereas 75 per cent of agricultural landholdings at the all India level are small or marginal, i.e. having less than 2 hectares of land, only 57 per cent of the holdings in Haryana are small or marginal. On the other hand, whereas only 23 per cent of the all India holdings are semi-medium/medium, i.e. having 2-10 hectares of land in Haryana, 38.5 per cent of the holdings belong to this category. The average size of operational holdings in Haryana is also considerably higher than the national average. In 1985-86, whereas the average size of operational holdings in Haryana was 2.76 hectares, the all India average was only 1.69 hectares. The distribution pattern of operational holdings in Haryana seems to have had a positive impact on productivity levels in agriculture. However, it is a matter of concern that the average size of holdings in Haryana has been contracting at a very rapid rate. Between 1980-81 and 1985, the average size of holdings in Haryana dropped from 3.52 hectares to 2.76 hectares, recording a 21.6 per cent decline, the highest in the country. Comparable with Punjab, registered a decline of only 1.3 per cent, from 3.82 hectares to 3.77 hectares. At the all India level the holding size became smaller by 9.1 per cent during this period.[5]

Most of the land is cultivable and under agriculture. The remaining land is either fallow land, land under forest cover, common land, land under trees and groves, cultivable wasteland and land not available for cultivation. There is also land that is taken up by ponds and rivers.

Although most of the cultivation is done by owner-cultivators, tenancy exists. Many landowners let out their lands on cash or sharecropping basis. But this is done in a fairly businesslike manner on a year to year basis. Tenancy is not regularly recorded or updated in the land records because of the cumbersome procedure involved. Moreover, since most of the letting is on a year to year basis, the tenant has no great interest in having the tenancy recorded in the *Jamabandi* or the Record of Rights.

Box 2.14
Land Use in Kakani Bhadri

Kakani Bhadri is a small village. Its area is 1510 acres out of which 1130 acres is cultivated. The remaining 380 acres is as follows:

Fallow land (*Banjar Jadid and Banjar Kadim*)	267.5 acres
Land under forest cover	25 acres
Grazing land	5 acres
Cultivable wasteland	50 acres
Not available for cultivation	212.5 acres
Land under miscellaneous trees and groves	7.5 acres

The common property resources of the village include community forest, forest under forest department, fishing pond (2.5 acres), a temple and 2 *chaupals*. The Panchayat takes little interest in maintaining these resources of the village. [Gupta, 1999: Kakani Bhadri (Sonepat)]

Box 2.15
Land Use and Land Distribution in Bibipur

Total area of village Bibipur is 452 Standard Acres out of which cultivable land is 408 acres, i.e. 89.8 per cent of total land. Irrigation is primarily through tube wells as the water level is very high due to the proximity of Yamuna River to the village. Village Bibipur has 29 acres of land categorized as Community and Panchayat Land. Net sown area is 411 acres and 3 acres of land has been left fallow. Land is very fertile and productive and has provision of assured irrigation. The Gram Panchayat also leases the cultivable panchayat land out for cultivation through open auction. 18 families were allotted cattle sheds under the 20-point programme that belong to the SC category.

Out of the total cultivable area, 347 acres, i.e. more than 90 per cent of the cultivable land is yielding two crops whereas 59 acres is under single crop and 5 acres under multiple cropping. These figures imply that in general two crop pattern is followed in cultivation.

The average landholding in the area is 5.6 acres which is much below the land ceiling limit and hence there was no surplus land declared in the village after the Land Ceiling Act came into force. The village is also located in the most fertile and irrigated area of the riverbed where traditionally agriculture has been the mainstay of the economy unlike in western Haryana where lands are barren and without irrigation facilities average landholdings are large. There is no *Benami* landholder in the village that came to my notice. Since the landholdings are small and none of them come close to reach the limit of Land Ceiling Act, it is not necessary for the people to have *benami* landlordism. In regular times it is counterproductive to have *benami* land as it involves lot of risk especially at times of transfer of land or mortaging of the land. Most of the cultivators in the village have medium landholding and hence prefer to have joint holding with joint liability.

There are 59 *Khewats* or ownership index in the record of rights and 70 *Khatoni* or tenant index. A tenant would be working for 8-10 landlords and the total number of tenants (as a family) are 29 with the coverage of 19 acres while the number of owners-*cum*-tenants are 27 with a coverage of 18 acres. In fact there is only one pure tenant who cultivates an area of 1 acre.

The land is highly fertile and most of the time can yield multiple crops, however, due to the lack of money for fertilizers etc. most of the cultivators stick to two crops a year, which is paddy and wheat. Some of them also grow sugarcane and vegetables. Cash crops like mustard oil etc. are also grown.

Table 2.14: In village Bibipur distribution of landownership household-wise

Category	*Land in acres*
Landless	120
< 1 acre	240
1-3 acres	160
3-5 acres	70
5-10 acres	52
10-20 acres	28
20 acres or more	7

Table 2.15: Distribution of Operational holdings

Category	*Number of holdings*
< 1 acre	16
1-3 acres	26
3-5 acres	8
5-10 acres	8
10-20 acres	6
20 acres or more	5

[*Yadav,2002: Bibipur (Karnal)*]

Box 2.16

Land Use and Land Distribution in Guskani

Out of the total village area of 1000 acres, cultivable land is 860 acres. Net sown area is 100 per cent of cultivable land. Land could be classified into the following soil types:

Sandy soil	100 acres
Fertile soil	700 acres

Land under forest cover is 40 acres. Community land put to common use is 300 acres. No land has been declared surplus. Apart from SC and BC families all other households have at least some land or the other. Although there are 210 persons belonging to the SC and 210 persons to BC, none of them possess even a single acre of land

(Contd.)

Box 2.16 (Contd.)

for cultivation.12 households have land less than 1 acre, 120 households have land between 1-3 acres and 7 households possess 20-30 acres of land, 33 per cent of the panchayat land is reserved for the SC and 10 per cent for the BC. Panchayat has 178 acres of land. The panchayat land as well as the land kept for community purposes is around 300 acres. The community land is being used for burial ground (*shamshan bhumi*), *Chaupals* or community halls or for cowsheds (*goshalas*) etc. [Suresh, 1997: Guskani (Rohtak)]

Box 2.17
Common Property Resources

The villagers are using common property resources like village ponds called *Johad*, streets and common drinking water taps without any discrimination on the basis of caste or religion. The other important common property of the village is panchayat land also known as *Shamlat Deh*. From time to time panchayat has donated land to the people of lower strata to construct their houses. However, agricultural land out of *Shamlat Deh* is leased out to the bidders for one year by the village panchayat. In bidding 30 per cent of the land is reserved for the Scheduled Caste population of the village.

The total land that is being auctioned is 8 acres, 6 kanals and 18 marlas of which 3 acres, 2 kanals and 3 marlas are reserved for the SC population, while the other, namely 5 Acres, 4 kanals and 15 marlas are for the general category. The reserved land had been auctioned for Rs. 15,000 while that of the general category had gone at Rs. 60,500, making a total amount of Rs. 75,500. The bidding process is fairly open though there are always complaints that proper publicity of the bidding was not done or that the officials required were not present. These allegations are serious, as there are clear guidelines that for land more than 20 acres, the District Development and Panchayat Officer is supposed to be present in the auctioning and for lesser area the Block Development and Panchayat Officer has to be present. This is often not done. The work is delegated to subordinate officers and this leads to problems. Also the timings of the auction is important as that would lead to change in the pattern of bidding, depending on whether there is a standing crop or not. During bidding the officer present at the auction should ensure that there is no collusion among the bidders. The village ponds are also auctioned to bidders for the production of fish.

(Contd.)

Box 2.17 (Contd.)

The *Shamlat* land is under the management and control of the Gram Panchayat. The panchayat sees to it that encroachments upon the *Shamlat Deh* by the villagers do not take place. [Yadav, 2002: Bibipur (Karnal)]

Box 2.18
Tenancy

As per the *Jamabandi* of the village for the year, there are tenants in the village comprising an area of 7 acres. This is hardly 2.27 per cent of the total cultivable area of the village. I obtained a list of these tenants and their respective landowners and met quite a few of them during my stay in the village. It is surprising that most of these entries are old and not even 10 per cent of them are true. Most of the persons indicated as tenants are in fact not tilling the land shown under tenancy. These lands are either being tilled by the owners themselves or by some other tenants whose names are nowhere in the records. Many people did not even know that their names feature as tenants of some landowners in the *Jamabandi.* Most of the problems exist because of the prescribed cumbersome procedure to amend the entries of tenancy.

If the entry has to be changed at the time of the *Girdawari* (crop survey which is done twice a year), then both the landowner as well as the tenant have to give written affidavits to the Patwari about the end of the tenancy and only then the Patwari can make necessary amendments in the *khasra Girdawari*. Otherwise, if any single party wants the entry to be changed, they have to give a petition in the court of the Assistant Collector Grade-II (*Durasti Girdawari* Case), who is authorised to order changes in the *Girdawari* after conducting a detailed inquiry. While most of the landowners were not aware of what has been shown regarding their land in the *Jamabandi*, the tenants even if they were aware of it, did not find any need to get it changed.

On the one hand, while the tenants recorded are not tenants, in actuality there are a large number of tenants, who are not recorded. As per the records, most of the land (97.73 per cent of the cultivable area) is under self-cultivation, while in actual practice more than a quarter of the cultivable area of the village is given under tenancy every year. The reasons for such a large extent of concealed tenancy are:

(a) In order to enable the tenant to get his tenancy recorded, there must be a written lease document. It is only when

(Contd.)

Box 2.18 (Contd.)

this document, signed by both the parties is there that the Patwari can show tenancy in the *Girdawari*. In the majority of the cases land is given on lease on year to year basis without any documentation.

(b) After getting possession, if the tenant wants to get his tenancy recorded without the written consent of the landowner, he has to give a petition in the court of Tehsildar for *Durasti Girdawari* (modification of crop survey), which will be contested by the landowner and it will create bad blood, which may antagonise the landowner. Besides, nobody in the village will give their land on lease to the petitioner thereafter.

(c) The entire transaction is seen in the village in purely commercial terms. Tenants do not see much reason in getting their tenancies recorded, because tenancies are in any case temporary, they seldom last beyond a year or two.

Terms of lease can be any of the following:

1. Cash lease (presently this is the only prevalent type)
2. Share cropping (*Batai*)
3. 20 per cent to 25 per cent share

[*Gupta 1999: Kakana Bhadri (Sonipat)*]

Box 2.19
Share Cropping

Generally share cropping is done on the basis of sharing of cost of seeds, fertilizer, revenue charges, tube well rate etc. on 50:50 basis. Labour costs are borne totally by the person who undertakes cultivation. By and large two crops are taken. [Suresh, 1997: Guskani (Rohtak)]

Box 2.20
Land Records

The most important record is the Record of Rights also called the *Jamabandi*. This record clearly mentions for each piece of land the

(Contd.)

Box 2.20 (Contd.)

status of ownership, the name etc. of the tenant, if any, the terms and conditions of tenancy, the area of the land, its type, including source of irrigation. In Kakana Bhadri, the latest *Jamabandi* is of the year 1993-94 and *Jamabandi* for the year 1998-99 is being prepared. The *Jamabandi* is revised after every five years and the changes which take place during these five years are recorded in the form of mutations by the village Patwari and these mutations are attested by the Circle Revenue Officer (CRO). These mutations are then duly incorporated in the next *Jamabandi* showing the charges in ownership which may have taken place by way of sale, gift, inheritance, will etc. Thus the records are kept up-to-date and correct. Other than the entries of tenants all the other entries are as per the ground reality. [Gupta, 1999: Kakana Bhadri (Sonipat)]

AGRICULTURE

Infrastructural development which began in the 1950s took positive shape with the agricultural policies of the 1960s and brought about the Green Revolution in Haryana. The Bhakra system provided water and electricity; roads provided access to the emerging markets for agricultural produce, finance and inputs. An effective agricultural extension system was put in place to transfer technology from the agricultural universities to the farmers. Consolidation of holdings made application of the high return technology feasible. And Haryana began to witness the spectacular yields and returns which were to put the state along with Punjab among the most affluent of the Indian states. Political and administrative will, the convergence of the efforts of the scientist and the administrator and the entrepreneurship and diligence of the farmer brought about this takeoff into a sustainable pattern of agricultural development.

With the availability of water and markets, cropping patterns began to change. Wheat and rice gradually began to replace the coarse grains. Hisar and Sirsa began to emerge as important cotton belts of the country. Because of the availability of water, the north east zone along with Hisar, Sirsa and Rohtak developed into the large cereal producing basket of the state. The semi-arid districts of Mahendragarh, Gurgaon, Rewari and Bhiwani have however lagged behind. But on the whole, rural Haryana has forged ahead, at least in terms of material prosperity.

Box 2.21
The Farmer

After coming to Haryana, my concept of a 'farmer' changed totally. Earlier, I use to take the actual tiller of land as the farmer. But in Haryana, the *Zamindar* (land owner) who hires agricultural labourers (mostly from Bihar and eastern Uttar Pradesh is called a farmer. The younger ones are actually averse to doing agriculture in this materialistic world. ... Many a youth took to easier way of making money during the period of prohibition. And now they indulge in petty crimes. [Gupta, 1999: Kakana Bhadri (Sonipat)]

Box 2.22
Agriculture and Animal Husbandry in Kherki Daula

Generally two crops are cultivated—wheat in Rabi season and paddy in kharif season. Other prominent crops cultivated in this village are Sarson, Gwar, Jowar, Arhar and Barley. Nearest grain market is located at Badshahpur and Gurgaon from where farmers also purchase farm inputs such as seeds, fertilisers etc. There are approximately 695 milch cattle in the village out of a total of 1201, the remaining obviously being non-milch. However, there is no land earmarked as pastureland in the village. The farmers produce cattle feed on a small patch of land and use it the year around to feed the cattle. [Singh, 1999: Kherki Daula (Gurgaon)]

Box 2.23
Agriculture in Kakana Bhadri

... due to availability of water in abundance, no land is left uncultivated for any part of the year. Approximately same area is sown during both kharif and rabi seasons ...

The seeds are mostly taken from the produce itself and at times it is brought from the seed traders at Gohana. The requirement of fertilizers is met from the traders at Gohana or from the local co-operative bank. The credit for the input requirements is met from the local cooperative bank or from the traders who supply the inputs.

Most of the sowing and ploughing is done through tractors. There are around 25 tractors in the village and the owners lend them to others during the sowing season. Harvesting is usually done by hand. [Gupta, 1999: Kakana Bhadri (Sonipat)]

Box 2.24
Agricultural Credit

All the seeds fertilisers and other inputs are usually bought from the city traders with whom the farmers have regular links. They also get credit from these traders. Although, there is no cooperative bank in the village, there is one 2 km away from the village and many villagers take loan from it. However, many other prefer relying of the city based trader because:

(a) The trader, although he charges more interest, is more flexible in adjusting the terms of repayment, e.g. he can easily reschedule the repayment if the crop of a particular farmer fails or if there is a marriage in the family etc.

(b) Non-payment of installment to the co-operative or commercial bank may result in officials or police coming to the debtor's house and may result in his arrest. This is considered to be a major insult and the farmer is ready to pay a higher rate of interest rather than bear this insult.

Marketing

For sale, all the crops are taken to the *mandi*. The transportation is usually done by the tractors of the village. The owner charges a flat rate of Rs. 15 for a bag of 100 kgs. of any grain. At the *mandi* there are licensed *arhtias* or the middlemen who help the farmer in getting the produce unloaded, getting it cleaned and organising an auction of the produce. At the time of the auction, representatives of the market committee and of HAFED and CONFED are also present. Sometimes produce such as wheat is auctioned at rates higher than the reserve prices fixed by the Government. Majority of the produce of the village is brought into the *mandi*. There is a small fraction which is brought by the traders who visit the village at the time of harvesting. These traders pay rates which are slightly less than those prevailing at the *mandi*. [Mishra, 1996: Kasumbhi (Bhiwani)]

Box 2.25
Institutional Credit

The institutional credit system seems to have failed in Guskani. A mere 20 per cent or so depend on institutional credit. 75 per cent of the village population lend between themselves. The villagers feel

(*Contd.*)

Box 2.25 (Contd.)

that it is every time consuming to obtain credit from banks and other similar institutions, demands by the banks for surety etc. not only leads to delay but also breeds corruption. [Suresh, 1997: Guskani (Rohtak)]

Rice

The North-eastern zone comprising the districts of Kaithal, Karnal, Kurukshetra, Panipat, Ambala and Yamunanagar are the principal rice producing districts of the state. The districts of the Central Zone comprising Rohtak, Sonipat and Jind are also rice producing. However in the South-western Semi-Arid Zone, only in limited areas of Hisar, Sirsa and Faridabad rice is produced. The districts of Rewari, Mahendragarh and Bhiwani produce no rice. Kaithal district is the largest rice producing district of the state, in terms of area

Table 2.16: Area under Rice, Rice Production and Yields (1990-91)

District	*Population (1991 census)*	*Area under Rice ('000 hectares)*	*Rice production in '000 tonnes*	*Yield (kg. per hectare)*
Kaithal	820685	119.4	312	2622
Karnal	885797	115.2	309	2690
Kurukshetra	641943	101.6	299	2959
Panipat	833501	76.8	196	2539
Ambala	1116878	58.8	149	2531
Yamunanagar	821880	43.9	137	3123
Hisar	1844634	37.1	136	3679
Jind	963104	43.2	119	2758
Sirsa	903536	26.3	78	3006
Sonipat	754866	19.9	51	2563
Faridabad	1477240	7.7	21	2673
Rohtak	1808606	9.7	21	2070
Gurgaon	1146090	1.6	6	2778
Rewari	623301	—	0	—
Mahendragarh	681869	—	0	—
Bhiwani	1139718	—	0	—
Average		*50.86*	*114.63*	*2768*
Total		**661.2**	**1834**	

Source: *Statistical Handbook of Haryana* (*1991-92*), Government of Haryana.

under rice and the total production of rice. However, in terms of yield, the performance of Kaithal is lower than Karnal, Kurukshetra, Yamunanagar, Hisar, Sirsa, Jind, Faridabad and Gurgaon. It is interesting to note that Hisar has the highest yield per hectare of 3679 kg, above the yield of 2622 kg per hectare in Kaithal. Hisar, Yamunanagar, Sirsa, Kurukshetra and Gurgaon have yield higher than the average yield for the state in 1990-91 of 2768 kg per hectare. Rohtak, Ambala, Sonipat and Panipat have the lowest yields.

Wheat

Hisar, Kaithal, Sirsa, Rohtak, Jind, Karnal and Panipat, in that order, produce the highest quantities of wheat. Hisar with a production of 9,78,000 tonnes produces more than double the average of the districts of Haryana. Significantly the area under wheat in Hisar is not double of the average area under wheat in the districts of Haryana. The semi-arid districts of Mahendragarh, Rewari, Bhiwani and Gurgaon, along with Yamunanagar have the lowest production of wheat. Kaithal,

Table 2.17: Area under Wheat, Wheat Production and Yields (1990-91)

District	*Area under wheat ('000 hectares)*	*Wheat production in '000 tonnes*	*Yield (kg. per hectare)*
Hisar	256.2	978	3820
Kaithal	176.5	688	3907
Sirsa	165.9	612	3685
Rohtak	185.5	573	3078
Jind	150.5	508	3364
Karnal	129.0	499	3870
Panipat	112.8	426	3774
Kurukshetra	105.2	400	3808
Faridabad	111.9	327	2922
Ambala	92.9	271	2909
Sonipat	80.5	266	3330
Gurgaon	98.1	258	2637
Bhiwani	59.3	197	3339
Yamunanagar	57.7	181	3120
Rewari	39.3	144	3701
Mahendragarh	28.8	108	3707
Average	*115*	*402.25*	*3436*
Total	**1965.1**	**6436**	

Source: Statistical Handbook of Haryana (1991-92), Government of Haryana.

Karnal, Hisar, Kurukshetra, Panipat, Mahendragarh, Rewari and Sirsa have an average yield of wheat which is higher than the average yield for the state as a whole. Thus the semi-arid districts of Mahendragarh, Rewari, Sirsa and Hisar are fairly productive areas, so far as yields are concerned. Kaithal and Karnal top the yields with productivity of 3907 and 3870 kgs. per hectare. The lowest yields are in Gurgaon, Ambala, Faridabad, Rohtak and Yamunanagar, in that order. Districts with the smallest area under wheat are Mahendragarh, Rewari and Yamunanagar.

Bajra

The semi-arid districts are by far the largest producers of Bajra. Except for Hisar, the districts which top the list in the production of Bajra are the ones which produce very little wheat or rice. Significantly the least producing districts are those located in the north-east comprising Kurukshetra, Karnal, Yamunanagar and Ambala. In fact Kurukshetra and Karnal do not report any area under Bajra. Bhiwani has the largest area under Bajra of 1,84,300 hectares. The production figure of

Table 2.18: Area under Bajra, Bajra Production and Yields (1990-91)

District	*Area under Bajra ('000 hectares)*	*Bajra production in '000 tonnes*	*Yield (k.g. per hectare)*
Bhiwani	184.3	113	616
Hisar	74.5	89	1193
Rewari	52.6	66	1250
Mahendragarh	95.2	65	687
Gurgaon	54.0	54	997
Rohtak	48.1	47	985
Jind	46.7	41	876
Faridabad	24.6	26	1025
Kaithal	11.8	10	869
Sirsa	8.3	8	938
Sonipat	3.4	4	1090
Panipat	2.4	1	500
Ambala	0.8	1	864
Yamunanagar	1.2	1	864
Karnal	0.5	0	—
Kurukshetra	0.2	0	—
Average	*38.04*	*32.88*	*911*
Total	**608.6**	**526**	

Source: *Statistical Handbook of Haryana* (*1991-92*), Government of Haryana.

1,13,000 tonnes is also the highest. However the yield in Bhiwani of 616 kg per hectare is among the lowest. Only Panipat with a yield of 500 kgs. per hectare has a yield lower than that of Bhiwani. Yields in Rewari and Hisar of 1250 kg and 1193 kg per hectare are almost double that of Bhiwani.

Cereals

Hisar, Kaithal, Karnal, Sirsa, Kurukshetra and Rohtak in that order are the largest producers of cereals. Hisar and Kaithal lead with 1.22 million tonnes and 1.01 million tonnes respectively. Of the total cereal production in 1990-91 of 9.01 million tonnes, wheat contributed 6.43 million tonnes and rice 1.83 million tonnes. Thus wheat contributed 71.4 per cent to the cereal production in Haryana. The contribution of Bajra was only 0.52 million tonnes. The production in Hisar, Kaithal, Karnal, Sirsa, Kurukshetra, Rohtak, Jind and Panipat was higher than the average district production of cereals of 0.56 million tonnes. Hisar and Kaithal produced more than double this average.

Table 2.19: Cereals Production (1990-91)

District	*Population (1991 census)*	*Rice production in '000 tonnes*	*Wheat production in '000 tonnes*	*Bajra production in '000 tonnes*	*Total cereals production in '000 tonnes*
Hisar	1844634	136	978	89	1220
Kaithal	820685	312	688	10	1014
Karnal	885797	309	499	0	811
Sirsa	903536	78	612	8	709
Kurukshetra	641943	299	400	0	703
Rohtak	1808606	21	573	47	682
Jind	963104	119	508	41	680
Panipat	833501	196	426	1	625
Ambala	1116878	149	271	1	451
Faridabad	1477240	21	327	26	398
Gurgaon	1146090	6	258	54	342
Yamunanagar	821880	137	181	1	330
Sonipat	754866	51	266	4	327
Bhiwani	1139718	0	197	113	317
Rewari	623301	0	144	66	230
Mahendragarh	681869	0	108	65	178
Average		*114.63*	*402.25*	*32.88*	*563.56*
Total		**1834**	**6436**	**526**	**9017**

Source: *Statistical Handbook of Haryana (1991-92)*, Government of Haryana.

Mahendragarh with 0.178 million tonnes and Rewari with 0.23 million tonnes produced less than half the average for the districts of Haryana. The districts of Ambala, Faridabad, Gurgaon, Yamunanagar, Sonipat and Bhiwani fall in between.

Pulses

In 1990-91 Haryana had a total production of pulses of 0.54 million tonnes. Of this 0.469 million tonnes was of Gram. Bhiwani, Hisar, Sirsa, Rohtak and Mahendragarh are the pulses producing districts of Haryana and produce more than the average for the districts of Haryana. Bhiwani produces 197,000 tonnes which is about six times the average district production of 33,800 tonnes. Hisar with 103,000 tonnes comes next. Kurukshetra, Karnal, Panipat, Yamunanagar produce about 5,000 tonnes or less, which is less than one-sixth of the average for the districts. In the total foodgrains production of 9.58 million tonnes in the state, the share of pulses of 0.54 million tonnes is however very low.

Table 2.20: Production of Gram, Total Pulses and Total Foodgrains (1990-91)

District	*Population (1991 census)*	*Gram production in '000 tonnes*	*Total pulses production in '000 tonnes*	*Total Foodgrains production in '000 tonnes*
Bhiwani	1139718	194	197.9	515
Hisar	1844634	98	103.0	1323
Sirsa	903536	59	59.6	769
Rohtak	1808606	26	38.1	720
Mahendragarh	681869	36	36.1	214
Jind	963104	23	31.5	712
Sonipat	754866	1	13.1	340
Rewari	623301	13	13.0	243
Ambala	1116878	3	10.0	461
Kaithal	820685	3	8.4	1022
Gurgaon	1146090	7	7.7	350
Faridabad	1477240	1	7.1	405
Yamunanagar	821880	2	5.1	335
Panipat	833501	1	5.0	630
Karnal	885797	1	3.7	815
Kurukshetra	641943	1	2.4	705
Average		*29.31*	*33.86*	*597.44*
Total		**469**	**541.7**	**9559**

Source: *Statistical Handbook of Haryana* (*1991-92*), Government of Haryana.

In the total foodgrains production, it is again Hisar, Kaithal, Karnal, Sirsa, Rohtak, Jind and Kurukshetra in that order, which top the list. Hisar and Kaithal together contribute almost 25 per cent of the total foodgrains production in the state. Hisar alone contributes about 14 per cent. On the other hand Gurgaon, Sonipat, Yamunanagar, Rewari and Mahendragarh together contribute only 15 per cent to the total foodgrains production of the state. Mahendragarh contributes as little as 2.2 per cent.

Oilseeds

The total oilseeds production in the state in 1990-91 was 638,000 tonnes. To this, Hisar and Rohtak being the highest producers, contributed 102,400 tonnes and 102,200 tonnes respectively. Their production was followed by Bhiwani, Rewari, Mahendragarh and Gurgaon. Together these six districts contributed 520,000 tonnes, i.e. 81.5 per cent of the total oilseeds production of the state. It is the semi-arid belt which contributes to oilseeds production. The north-eastern zone contributes very little. Kaithal, Ambala, Sonipat,

Table 2.21: Oilseeds Production (1990-91)

District	Total oilseeds production in '000 tonnes
Hisar	102.4
Rohtak	102.2
Bhiwani	83.2
Rewari	80.1
Mahendragarh	79.0
Gurgaon	73.4
Sirsa	59.1
Faridabad	25.4
Jind	15.2
Kaithal	4.2
Ambala	4.2
Sonipat	4.0
Yamunanagar	2.6
Karnal	1.0
Kurukshetra	1.0
Panipat	1.0
Average	*39.88*
Total	**638**

Source: *Statistical Handbook of Haryana (1991-92)*, Government of Haryana.

Yamunanagar, Karnal, Kurukshetra and Panipat together contribute only 18,000 tonnes, which adds up to only 2.8 per cent of the total oilseeds production in the state.

Sugarcane

Yamunanagar is by far the largest producer of sugarcane in the state. Of the total production of sugarcane (*Gur*) in 1990-91 of 780,000 tonnes, Yamunanagar alone contributed 256,000 tonnes, i.e. 32.8 per cent. Yamunanagar and Rohtak together contributed about 50 per cent to the total production of *gur* in the state. Only four districts, Yamunanagar, Rohtak, Kurukshetra and Jind had production figures higher than the average for the districts of Haryana. The semi-arid areas of Mahendragarh, Rewari and Sirsa do not grow any sugarcane. In terms of productivity, Kurukshetra recorded the highest yields of 6100 kg per hectare, substantially higher than that of Yamunanagar with only 5699 kg per hectare.

Table 2.22: Sugarcane Production and Yields (1990-91)

District	*Total Sugar cane (Gur) production in '000 tonnes*	*Yield (Kg. per hectare)*
Yamunanagar	256	5699
Rohtak	126	4845
Kurukshetra	73	6100
Jind	67	5598
Ambala	46	4569
Karnal	44	5451
Panipat	39	4930
Sonipat	39	5509
Faridabad	37	4133
Kaithal	25	5059
Hisar	20	4929
Gurgaon	5	5273
Bhiwani	3	3279
Sirsa	0	—
Mahendragarh	0	—
Rewari	0	—
Average	*48.75*	*5028*
Total	**780**	

Source: *Statistical Handbook of Haryana (1991-92)*, Government of Haryana.

Cotton

Hisar and Sirsa with a production of 997,000 bales of cotton lint account for 86.3 per cent of the total cotton production of the state. Hisar leads with 597,000 bales, followed by Sirsa with 400,000 bales. The other cotton producing districts are Bhiwani, Jind, Rohtak and Kaithal. Ambala, Panipat and Sonipat produce 1,000 bales each. The rest of the districts do not produce any cotton. The total production of cotton in the country in 1990-91 was 9,759,000 bales. It is interesting to note that of this total production, 10.21 per cent was contributed by Hisar and Sirsa, with Hisar alone contributing 6.1 per cent of the total cotton production of the country.

Table 2.23: Cotton Production (1990-91)

District	*Cotton lint production in '000 bales of 170 kg each*
Hisar	597
Sirsa	400
Bhiwani	64
Jind	63
Rohtak	17
Kaithal	11
Ambala	1
Panipat	1
Sonipat	1
Mahendragarh	0
Rewari	0
Gurgaon	0
Yamunanagar	0
Karnal	0
Kurukshetra	0
Faridabad	0
Average	*72.19*
Total	**1155**

Source: *Statistical Handbook of Haryana (1991-92)*, Government of Haryana.

Irrigation

Of the total net area sown in the state, the net area irrigated is 72.7 per cent. Sonipat tops the list at 99.1 per cent, followed by Karnal with 98.7 per cent, Kaithal with 98.6 per cent, Panipat with 97.4 per cent, Kurukshetra with 95.7 per cent and Jind with 95.3 per cent. Hisar, Rewari, Yamunanagar and Sirsa range between 70-80 per cent, with Hisar at 80.4 per cent and Sirsa at 71.3 per cent. Mahendragarh and Bhiwani have less than 50 per cent irrigation of the net sown area. Bhiwani is at the bottom of the list with 39.8 per cent. The agricultural productivity of the state follows this broad pattern of irrigation. However, it is worth noting that Hisar, which, without being at the top of the charts in irrigation, is definitely at the top of the charts in agricultural production in the state.

Table 2.24: Net Area Irrigated (1990-91)

District	*Government canals*	*% irrigated by Government canals*	*Tubewells*	*% irrigated by tubewells*	*Total*	*Percentage of net area irrigated to net area sown*
Hisar	385	87	58	13	443	80.4
Sirsa	234	88	32	12	266	71.3
Rohtak	184	71	75	29	259	69.1
Jind	125	61	80	39	205	95.3
Bhiwani	104	66	54	34	158	39.8
Kaithal	99	47	103	49	212	98.6
Sonipat	53	50	52	50	105	99.1
Panipat	46	30	105	70	151	97.4
Faridabad	39	49	40	51	79	50.3
Karnal	27	18	126	82	153	98.7
Kurukshetra	19	14	114	86	133	95.7
Gurgaon	12	13	82	87	94	51.9
Rewari	3	3	90	97	93	72.7
Yamunanagar	3	3	88	97	91	72.2
Mahendragarh	3	4	72	96	75	48.1
Ambala	1	1	77	93	83	56.8
Total	**1,337**		**1,248**		**2,600**	**72.7**

Source: *Statistical Handbook of Haryana* (*1991-92*), Government of Haryana.

Of the 2.6 million hectares of net area under irrigation, 1.33 million hectares are irrigated by Government canals and 1.24 million by tubewells. Most of the area in Hisar, Sirsa and Rohtak is irrigated by Government canals. In Sirsa 88 per cent of the irrigation is by Government canals. In Hisar 87 per cent is by Government canals. In contrast, over 80 per cent of the irrigation in Karnal, Kurukshetra, Gurgaon, Rewari, Yamunanagar, Mahendragarh and Ambala is through tubewells, most of which are privately owned. Individùal initiative has contributed as much to irrigation in the state as governmental effort. The magnitude of the private initiative can be gauged by the fact that in 1991-92 there were over 2.08 lakh diesel pumping sets and over 3.02 lakh electric pumping sets operational in Haryana.

Box 2.26
Irrigation in Kakana Bhadri

Kakani Bhadri has got no problem as regards the availability of water for irrigation. Almost 87.6 per cent (i.e. 900 acres) of cultivated land is irrigated by canal irrigation. Around 140 acres of land is irrigated by private tubewell. A canal flows through the village. Here, the problem is of a different kind, i.e. excess use of water resulting in high water table and water logging. This problem is being faced in many areas of west and south-west Haryana. The ignorant farmers use a lot of water without thinking about the negative fallout of this. Already the water table is too high. It is well known that in Moga and Muktsar districts of Punjab and Hisar, Sirsa, Rohtak and Bhiwani districts of Haryana, many well-to-do farmers have lost all their sources of livelihood due to this problem. The ongoing research at Haryana Agricultural University, Hisar shows that reclaiming land is a very costly proposition. Recently Government of Haryana made an ambitious plan of Rs. 2200 crore to tackle this problem in a big way. Any progress in this project seems unlikely in the near future due to the non-availability of funds. [Gupta, 1999: Kakana Bhadri (Sonipat)]

Box 2.27
Irrigation in Guskani

One minor irrigation project of the State Government provides irrigation to the 800 acres of cultivable land in the village. This is more than 90 per cent of the total cultivable land of the village. About 10 per cent farmers depend for irrigation on individual tube wells. Irrigation costs (water rates) work out to approximately Rs. 90 per acre per year. [Suresh, 1997: Guskani (Rohtak)]

Fertilizer Consumption

Consumption of fertilizer per hectare of cropped area was highest in Kurukshetra in 1990-91 with a figure of 189 kg per hectare. This was followed by Panipat at 180 kg, Karnal at 171 kg and Kaithal at 148 kg. Although Hisar consumes the highest quantity of fertilizer in the state, the high figure is partly on account of the very large cropped area in Hisar. Hisar has a total cropped area of 950,000 hectares, much above the average of 370,000 hectares for the districts of Haryana. Bhiwani has the lowest fertilizer consumption of only 19 kg per hectare. Faridabad, Rewari, Rohtak, Mahendragarh and Gurgaon have fertilizer consumption less than 100 kg per hectare, lower than the average for the state.

Table 2.25: Fertilizer Consumption (1990-91)

District	*Total fertilizer consumption in tonnes*	*Total cropped area ('000 hectares)*	*Consumption of fertilizer per hectare in kg*
Kurukshestra	48,299	255	189
Panipat	44,282	246	180
Karnal	50,172	294	171
Kaithal	55,976	379	148
Yamunanagar	26,275	195	135
Sonipat	19,656	160	123
Sirsa	70,819	591	120
Ambala	28,533	240	119
Jind	45,394	417	109
Hisar	97,828	950	103
Faridabad	20,889	254	82
Rewari	12,074	199	61
Rohtak	27,533	523	53
Mahendragarh	13,791	263	52
Gurgoan	12,274	295	42
Bhiwani	12,497	658	19
Total	586,292	5919	
Average		370	107

Source: *Statistical Handbook of Haryana (1991-92)*, Government of Haryana.

Agricultural Machinery

The data in Table 2.26 pertain to the 12 districts that existed in 1988. The ownership and use of agricultural machinery shows wide variation within the states. Whereas Kurukshetra has 38 tractors per 1000 population, Gurgaon and Bhiwani have only 4 tractors per 1000 population. The use of tractors is highest in Kurukshetra, Karnal, Sirsa, Sonipat, Jind and Ambala, in that order. Mahendragarh, Faridabad, Bhiwani and Gurgaon have less than 6 tractors per 1000 population. The agricultural prosperity of the north-eastern belt is once again reflected in the distribution of agricultural machinery.

Table 2.26: Tractors (All Types), 1988

District	Population (1991 census)	Tractors all types	Tractors per 1000 population
Kurukshetra	641943	24262	38
Karnal	885797	21348	24
Sirsa	903536	16403	18
Sonipat	754866	13479	18
Jind	963104	13328	14
Ambala	1116878	14671	13
Hisar	1844634	22923	12
Rohtak	1808606	19167	11
Mahendragarh	681869	3893	6
Faridabad	1477240	7550	5
Bhiwani	1139718	4313	4
Gurgaon	1146090	4311	4

Source: *Statistical Handbook of Haryana* (1991-92), Government of Haryana.

Box 2.28
Agricultural Implements used in Village Khanna Majra, District Ambala

Any improvement in agriculture is inconceivable without a corresponding improvement in the implements used. Modern implements are being gradually adopted by the farmers in accordance with their utility and scope for use. These are popularised by the Government through different schemes. The agricultural implements used in the district are given below:

Traditional Implements

Baguri	Small *Khurpa* like implement used for the hoeing of sugarcane at the time of the first and the second hoeing
Balan	Hand ginning mill, also sugar-press
Behli	Bullock cart
Bijoudi	Seed bag
Charsa	Leather bucket
Chhaj	Winnowing basket
Damcha	Watchman's controlling station
Datrali	Used for water bandi in the irrigation areas

(Contd.)

Box 2.28 (Contd.)

Dhainkli	Appliance for manual water-lifting suitable for small holdings
Dranti	Sickle
Gadi	Cart
Gandasa	Hand fodder cutter
Gandasi	Long handled chopper used for cutting sugarcane, cotton sticks and bushes
Gandola or Khodna	Digging tool
Garhi-ki-machine	Wheat thresher
Gharaunchi	Stand for oiling card
Gopia	Bird scarer
Gori	Leveller
Gulail	Bird scarer
Hal	Plough
Jali	Four pronged fork
Jua	Yoke
Kasola	Large mattock for weeding and hoeing
Kasoli	Smaller mattock for weeding and hoeing
Kassi	Spade
Khurpa	Grass spade
Kohari	Hatchet
Kolhari	Axe
Kolhu	Round cold-crusher
Kuthla	Seed storage
Kutti-ki-machine	Chaff cutter
Maij or Sohaga	Flat cold-crusher
Orna	Seed drilling tube
Phala	Large mattock spade
Rahat	Persian Wheel used where water table is not low
Rath	Chariot
Rehru	Small cart
Santa	Ox goad
Tat	Bird scarer
Thela	Four wheeler bullock cart
Tipaya	Stand for winnowing
Untgadi	Camel cart

Box 2.29
Modern Implements

Anaj Nikalney ki machine	Power Thresher
Beej-aur-Khad Boney-ki-machine	Fertilizer-*cum*-seed drill
Cultivator	
Harrow	
Mitti Palatney wala hal	Soil inverting plough
Nalai gudai wala hal	Hoe
Panch datta	Five tined cultivator
Pumping Set	
Sooki-davai-ki-machine	Duster
Tar-davai-ki-machine	Sprayer
Tractor	
Triphali	Three tined tiller
Trolly	
Tube well	

The Plough

The plough consists of three major parts: the beam (*halas*), wooden body (*hal*) and the coulter (*panhiari* and *kuis*). It may be of wood or iron but one in common use is generally of *kikar* wood, made by the village carpenter. It merely scratches the soil up to 4-5 inches and does not really serve the purpose of a plough. The chief defect in it lies in the fact that it leaves ridges of unploughed land between the V-shaped furrows which it makes. The plough also fails to eradicate the weeds properly. However in the small landholdings and fragmented and non-contiguous plots, the plough is very much suited and it does not disturb the level of the land. [Gulati, 1987: Khanna Majra (Ambala)]

Box 2.30
Common Crop Pests and Diseases

Rice Bug

This is the most destructive pest of the paddy crop. It appears generally in August and does maximum damage during August and September. The insect is essentially diurnal and is active in morning and evening. Both adults and nymphs suck the juice from grains in milky stage.

(Contd.)

Box 2.30 (Contd.)

Loose Smut of Wheat

This is a serious disease of the wheat crop. It burns the grain ears completely into a black powder. Infection is carried through the seed.

Earcocle of Wheat

In young plants, the disease is characterised by wrinkling, rolling, twisting and distortion of the leaves, all these symptoms tending to make the plants bushy and considerably dwarfed in size. Plants may die in the seedling stage. Earcockle galls being lighter than water can be separated from wheat seed by the floatation method combined with solar treatment.

Downy Mildew

The infected plants remain stunted and unthrifty. Leaves turn yellowish and undersurface of the leaves covered with white powdery mass. The ears transform wholly or partially into leaf like structures which remain green for longer period.

Ergot

Pinkish or light coloured thick gummy fluid starts dropping from spikelets of the infected earhead, later on brown to dark coloured sclerotia appears on these spikelets in place of normal grains due to the invasion of ovary by the fungus.

Stored Grain Pests

To guard against the damage caused to stored grains by Khapra, Susri and Dhora, the stores are dusted or sprayed with B.H.C. The infested stored grain could be saved by fumigation by making the stores completely air tight. The fumigation is very commonly done by Aluminium Phosphide tablets at the rate of one tablet per metric tonne of grain.

Emerging Trends in Agriculture

The Green Revolution has taken place in Haryana, about this, there can be no dispute. Awareness of scientific farming has been on the ascendancy all over the state. Progress may have been faster in the traditionally richer agricultural belt and where water has reached, but there can be no doubt, that the entire state has witnessed dramatic changes in agricultural practices. The role of the state and the agriculture scientists has been central in this process of transformation. Apart from the consolidation of holdings, the critical factor contributing to this change, has been the increase in the availability of surface irrigation and tube well irrigation. Extension work, whether through the Krishi Gian Kendras, the extension workers or through the media has also been an important factor contributing to the adoption of improved practices. The availability of improved seeds, chemical fertilizers, pesticides and weedicides through cooperatives and private trade, made possible the widespread adoption of the techniques taught by the agricultural scientists. Electrification of villages and building of village road networks emerged as the next important landmark in the changes that were to sweep this region. Villages which could not get water from surface irrigation, now, found alternative irrigation in tubewells. Roads brought the tractor and the combine harvester to the village. Improved cultivators, tillers, harrows, seed drills, threshers all became part of the plant and machinery of the emerging modern farmer. Those who could not afford tubewells or tractors could nevertheless, hire these services from those who had them. The road system led to a growing network of "*Mandis*"—agricultural markets, where farmers could sell their produce, obtain loans and buy inputs. Also at the village level, in addition to the money lender, institutional finance became available through the Cooperative Societies and Banks, Land Mortgage Bank, Gramin Banks and Commercial Banks. And, finally, to assure a good price for the produce to the farmer, the national food policy provided reasonable support prices and a network of purchasing centres through the Food Corporation of India.

So far as the cropping pattern is concerned, wheat and rice have, over time, replaced the coarse grains in most of the districts. In Hisar and Sirsa, cotton has emerged as an important cash crop. Sugarcane continues to remain important in Yamunanagar and Rohtak. The new set of developments, however, are beginning to focus on commercial crops. Garlic, Onion, Coriander, Potato, Ajwain, Sunflower, Mustard, Vegetables, Chillies, Pulses and fodder crops like Barseem, Guar, Jowar and Chari are already becoming popular. Farm forestry especially of Eucalyptus and Poplar has come to stay. Horticulture is picking up and as global markets open up, floriculture may well define the road to prosperity in the 21st century. As the less developed states catch up with the Green Revolution, the pioneering states are likely to advance into activities with higher returns. And as information technology brings the world to the doorstep of the villager, the gulf between rural and urban India is likely to be bridged in a future that may not be too far away.

Box 2.31
Cropping Pattern

The total cultivable area of 2843 acres is cultivated for two crops. After discussions with the villagers, local people and revenue Patwaris, the following pattern of cropping was found in the village.

Kharif Crop

It is sown in the month of April and harvested in the month of October. Since the area has an assured water supply and low water table, the farmers can afford to go for crops with very high water requirement. Most common crops in Kharif or *sawani* season are that of Sugarcane, Paddy and Makka or corn. The normal source of irrigations are that of Private Tubewell as a 3-5 BHP engine motor would easily lift enough water as the water table is not a problem in the area.

Another, Kharif crop which is widely cultivated in the village is Paddy. It is sown in the month of July and is harvested in the month of September and October. Paddy cultivation has been the traditional crop of the place being close to the river bed. The district *per se* is the largest producer of rice in the state. There are also some farmers who produce Basmati Rice which is procured by private rice millers to be exported. These fetch good prices in the market though they also require heavy investments. The main centres in which the farmers sell their produce are Indri, Yamunanagar, Tarawadi, Nilokheri and Karnal.

Sugarcane is an important cash crop. It also yields a good price for the farmers especially the early maturing varieties of sugarcane. The production has been especially profitable after the setting up of the Karnal Sugar Cooperative Mill, situated in Karnal. Also the advancement in technology leading to better varieties which are resisitant to the Red-rot disease has helped increase the yield.

Rabi Crop

During the Rabi season all the cultivable land is sown either for wheat or mustard. Wheat is the major rabi crop and it is sown in the month of October or November and is harvested in the month of April generally after the festival of Baisakhi. The average yield of wheat is nearly 2812 quintals per hectare, which gives a handsome remuneration to the farmers though the input costs especially in pesticides is high. Mustard or *Sarson* is not so widely sown. The farmers prefer wheat over mustard because of their household consumption needs. *Sarson* is generally cultivated in conjunction with wheat. The average output

(*Contd.*)

Box 2.31 (Contd.)

is 8 quintals per acre and net profit is nearly Rs. 7000 per acre after deducting the cost of seeds, fertilizers and labour.

For activities like sowing and harvesting, farmers engage labourers and they are generally paid in cash at the wage rates fixed by the government of Haryana. None of the respondents complained of underpayment by the landowners and tenants. During off season landless labourers go to Karnal as daily wagers and most of them said that they get 15-20 days of work in a month, either at village or at district headquarters. Most of the landless people in the village are employed as agricultural labour and since there is general lack of labour, their rates are on the higher side, in fact more often labourers from UP are engaged. The local labourers were given wage rate of about Rs. 2430 as monthly wage, while the minimum wages were of Rs.1975 per month.

The majority of farmers get credit from their respective private traders in the village or near villages called *Arhati*. Although a rural bank is available within 7 km from the village often farmers take credit from the *Arhati* because of many reasons. First of all, it is not always easy to get loan from banks as and when required. Getting loan from a bank is not a easy task for poor and illiterate villagers and the lower staffs of banks keeps on harassing them. There is also the demands of the lower staff for bribes, which along with other hidden costs, compensates for lower rate of interest provided by the bankers over private money lenders.

Moreover, the farmers have flexibility in getting loan from private moneylenders. Surplus agricultural produce, i.e. wheat and paddy is marketed in the *mandi*. Other agricultural produce like vegetables is marketed in open markets. Haryana has a very wide network of procuring agencies that procure grains from the farmers through Market Committees. The *mandis* are one point place for the farmers to sell their products and get instant payment from the *Arhatis* who are the auctioneers. The *Arahtis* auction the grain to various government agencies like the Food Supply Department, Agricultural Cooperatives and the Haryana Agriculture Federation. The activities like loading, cleaning of grains, filling them in gunny bags etc. is done by the *Arahti*. [Yadav, 2002: Bibipur (Karnal)]

Box 2.32
Command Area Development

CADA is a beneficiary oriented scheme for the benefit of small and marginal farmers. The scheme covers installation of shallow tube wells, sprinkler sets, underground pipelines and land levelling for which bank loan is arranged and subsidy provided. The people of Guskani are quite happy with the work of Command Area Development. [Suresh, 1997: Guskani (Rohtak)]

ANIMAL HUSBANDRY

Second only to agriculture, animal husbandry is the most important occupation of the villagers in Haryana. Most households possess livestock of some kind. Cows and buffaloes constitute the main livestock in the state. The poorer households go for pigs, sheep and goats. Poultry units varying in size are also becoming popular. Cross-bred varieties in cows, pigs and poultry are fast becoming popular in the state.

Veterinary care facilities are gradually coming up to cover most villages. The Pasudhan Centres (Veterinary care centres) are coming up to provide veterinary cover to groups of villages. Although all the villages have not been adequately covered by these centres, most villages now have access to veterinary care in some form or the other. Many villages still practice local remedies for the common diseases, however, once the animal is found to be in an incurable state, most villagers seek the assistance of a veterinary doctor or compounder, who visit villages and attend to the animals on payment basis.

Cattle breeds are gradually responding to artificial insemination. This facility is available at the Pasudhan Centres and Veterinary Hospitals. Consequently, bovine animals are becoming more productive. Although the average yield of buffaloes is still about 8 litres of milk a day, the maximum yields are going up to 15 litres. Similarly, maximum yields of Jersey and Holstein cross-breds are going above 20 litres of milk per day.

Grazing lands which were common property resources are gradually offering very limited service for animal grazing. Moreover, the cross-bred cows and buffaloes respond much better to stall feeding. This has led to an important focus on fodder cultivation. Barseem, lucerne, chari, jowar and other greens are being grown by farmers as fodder. This is being supplemented by dry fodder in the summer months. Concentrates are also increasingly being resorted to for improving yields.

Much of the milk is still used up in the villages as fluid milk or as ghee, butter, paneer or lassi. However, in many villages, especially those near urban centres, surplus milk is being generated for marketing. Milk Cooperative Societies have come up in a large number of villages. These societies procure the milk on the basis of fat content and S.N.F. content. A reasonable price is thus made available to the farmers. These societies sell their milk to the Cooperative Unions of the districts. For further processing, the Milk Federation procures the milk from these Unions. Along with the cooperatives, private dairies and private vendors also collect milk from the villages.

Poultry farms are also emerging as profitable units. Apart from the small poultry units financed by the District Rural Development Agencies and the local banks, larger and more profitable units are also coming up in villages of Haryana, especially in villages located on highways and near urban centres.

Haryana has been doing well in animal husbandry. However, there is still need to further develop veterinary care facilities closer to the villages. Cooperative societies for marketing of milk also need to be strengthened in terms of coverage. With the white revolution already underway in Haryana, there is now need to develop an increasing focus on piggery, sheep and goat rearing and processing of livestock products in the villages.

Cattle

The tables containing livestock statistics are again limited to the 12 districts that existed prior to 1989. The population of cattle per '00 rural households is highest in Kurukshetra with 438 cattle, followed by Ambala with 294 cattle, Karnal with 284 cattle and Jind with 232 cattle. In contrast Sonipat has only 89 cattle per '00 households against an average for the state of 195 cattle per '00 households. Hisar, Sirsa, Bhiwani, Gurgaon, Faridabad, Rohtak and Mahendragarh all have cattle population per '00 rural households lower than the average for the state.

Table 2.27: Cattle, 1988

District	*Number of rural households (1981)*	*Cattle in '00*	*Cattle per '00 rural households*
Kurukshetra	59733	2618	438
Ambala	88275	2599	294
Karnal	80245	2282	284
Jind	97323	2257	232
Hisar	176938	3253	184
Sirsa	82997	1311	158
Bhiwani	110738	1736	157
Gurgaon	100447	1287	128
Faridabad	83862	1070	128
Rohtak	140407	1787	127
Mahendragarh	70123	872	124
Sonipat	104483	929	89
Average			*195*

Source: Derived from *Statistical Handbook of Haryana* (*1991-92*), Government of Haryana and Census of India (1981).

Buffaloes

Kurukshetra with 739 buffaloes per '00 rural households has a density of population of buffaloes which is double that of the state average of 344. Karnal follows with 527 buffaloes per '00 households, to be

Table 2.28: Buffaloes (1988)

District	*Number of rural households (1981)*	*Buffaloes in '00*	*Buffaloes per '00 rural households*
Kurukshetra	59733	4417	739
Karnal	80245	4232	527
Jind	97323	3815	392
Ambala	88275	3206	363
Faridabad	83862	2917	348
Mahendragarh	70123	2068	295
Rohtak	140407	3882	276
Gurgaon	100447	2676	266
Sirsa	82997	2135	257
Hisar	176938	4459	252
Sonipat	104483	2572	246
Bhiwani	110738	1906	172
Average			*344*

Source: Derived from *Statistical Handbook of Haryana* (*1991-92*), Government of Haryana and Census of India (1981).

followed by Jind (392), Ambala (363) and Faridabad (348). Bhiwani has the lowest population of buffaloes as also the lowest population per '00 households of 171. The other districts fall in between. It is essentially the Ambala, Karnal, Kurukshetra and Jind belt which is rich in buffaloe rearing.

Sheep

Sheep rearing is mainly in the districts of Sirsa, Bhiwani, Kurukshetra, Mahendragarh and Jind. Sirsa has 168 sheep per '00 rural households, Bhiwani follows with 112 and Kurukshetra with 107. Gurgaon, Faridabad and Sonipat have less than 40 sheep per '00 households against an average for the state of 77 sheep per '00 households.

Table 2.29: Sheep (1988)

District	*Number of rural households (1981)*	*Sheep in ('00)*	*Sheep per '00 rural households*
Sirsa	82997	1395	168
Bhiwani	110738	1244	112
Kurukshetra	59733	637	107
Mahendragarh	70123	696	99
Jind	97323	948	97
Hisar	176938	1439	81
Karnal	80245	632	79
Ambala	88275	428	48
Rohtak	140407	602	43
Gurgaon	100447	341	34
Faridabad	83862	256	31
Sonipat	104483	293	28
Average			77

Source: Derived from *Statistical Handbook of Haryana (1991-92)*, Government of Haryana and Census of India (1981).

Goats

Mahendragarh, Bhiwani, Gurgaon and Sirsa are the main goat rearing districts of Haryana. Mahendragarh with 136 goats per '00 households is way above 8 districts which have 50 or less goats per '00 households. By and large goat rearing in the north eastern belt is not so popular, perhaps because of the switchover to stall feeding of buffaloes.

Table 2.30: Goats (1988)

District	*Number of rural households (1981)*	*Goats in '00*	*Goats per '00 rural households*
Mahendragarh	70123	951	136
Bhiwani	110738	1098	99
Gurgaon	100447	944	94
Sirsa	82997	729	88
Ambala	88275	462	52
Kurukshetra	59733	281	47
Faridabad	83862	387	46
Hisar	176938	700	40
Jind	97323	335	34
Rohtak	140407	457	33
Karnal	80245	202	25
Sonipat	104483	206	20
Average			*59*

Source: Derived from *Statistical Handbook of Haryana (1991-92)*, Government of Haryana and Census of India (1981).

Poultry

The districts of Ambala, Gurgaon and Mahendragarh are the main poutry producing districts of the state. Ambala led in 1988 with 1661

Table 2.31: Poultry (1988)

District	*Number of rural households (1981)*	*Poultry in '00*	*Poultry per '00 rural households*
Ambala	88275	14660	1661
Gurgaon	100447	11852	1180
Mahendragarh	70123	8109	1156
Karnal	80245	4791	597
Kurukshetra	59733	3434	575
Sonipat	104483	2514	241
Jind	97323	2256	232
Sirsa	82997	1280	154
Faridabad	83862	1055	126
Rohtak	140407	1730	123
Hisar	176938	1429	81
Bhiwani	110738	280	25
Average			*512*

Source: Derived from *Statistical Handbook of Haryana (1991-92)*, Government of Haryana and Census of India (1981).

birds per '00 rural households, followed by Gurgaon (1180) and Mahendragarh (1156). Karnal and Kurukshetra had between 500-600 birds per '00 households, whereas the other districts had less than 250 birds per '00 households. Hisar and Bhiwani had less than 100 birds per '00 households.

HEALTH AND SANITATION

Health care and family welfare in rural Haryana is largely the responsibility of the Government. Although private doctors, especially Registered Medical Practitioners are gaining popularity on account of the poor functioning of governmental health institutions, the government health centres and hospitals because of their infrastructural strengths, continue to remain the backbone of health care in the state. The facilities in the state are, however, unevenly distributed. Table shows district-wise hospital facilities in the state. Bhiwani, Rohtak, Ambala and Hisar have more than 85 hospital beds per lakh of population, whereas Gurgaon, Panipat, Kaithal and Rewari have less than 37 beds. The skewed nature of health infrastructure is best demonstrated by the fact that, whereas Bhiwani has 124 beds per lakh of population, Rewari has only 32 beds.

Table 2.32: Hospital Beds per lakh of Population (1990-91)

	Beds per lakh of population
Bhiwani	124
Rohtak	107
Ambala	86
Hisar	85
Jind	75
Yamunanagar	56
Karnal	49
Faridabad	48
Mahendergarh	44
Sirsa	42
Sonipat	41
Kurukshestra	38
Gurgoan	37
Panipat	35
Kaithal	34
Rewari	32

Source: Statistical Handbook of Haryana (1991-92), Government of Haryana.

At the village level, the Sub-Health Centres and the Primary Health Centres (PHC) are the key health care institutions. Whereas the PHC are staffed with doctors, compounders and nurses, the Sub-Health Centres have the key village level field functionaries in the form of Lady Health Visitor, Auxiliary Nurse, Multi-purpose Workers and Field Workers. These institutions exist to provide health cover for common ailments, immunization against communicable diseases, and also function as the family planning centre for the area.

Although diseases like Tuberculosis (T.B.), Polio, Diabetes, Heart ailments, Tetanus continue to take toll of human life, the common diseases afflicting most villages are Malaria, Gastroenteritis, Diarrhoea, Dysentery, Cholera, Respiratory Tract Infections, Asthma and skin infections like Scabies. For the communicable diseases immunization is done by the PHCs, the staff of the sub-centres and most important of all, by the Anganwadis. For treatment, where the governmental institutions are properly managed, people visit them. However, most of the institutions are badly managed. Medicines are often in short supply and people are unable to get medicines from the governmental institutions. Even civil hospitals are unable to provide the attention that patients desire. Private doctors, despite their fees are able to fulfil these needs and are thus being preferred to government health centres. For minor ailments, people still resort to local (*desi*) home remedies. Only when these cures do not succeed they visit the doctor.

Government maternity centres do not have a wide enough coverage. For most deliveries, the midwives (*dais*) continue to provide service to the villagers. Upgradation of their skills by suitable training in government institutions has improved their service.

Sanitation is another important area of concern in the villages of Haryana. Open drains, poorly paved streets with poor drainage, cause stagnant pools which not only stink, but become breeding grounds for mosquitoes and other pests. Poor management of solid wastes especially dung heaps add to the unhygeinic environment. With the depletion of wastelands for defecation, human excreta is developing into another major problem. Apart from the unhygeinic aspect of defecation, the embarrassment of defecating in limited open spaces is becoming a human problem. Subsidized latrines are being encouraged, but the programme has not been followed up with the pursuastion required for such a programme.

Drinking water facilities are more or less satisfactory in the state. Tap water, handpumps, tubewells and wells are able to fulfil the requirements. However, for many, the drinking water facility is unable to cater to the requirement of bathing and washing. For the latter, villagers still depend on the village pond, where villagers not only bathe and wash, but also take their livestock for bathing and drinking water. These ponds thus become sources of skin infections.

Family planning is gradually being accepted in principle by the villagers. However, the concern for having the male child, and generally more than one male child, often leads to large families with 4-6 children. Contraceptives like the condom, oral pills, copper-Ts, IUCDs have still not been popularised. Family planning is still dependent largely on sterilization and that too on tubectomy. With Laproscopic tubectomy, the operation has become more friendly, but the simpler vasectomy is still to get the acceptability that it deserves.

Box 2.33

Health Care and Family Planning in Ransika

There have been 5 cases of male sterilization and 7 cases of female sterilization in the village. By and large the acceptability of family planning measures has been satisfactory in the village and people are aware of it.

There is a Primary Health Centre in Ransika. Sanitation is cause for concern in the village as lack of dry land makes it difficult to defecate with sufficient hygiene. [Tayal, 2000: Ransika (Gurgaon)]

Box 2.34

Health Care, Sanitation and Family Welfare in Bibipur

Being located on the riverside, the village is very vulnerable to water borne disease. The prime sanitation issue in the area involves issues of wastewater disposal, defecation place, safe drinking water, and toilets.

While the village has a Primary health care sub-centre, it is severely understaffed though the ANM is found to be playing a positive role in the village, as she belongs from the adjoining village. The PHC is located in the town of Garhi Birbal, which is 8 kms from the village, and so it acts like the referral place for the patients after the ANM gives them basic treatment. The PHC was offering all the basic health services like Immunization, Ante-Natal care, Treatment of minor illness, Pediatric care, Availability of contraceptives and IUD insertion.

The sub-centre however is very poorly equipped and requires to be upgraded specially as far as storage of medicines is concerned. The furniture was lacking and the doctors visited the sub-centre very irregularly as there were not many cases, which would come to them even when they came. However being a relatively remote, small village, there were not any private practitioners in the vicinity. Most of the people either went to the local quake or to the PHC located in the nearby town, as conveyance was not a problem.

The Births in the village was 53 in the last year while the number of deaths was only 13. The number of infant deaths was 5 and most of them were due to malnutrition of the mother leading to premature babies. There were only 2 births that took place in the civil hospital in Karnal, which had got complicated, while the rest had been domestic births.

As far as family care was concerned, the number of persons in the reproductive age group was 410 among men and 356 among women. The total number of married couples was 276. The number of men who had adopted the planning methods was only 7 while women had to adopt most of the time the family planning method that was 112 in case of this village.

Clearly showing the discrimination in case of women, most of the time Tubectomy was used while after that IUD was most popular and then contraceptives and finally, vasectomy which was used by only a few people. [Yadav, 2002: Bibipur (Karnal)]

EDUCATION

According to the 1991 Census, percentage literacy in Haryana was reported as 55.5 per cent against the national average of 52.1 per cent. Male literacy was reported as 68 per cent and female literacy as 41 per cent. The figures have improved over the period 1991-2001. Literacy in Haryana in 2001 has been reported at 57.98 per cent as against the national average of 55.17 per cent Literacy in Haryana is lower than in the neighbouring states of Himachal Pradesh and Punjab. A district-wise analysis based on the number of literates and the total population (not population above a particular age group) shows that literacy levels are highest in Ambala, Rewari, Sonipat and Rohtak (Table 2.16). Although in male literacy Rewari is highest, the proportionately higher female literacy level in Ambala puts the latter on top. The lowest performers are Kaithal, Sirsa, Jind and Hisar, in that order. In total literacy, Kaithal has only 34 per cent literacy compared to 55 per cent in Ambala. So far as female literacy is concerned Kaithal has only 23 per cent literacy, compared to 47 per cent in Ambala.

Table 2.33: Literacy in Haryana as per cent of Total Population (1991)

(*in per cent*)

District	Male literacy	Female literacy	Total Literacy
Ambala	63	47	55
Rewari	66	38	53
Sonipat	64	38	52
Rohtak	63	37	51
Yamunanagar	56	42	50
Kurukshetra	57	39	48
Faridabad	60	33	48
Mahendragarh	62	30	46
Karnal	54	35	45
Panipat	54	33	44
Bhiwani	57	28	44
Gurgaon	53	27	41
Hisar	50	26	39
Jind	49	24	38
Sirsa	47	28	38
Kaithal	44	23	34

Source: Data on Total Population, Sex-ratios, literates male and female derived from the *Statistical Handbook of Haryana, 1991-92*. per cent literates as proportion of total population derived from this data.

Chart 2.1: Total Literacy in Haryana as per cent of Total Population

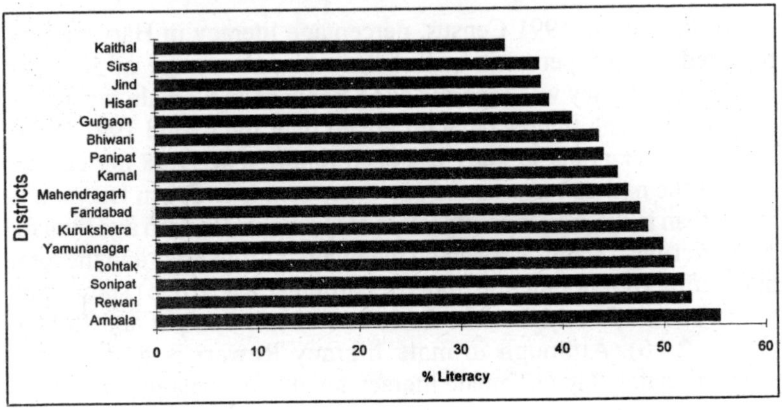

Despite rapid material progress in Haryana, literacy especially among women has lagged behind. Although the villages of the state have been well covered by an expanding network of primary schools, middle schools, high schools, balwaris and adult literacy centres, the quality of education has not kept pace to attract the down to earth, pragmatic villagers to the desired extent. The intrinsic value of education has not been successfully popularised. At best, education is considered as a commodity to be consumed for the purpose of gaining qualifications to get jobs, especially government jobs. And when this education is unable to promise even these jobs, its worth is questioned. With regard to education of girls in Haryana, it is a common refrain that what the girl practically needs to learn is management of household jobs, so as to be a successful wife and mother. With such a world-view, especially so, when opportunities for female careers are extremely limited in rural areas, and when urban areas are already teeming with unemployed populations, it is very difficult to convince the earthy and common sensical villager about the worth of the kind of education being imparted, in the schools of today.

The perception about the lack of adequate relevance of education is compounded by the low motivation and competencies of the teachers and administrators of education. The situation becomes worse when infrastructural facilites are also lacking. Although primary schools have sprung up in almost all the villages of Haryana, most of them do not have adequate accommodation facilites for the growing number of students.

The low quality content, the indiscipline and lack of motivation of the teachers and the lack of facilites to engage the youth in productive and creative work, often makes the total environment of the schools indisciplined and meaningless. The village surveys repeatedly noted the complaints regarding lack of discipline, reflected most significantly in the rampant copying in examinations.

Within this general environment of inefficiency, cynicism, lack of motivation and conviction, there do exist islands of excellence. Some headmasters are able to lead their institutions and channelize the youth along creative and productive lines. Such schools not only display exteriors of well managed institutions, with lawns, flowers and general upkeep, but also demonstrate their excellence in the academic and extra-curricular achievements of the students.

Observing different sections of society, it remains a fact that in villages, the Scheduled Castes are still the most illiterate. Their children are required to assist their families at home and in the fields. The incentives of stipends, free books and free uniforms for girls and prizes for attendance do help in attracting students of these backward communities, but unless society is able to demonstrate the utility of education, the impact of this education may not be sustainable. It is a fact that many literates often slip back into illiteracy for lack of practice and follow up. And this follow up comes best, when the life styles that follow education, demand the use of an ever growing body of knowledge which can be best acquired through the written word.

Maximum dropouts occur after Class V. Among the dropouts, Scheduled Castes and girl students figure most prominently, followed by the Backward Classes. The demands on these children for assistance in the work place of the parent or at home pulls them back to their homes. In addition, when the middle school or high school is not located in the student's village, there are many dropouts, especially girls. Parents do not generally approve of the female child going out of the village for schooling.

Since 1983, there has been a general upswing in the enrollment in primary schools, this increase appears to be sharper in the case of girls. General awareness on account of various factors seems to be responsible for this. From this trend it appears that the demand for good education is likely to grow.

To meet the growing demand of quality education, private schools are beginning to come up in the villages. With suitable support from the local bodies and the government, these could help in bringing competition into education, thereby raising the standard of even the government schools.

The District Primary Education Programme which has been launched in Haryana is likely to bridge the gaps that exist in infrastructure, teachers, syllabi and curriculum. The focus of the programme in attracting the girl child and the weaker sections may push up enrollment further. As the need for education is propagated in the villages, the demand for relevant quality education is likely to increase. For this, the motivation and competence of the teachers would have to become a focus. Alternatively, private schooling would come in to meet the demands. The way private clinics of Registered Medical Practitioners are beginning to gain preference over government dispensaries and health centres, the same kind of story may get replicated in the case of education.

Box 2.35
Enrolment in Kakana Bhadri

The enrolment in the private primary school is greater than the Government primary school. Most of the enrolled children attend the school regularly. Around 254 children are not enrolled in any of the two schools. Normally the elders of the village take interest in running of the schools. They ensure that the teachers attend the school regularly. [Gupta, 1999: Kakana Bhadri (Sonipat)]

Box 2.36
Literacy and Education in Ransika

There is a primary school in the village. Literacy figures show that around 33 per cent of the population has an education of high school or above. However, it also emerges that 39 per cent of the people are illiterate. Child education figures have not come out very encouraging. Around 33 per cent of the children seem to be out of school. [Tayal , 2000: Ransika (Gurgaon)]

Box 2.37
Education in Bibipur

Education is one of the most neglected of the social sectors in the State. There is a Primary school in the village with total 474 children enrolled in it out of which 246 are boys and 228 girls. There are 3 sanctioned posts in the school and only 2 of them have been coming regularly as the other teacher is on deputation to another school. The Attendance in the school is fair (59.6 % for boys and 53 % for girls) considering that almost half of the population migrates to other places to sell their products and most of them being nuclear families take their children along. In fact the percentage of the children that were attending school as a proportion of those present in the village was as high as 87 percentages. This was result of the serious efforts by the administration to bring the children of the age of below 14 years old into the fold of regular education system as the district was to be considered for the PLP project. However the literacy rate remained low at 38.31 per cent for men and 24.14 per cent for females as per 2001 Census.

(Contd.)

Box 2.37 (**Contd.**)

> **The primary reason for this is the village has a population, which had migrated from Pakistan and had settled in the riverbed of Yamuna, and then was settled, in the village panchayat land. As they migrate during off-season their children are not able to get regular education and hence the drop out ratio is large. Also the parents themselves were not educated as their status as refugee was not settled. The number of children that had yet to cover under the education system was 74 among boys and 111 among girls bringing the total to 185. The PDS system in the village was functioning satisfactorily and so was the Mid Day meal, though it was not followed in its right spirit and a bulk quantity of cereals were given to the children at the end of the month instead of giving them cooked food in the school.**
>
> **Though the Mid Day meal scheme helped in retaining the children in school, it was not incentive enough for the families who migrate, to let their children stay back in other's place while they are outside selling their products. Under operation Black Board and Chief Minister's "Government at your doorsteps" programme, two school rooms were constructed and also uniforms and textbooks were being distributed free of costs to the children. Though there were complaints of irregularities, by and large the performance in this regard was satisfactory and the teaching staff was a motivated lot, who also participated in other social awareness programme like rural sanitation. The school had a hand pump, which provided drinking water supply to the school and also a public health department connection was provided along with a sanitary toilet, which was setup under school sanitation project.**
>
> **The school however was located in a low-lying area and was prone to water logging. Hence it was suggested that the soil which dug out from ponds as part of works undertaken under SGRY be used to fill the low lying area and during these months, almost all of the school complex's low lying area was raised. This would certainly help the children in the rainy season.**

The children also complained of the noise from the workshop, which was constructed nearby in order to promote the skill development for the various craftsmen present in the village. The Headman explained that there was lack of space in the village and hence the site had to be chosen, though they tried to ensure the workshop starts only after the children had left the school. [Yadav, 2002: Bibipur (Karnal)]

POVERTY ALLEVIATION PROGRAMMES

"People look forward to the government to help improve the conditions of their living and in turn, the government has to yield results, may be by extending grants only."

—Kumar, 89: Hisar

The Programmes

In the last two decades a number of programmes were launched all over the country by the Government of India for alleviation of poverty in rural areas. The Integrated Rural Development Programme (IRDP), Rural Landless Employment Guarantee Programme (RLEGP), National Rural Employment Programme (NREP), Jawahar Rozgar Yojana (JRY), Training of Rural Youth for Self-employment (TRYSEM) and Development of Women and Children in Rural Areas (DWCRA) being the most prominent. IRDP in its present form was launched in 1978-79 in selected blocks all over the country. District Rural Development Agencies were set up in all the districts to implement IRDP, TRYSEM and DWCRA to begin with. Later other rural development programmes were also brought under the DRDA. Prominent among these are the Indira Awas Yojana (IAY), Swaranajayanti Gram Swarojgar Yojana (SGSY), Sampooran Gram Rojgar Yojana (SGRY) and Employment Assurance Scheme (EAS). There is also a concerted effort to organize and develop Self Help Groups (SHG). The District Rural Development Agency is headed by the Deputy Commissioner as Chairman and a Senior scale IAS officer as Chief Executive Officer.

The employment generation and community works taken up in Haryana under the rural employment schemes include the following:

- Making of pucca roads
- Gali construction
- Johad repair
- Installation of street lights
- Construction of school buildings
- Renovation of school buildings
- Residential plots and low-budget houses with sanitation facilities for the Scheduled Castes
- Smokeless chullahs
- Gobar gas plants

Under IRDP loans have been distributed for income generating activities mainly for the following:

- Tubewell
- Buffalo unit
- Pair of bullocks
- Horse Tonga
- Sheep unit
- Camel unit
- Jhota Buggi
- Cycle rickshaw
- Kirana shop
- Motor mechanic shop
- Leather work
- Knitting machine
- Durree carpet making

Although the data base is inadequate, specific data relating to financing of different trades from villages of 9 districts of Haryana throws up the following picture:

Buffaloes	93
Pair of bullocks	30
Sheep Unit	3
Camels	5
Cycle shop	1
Cycle rickshaws	2
Horse Tonga	7
Jhota Buggi	8
Leather work	1
Knitting machine	1
Durree carpet	8
Motor mechanic shop	1
Shop	2
Tubewells	3
Total	165

Although the sample is small the picture that emerges is very clear. Animal Husbandry seems to be the most popular trade and within animal husbandry financing of Buffaloes is by far the most attractive option. This is followed by the service sector in which transportation seems to be the most popular activity. In the above sample 17 cases have been financed for cycle rickshaws, horse tongas and jhota buggis (buffalo carts). Cottage industry which would include leather work, knitting machines and durree, carpet making is also popular. Financing of shops was not found to be very popular. This could be on account of the larger capital requirements for this trade.

Box 2.38
Poverty Alleviation Programmes

The various poverty alleviation programmes are classified into the one, which increase employment opportunity or increase the quality of life. The two schemes which provide employment are classifiable into the self-employment scheme, namely SGSY and the wage employment scheme, namely JGSY whose funds are directed straight to the panchayats, while that of Employment Assurance Scheme goes through the Panchayat Samiti and Zila Parishad. Apart from these, there are other schemes for improvement of quality of life like that for providing housing through IAY or PMGY.

The population of the village that comes under the BPL list has 61 families. Most of them belong to the SC families which is that of the Sikligar. Though there are families which belong to other castes who deserve to be brought into the BPL since the Sarpanch is from the Sikligar caste, he has ensured that most of the beneficiaries of the scheme are that of the Sikligar caste. After a test case was done on 15 of such families they were all found to be genuine in terms of their total income and their standard of living.

Self Employment Scheme

The Swaranajayanti Gram Swarojgar Yogana was started in the village on 1st of April 1999. The major activities that are performed in the village include that of dairy farming while the Sikligars are involved in the activities of iron works for which a workshop has also been constructed.

Since these trades have been traditional to the Sikligars, they have a well established network of marketing and input supply network like the iron scrap-yards. The tools that are used are very basic and hence most of the products that are produced are for small consumption and cannot enter the market on a big scale. They represent the unorganized sector of the industry.

Wage Employment Scheme

Wage employment was being provided under the JGSY scheme. Since the funds for the EAS were allotted by the Panchayat Samiti and the Zila Parishad, and the village did not have any person elected to either of these bodies, there was no work that was sanctioned under the EAS.

The JGSY was started in the village in 1998, and during the financial year, Rs. 50,787 was allocated to the panchayat. The labourer for the works were taken from the village itself since there were quite a few landless labourers in the village and there was no need for labour contractors to be hired for the purpose. There was no discrepancy in the labour rates between men and women. The rates that were given were at the market price of Rs. 2400 per month which was way above the Minimum Wage Rate in the state at Rs. 1975 per month. Also there was no discrepancy between the actual wages paid and that entered in the Muster Roll, though some bogus names were added to adjust the expenditure in the works.

Table 2.34: Wage Employment Scheme

Physical Asset	*Total Expenditure*		*Employment Generated (Mandays)*			
	Wage	*Non-wage*	*SC*	*Women*	*Others*	*Total*
Hand Pump	880	1800	8	—	2	10
Boring	3300	—	24	—	8	32
SC Chaupal	1100	2416	34	—	9	43
Boundary wall of School	1200	1850	34	—	5	39
Community Centre repair	300	1275	3	—	1	4
Pavement of Street	800	1210	40	—	2	42

Though no specific training was given to the labourers for the work, the labourers were engaged according to their known skills.

The decision for the works were taken by the panchayat itself and almost all of the village was involved in the decision. As the works were few, there was general awareness among the villagers about the activities that were taken up by the panchayat.

Indira Awas Yojana

In general houses were made according to the requirements of the beneficiaries. Though there is a provision for the latrines, they were not made in proper manner like lack of water discharge was noticed. However, after the Rural Sanitation Project was sanctioned in the district, all the new houses were fitted with the latrines with single soakage pit. Under the Scheme 7500 bricks, 20 bags of cement, two window frames and one gate frame is provided to the beneficiary. Sometime people ask for the linters instead of window and gate frames. There do arise certain complications in construction of houses like a house may require some earth work for filling up the basement, so that the foundation is strong enough to hold the house. However, being a waterlogged area, it is very costly to have such earth work done. Also the wood work sometimes is cheaper than the standard design of iron frames on the roof, so these escalate the cost, balance of which has to be borne by the beneficiary. Under upgradation only Rs. 10,000 is allocated while for new houses Rs. 20,000 is provided. Many people play fraud in getting their house constructed. For example, there was a case in the village where the person had already been allotted the IAY house, however, he continued to stay in the old house and gave the IAY house to his son and then again claimed benefit on the ground that his son and he had different family and that they also had different BPL numbers.

In the village 14 houses were constructed or upgraded under the IAY and PMGY, giving a total expenditure of Rs. 2,70,000 in which 315 mandays were generated. As a policy, the houses are given in the name of the women so that they have right of property.

A new scheme called Sampooran Gram Rojgar Yojana was started after merging different wage employment schemes from December 1, 2001. Since the regular budget allocation was to start from the next financial year of 2002-03, the balance amount of the EAS and JGSY schemes were diverted to this scheme. The amount under the JGSY

(Contd.)

(Contd.)

was given directly to the panchayats for carrying out earth works in the village while those under the EAS were selected by the Zila Parishad and Panchayat Samiti. Under the new scheme an amount is released to the panchayat according to its SC population for carrying out earthwork in the village. It has wheat and wage component. Under this scheme, total fund of Rs. 13,050 was released to this panchayat for earth work. This work is being done under the general supervision of Village Development Committee and on inspection the work was found to be according to specifications and satisfactory.

Along with these development schemes, welfare schemes are also undertaken in the village. Tau Devilal Old Age Pension Scheme, Widow Pension, Handicap Pension are also given in the village to the eligible persons. Various welfare activities for Backward and Scheduled Caste are also being implemented in the village like Kanyadan Yojana, educational scholarships and assistances. The villagers did not report anything against the pension scheme and they were regularly receiving the pension before 7th of every month. [Yadav, 2002: Bibipur (Karnal)]

Box 2.39
Poverty Alleviation Programmes

Jawahar Rozgar Yojana

The various development works carried out in the village under various Central and State schemes such as Employment Assurance Scheme (EAS), Indira Awas Yojana (IAY), Panchayati Raj Institutions (PRI), Decentralised Planning (DCP) and MLA Scheme are as follows:

Sl. No.	*Year*	*Scheme*	*Work Done/Beneficiary*	*Funds allotted*
1.	1998-99	EAS	Minor Irrigation	192710
2.	1998-99	EAS	School Room	107000
3.	1996-97	DCP	Pavement of street	25000
4.	1995-96	MP LADS	Construction of building of community centre	31000

(Contd.)

Box 2.39 (Contd.)

5.	1995-96	MP LADS	Pavement of B.C. street	10000
6.	1995-96	MP LADS	Pavement of S.C. street	10000
7.	1996-97	MP LADS	Repair of B.C. Chaupal	27000
8.	1996-97	MP LADS	Street/Phirni Bust stand towards Chaupal	32700
9.	1998-99	MP LADS	Pavement of street of Raj Master	30000
10.	1998-99	IAY	Anil	20000
11.	1998-99	IAY	Dhanpati	20000
12.	1998-99	IAY	Barpai	20000
13.	1998-99	IAY	Jajbala	20000
14.	1998-99	IAY	Chandro	20000
15.	1998-99	IAY	Krishna	20000
16.	1998-99	IAY	Santosh	20000

When we look at the above pattern, we find that while some investments have been made in the village, there are only three kinds of assets which have been created. They are the school rooms, minor irrigation works, IAY houses, works of the streets.

While the investment made in the school room is visible, expenditure made on the streets are not much visible. Two kinds of works have been done on the streets:

1. Filling the Phirni (the circular path around the village residential area) with mud.
2. Brick paving of some streets.

The work under category (1) cannot be seen as the earth filled is washed away every year. Some of the streets did have brick paving. The quality of brick paving work was perceived to be very poor as there were no proper arrangements for drainage. While the streets which were not paved were cleaner because the sandy earth absorbed all the waste water which came out of the houses, in the brick paved street there was a lot of filth as the waste water was running through the streets and gathering at certain lower areas. Improper planning and poor masonry work was visible.

The development works undertaken in the village are highly stereotyped. They lack imagination and do not appear to be achieving any of the objectives of the scheme. The basic 60:40 wage material ratio is also not achieved because of this. Land development work of small or marginal farmers below poverty line can easily be undertaken under this scheme and will be very successful. Even other individual programmes can be undertaken. However, the problem remains that of identification of beneficiaries. Even the government instruction provides that works of roads and buildings should not exceed 17.5 per cent of total allocation.

When we attempt to analyse the performance of the schemes on the basis of their primary objective, i.e. "Generation of additional gainful employment for unemployed and under-employed persons in rural areas" we find that it totally fails to achieve this objective.

The first reason for this is the paucity of funds. For a village with such large scale under-employment, the funds available have generated 150-300 mandays of employment per year. Secondly, the nature of works undertaken is such that labour wage component is very low.

Impact of JRY on poverty situation of the village is absolutely minimal. No one in the village looks forward to any kind of employment under JRY, nor are they aware of the programme. Wage rates are as per the Minimum Wages Act. Wages in this block are paid only in cash and on weekly basis.

I met and talked to two beneficiaries under the IAY scheme. While one of them was a deserving recipient of the help offered under the scheme, the other one, was not in need of the help at all. The first one was actually making use of the house and was living in it with her son. The second one, on the other hand was living with her sons in a four room *pucca* house and was using the IAY house as a shed for storing fodder and grains. She apparently got the house under the pretext that her sons had turned her out of the house and that she had no place to go to. After the house was constructed with the help of a mason, she lived there for only 15 days and then declared that she had patched up with her sons and again moved in their *pucca* house to live with them. This was surely a case of a wrong selection of beneficiary.

I.R.D.P.

As per the instructions and guidelines of the Government of India, the beneficiary should have a family income upto Rs. 11,000 from all sources. Such beneficiaries are selected through a survey conducted by the Government personnel. Village-wise list of "Below Poverty Line (BPL)" people is prepared at the District Rural Development Agency's level.

After the selection of BPL, Credit Camps are organised in villages. In these camps, besides rural development officers, field functionaries from the banks, development and revenue departments are also present. The aims and objectives of the schemes are explained in these camps. These camps are held in public places and the forms of needy persons are filled there. Since most of the required field functionaries are present, all formalities are completed in these camps. After due processing and checking, the eligible forms are sponsored to the concerned bank which is supposed to convey sanction within 15 days.

Although these banks are supposed to mandatorily give sanctions to those loans approved in the camp, most of the times they reject the beneficiaries' claims on frivolous grounds and do not give sanction for the loans. This is a practice that needs to be checked.

After the loan is sanctioned by the bank, the assets are got purchased through a committee in non-cash Blocks, which advances loan plus subsidy to the beneficiary who creates assets on his own. After the establishment of the venture, the beneficiary is required to repay the loan in installments to the bank within a stipulated period ranging from 3 to 5 years.

> In this way, the IRDP helps the indigent persons to supplement their income by way of providing them financial assistance. With a view to providing marketing facilities to the IRD beneficiaries, a District Supply and Marketing Society (DSMS) has been created. This Society is open to all IRDP beneficiaries to avail marketing and other facilities for their products.

While the above is the official version of the implementation of IRDP in Sonipat, the ground realities as observed in village Kakana Bhadri were quite different.

The village has names of 72 persons in the BPL list but everyone believes that the BPL survey is incomplete and incorrect as a result of which it remains a paper document only. It is proposed to undertake a drive to correct the deficiencies in the BPL list. Till now IRDP loans were advanced to individuals identified by the BDO or the Gram Sachiv.

Table 2.35: List of Beneficiaries Who were Granted Loan

Sl. No.	Name	Sex	Category	Income	Purpose of Loan	Loan	Subsidy
1.	Rattan	M	BC	8900	Pneumatic Cart	12900	4000
2.	Gulab	M	BC	9000	Tailoring	3000	1000
3.	Om Prakash	M	SC	8800	Buffalo	7600	2533
4.	Dharam Singh	M	SC	8700	Sheep	10400	5200

Another factor noticed among IRDP beneficiaries was that they were not aware that the asset given to them was meant to increase their incomes and that they were expected to pay the installment out of the increased income. A majority of them told that the asset has not resulted in any increase in income. For most of them, the loan was welcome only because it provided them easy availability of instant cash as they immediately sold off their assets and pocketed the subsidy minus the amount paid as bribe to the bank officials to get their cases sanctioned. None of them had the asset with them presently. While most had sold off their assets immediately, some had taken care of it for a year or so and had derived more benefits from the loan. However, none of them had repaid the loan fully and none even had the slight intention of doing so. One of them even said that he did not want to avail of any further loans as in his opinion, they were more of a trouble than an advantage.

Thus, the IRDP programme is not generating the necessary results because of improper planning, faulty identification procedure and lack of follow up. [Mishra, 1996: Kasumbhi (Bhiwani)]

Box 2.40
SHG in Ransika

There have been no poverty alleviation programme in Ransika under IRDP, MWS, TRYSEM etc. for the past several years. The IAY scheme too has not yet been grounded. The group members of the SHG have conveniently split the money amongst them and are not engaged in any economic activity. The new SHGs that have come up however have been formed with the right kind of spirit and motivation. None of these groups has received the revolving fund and they are not counting on it either. Their main idea is to get linked to banks and raise loans directly. [Tayal, 2000: Ransika (Gurgaon)]

Box 2.41
Poverty Alleviation Programmes in Sikarpur

Under JGSY, i.e. Jawahar Gram Samridhi Yojana not much work has been done in the village. In 2000-01 total funds allocated under this scheme were only Rs. 27,914 and out of it Rs. 12,561 was reserved for Scheduled Castes. Construction of village street and digging of village pond were the two activities carried out by the village panchayat out of these funds. Labourers were engaged from the local village only and no contractor was engaged for this purpose. There was no disparity in the payment of wages to male and female workers.

SGSY was implemented in January 2001 in block Hisar-1 in which Sikarpur is situated. Buffalo rearing, dairying, grocery shops, carpentry, sheep rearing, tailoring, bead making have been identified as the key activities under SGSY in the district. Individual loans under SGSY for self-employment are given to BPL population of SC and general category. In the village I have selected ten persons who have been benefited by the scheme. In general, people take loan for 2 buffaloes, out of 10 cases studied, 8 took loans for buffaloes, one for furniture store and one for general store.

Table 2.36: List of Beneficiaries of Loans under SGSY (Individual)

Sl. No.	Name	Caste	Year	Activity	Total Amount	Subsidy
1.	Sugani W/oJita	SC	1998-99 1999-00	Two Buffaloes	26700	3270 3270
2.	Vidhya W/o Bhagchand	General	1998-99 1999-00	Two Buffaloes	26700	2770 2770
3.	Savitari W/o Rambhagat	General	1998-99 1999-00	Two Buffaloes	26700	2770 2770
4.	Devi Lal S/o Sheochand	SC	1998-99	Furniture Store	25000	6000
5.	Rarnchander S/o Molu Ram	General	2000-01	Shop	50000	7500
6.	Karambir S/o Lilu Ram	Others	2000-01	Two Buffaloes	31600	8130
7.	Charan Singh S/o Muodi	OT	2000-01	Two Buffaloes	31600	8130
8.	Sita Ram S/o Polu Ram	General	2000-01	Two Buffaloes	31600	8130
9.	Ram Kumar S/o Raju Ram	General	2000-01	Two Buffaloes	31600	8130
10.	Nar Singh S/o Kirpa Ram	General	2000-01	Two Buffaloes	31600	8130

In the village Shikarpur there was no SHG formed under SGSY Scheme up to January 2002. So the study of SHGs in the village cannot be made. But for studying the status of SHGs. in the villages of the district, I made the study of SHGs formed in the Hisar II block of the district. In total 19 SHGs have been formed in the block in 2000-01. Subsidy component has been released only for 11 SHGs to the bank, i.e. that too after a delay of 4-6 months from the due date. Moreover, so far the revolving fund of Rs. 25,000 has been released to only 4 SHGs in the block. Only one group have received the sanction for the loan of Rs.2,50,000 but disbursement is still awaited. Thus, it can be concluded that progress of SHGs is not satisfactory in the district and more concentrated efforts is required for forming SHGs. NGOs can be of great help in propagating the concept of SHGs and thus leading to their formation. One reason that is given by many villagers for reluctance on the part of villagers is that generally they are not so poor and lack of faith and co-ordination among the rural people due to caste and politics. Banks should also play a leading role in it as monitoring and recovery of loans is easy in case of SHGs.

In the village I have selected ten persons who have been given financial assistance to construct their houses under Indira Awas Yojana. In general houses were made according to the requirements of the beneficiaries. But the modern latrines were missing in most of the cases and smokeless *chullahs* in some cases, as people were interested in construction of two room instead of one room, a latrine and a smokeless *chullah*. They generally complained that the amount of Rs. 20,000 is less. Under the scheme as said by BDO 7500 bricks, 20 bags of cements, two window frames and one gate frame is provided to them. Sometimes people ask for the linters instead of window and gate frames. In general IAY houses were constructed according to specifications and are more or less fulfilling its objective of providing shelter to the BPL population of both SC and general, category.

Table 2.37: Details of Beneficiaries of IAY houses of Village Shikarpur

Sl. No.	*Name*	*Caste*	*Amount*	*Year*
1.	Shadu Ram S/o Arjun	SC	14,000	1994-95
2.	Chameli Devi W/o Hari Ram	SC	14.000	1994-95
3.	Seria W/o Balbir	Others	14,000	1994-95
4.	Purani Devi W/o Hari Singh	Others	14,000	1995-96
5.	Ramvir W/o Birbal	General	12,500	1995-96
6.	Banti W/o Rameshwar	General	12,500	1995-96
7.	Cherria Devi W/o Datta Ram	SC	14,000	1995-96
8.	Sher Singh S/o Lilu	SC	20,000	1998-99
9.	Inder Singh S/o Lalji	SC	20,000	1996-97
10.	Ram Chander S/o Jita Ram	SC	20,000	2001-02

In this financial year 2001-2002, a new scheme called SGRY, Sampooran Gram Rojgar Yojana was started after amalgamation of different wage employment schemes. Under this scheme an amount is released to the panchayat according to its SC population for carrying out earthwork in the village. It has wheat and wage component. Under this scheme, total fund of Rs.18,439 was released to this panchayat for excavation of earth from the village pond and only labourers from the village were employed for this purpose. This work is being done under the general supervision of Village Development Committee, i.e. V.D.C. and on inspection the work was found to be according to specifications and satisfactory.

Along with these developmental schemes welfare schemes are also being undertaken in the village. Tau Devilal Old Age Pension Scheme, Widow Pension, Handicap Pension are also given in the village to eligible persons. Various welfare activities for backwards and Scheduled Castes are also being undertaken in the village like *kanyadan yojana*, educational scholarships and assistances. The villagers did not report anything against the pension scheme and they were regularly receiving it before 7th of every month. [Agarwal, 2001: Sikarpur (Hisar)]

The observations of the probationers when aggregated reveal the broad truths of the poverty alleviation programmes in Haryana.

IRDP

It should be considered a substantial gain that the poor have been identified and programmes targetted at them. The fact that most probationers have reported that the beneficiaries of the programmes have been largely the poor, is also a significant gain. It has also been reported that as a result of IRDP, income generating assets have reached the poor. Moreover, in a state where the animal husbandry and tertiary sectors are fast growing, the fact that most of the loans have been provided for these sectors, aligns the programme to the general developmental processes in the state.

Under TRYSEM, unemployed youth have received training in *Mudha* making, blacksmithy, light engineering, carpet-*cum-durri* weaving, handloom and jute *tat patti* making etc. Other agencies like the Mewat Development Agency, in collaboration with the Haryana Small Scale Industries and Export Corporation, the Haryana State Handloom and Handicrafts Corporation and the Haryana State Industrial Cooperative Federation etc. are also having training centres for various trades, e.g. *Mudha* making, carpet weaving, *tat patti,* handloom, leather tanning, blacksmithy, pottery and hosiery. On completion of training arrangements are being made for financing the trainees for setting up these trades there.

On the negative side, malpractices, cumbersome procedures and non-repayment of loans seem to be the major weakness of the programme. Malpractices sometimes begin right at the beginning with the identification process. They get followed up as loan applications are processed and reach their peak at the time of disbursement. Not only is the machinery corrupt, but gradually the beneficiaries, in search of short term monetary gains go for the subsidy element of the loan, thereby sacrificing the income generating asset creation. This sacrifice puts the brakes on generation of additional income which results in non-repayment of loans. The atmosphere of loan waivers further vitiates this tendency of non-repayment of loans. The end result of this process is often quite bitter for the defaulter. Failure stories of this kind finally discredit the programme.

Community Assets

Employment generation programmes like NREP, RLEGP and JRY have been perceived by most of the probationers as primarily programmes for creation of community assets, rather than as programmes for employment generation. The assessment of these programmes is thus done not against the criteria of employment generation for the poor, but against the criteria of successful creation of community assets.

On the plus side it has been reported that pavement of streets, construction and repair of school buildings and street lighting works have been taken up with a fair degree of success. Success in bio-gas plants and smokeless *chulhas* has been limited. Many of the smokeless *chulhas* have been dismantled and their pipes used for alternate domestic purposes by the beneficiaries. Construction of low budget houses for the Scheduled Castes has to face constraints of availability of land and approach roads.

Though the demand for civic amenities is there, especially the need for proper drainage in the villages, the voluntary effort required of the villagers is usually not forthcoming. There is dependence on the Government, but the latter is not having the wherewithal to plan and execute such works to the extent that they are required.

Impact of Poverty Alleviation Programmes

Taking into account the successes and failures of the programmes, it must be admitted that the impact of most of these programmes is very limited and that, primarily on account of the limited financial resources. During the Seventh Plan period (1985-1990) the total expenditure incurred on Rural Development in Haryana was Rs. 7148 lakhs[6]. This works out to an average of Rs. 21,000 per annum for the 6759 villages of Haryana. Within this meagre amount not only were the poor to be directly assisted by way of subsidies under the IRDP, but employment generating community works had also to be taken up. The limitations of the programme become obvious. Even for the subsequent years the outlays have not been impressive. In the Annual Plan for 1993-94, the approved outlay for Rural Development was Rs. 1917 lakh. This works out to an average of Rs. 28,000 per annum for each village of Haryana. Wonders cannot be achieved with this level of investment. These programmes can only play a marginal, though an important role in providing some safety net for the poor, in the broad developmental dynamics of the state. So far as development of civic amenities of villages are concerned, these need a definite and independent focus and should not remain a byproduct of the poverty alleviation programmes.

Box 2.42

Local Employment Conditions in Guskani

The employment oriented programmes like the JRY provide employment to about 50 per cent of the village population. The labour rate is Rs. 70 for unskilled worker and Rs. 150 for the skilled worker. This is much higher than the national rate as fixed by the Government of India. It has however been noticed that some workers get lower wages when employed by contractors. Also workers belonging to the weaker sections receive lower wages as compared to the workers belonging to the upper castes. Members of SC and BC received wages of about Rs. 55 for both skilled and unskilled work. Persons belonging to these weaker sections are aware of this lower wage but they cannot do anything about it. The panchayat is hijacked by the dominant caste, i.e. the Jats. The SC and BC population is also much less. This creates a feeling of insecurity which is compounded by their landless position. [Suresh, 1997: Guskani (Rohtak)]

THE VILLAGE PANCHAYAT

The Village Panchayat system in its evolution is experiencing divisions on the basis of caste and politics. Now with reservation for women and the weaker sections under the Haryana Panchayati Raj Act, 1994, there are social processes at work hindering and strengthening the voice of these traditionally silent segments of society. Whereas real power still seems to be with males and the dominant castes, the balance of power is shifting. There are also questions of the funds required for undertaking village works. Dependence on state grants continues. The Panchayats have still not geared themselves for mobilizing local resources through fees and taxation. With the dependence for funds on the state agencies there is the corresponding dependence on state officials with regard to many of the processes for release of funds and verification of works. There is also the emergence of Village Development Committees for executing works under various state programmes. The comments of the probationers on these issues follow.

Box 2.43
The Panchayat in Kakana Bhadri

There is a separate Panchayat for village Kakana Bhadri. It has eight elected members including the Sarpanch. The post of Sarpanch was reserved for women this time, under the new Panchayati Raj Act. In fact, this is for the first time that village women are being represented in the Panchayat, which was till now a dominion of males only. Other than the Sarpanch there are two more female members of the Panchayat.

Most of the times, Sarpanches were from either of the two groups—Brahmins or Jats/Rajputs. However, in the last Panchayat elections, Sheela whose family was more or less neutral in political matters contested the elections and won against the wife of one of the ex-Sarpanches. It is, however, another matter that Sheela's husband also introduces himself as the Sarpanch and he too has become a type of power centre in village affairs.

However, the irony of the matter is that it is easier for Sheela to meet the officials and get her work done rather than trying to ensure order within the Panchayat and get some meaningful work done by it. The Panchayat is hopelessly divided, some of the members belonging to one of the ex-Sarpanch's group or to the other. In this situation the Scheduled Caste members find their position of critical importance as their's is the deciding vote. However, on very few occasions the matters come to voting stage. The effort usually is to do things by consensus. [Gupta, 1999: Kakana Bhadri (Sonipat)]

Box 2.44
Panchayat in Ransika

Though most of the respondents are aware of the existence and functions of the Panchayat and have even cast votes in the elections, they rarely ever approach the local body for any problem. Most of the respondents felt that there was no use of approaching the Panchayat. [Tayal, 2000: Ransika (Gurgaon)]

Box 2.45
Kherki Daula Panchayat

There are totally 12 members of the panchayat. The Sarpanch is a Harijan (Balmiki) as this panchayat was reserved for the SC candidates. The Sarpanch's name is Dev Karan and he is 55 years of age. He does not own any land and works either as farm labour or on some daily wage work. Out of the total strength of 12 of the village panchayat, there are 4 women and 4 members belonging to the SC. The details of other 11 members are as follows:

Name	*M/F*	*Age*	*Caste*	*Land Ownership*
Dinesh Kumar	M	30	Khati	landless
Kanta Devi	F	32	Ahir	2.5 acres
Chatter Singh	M	48	Ahir	3 acres
Harish Kumar	M	30	Ahir	2.5 acres
Azad Singh	M	32	Ahir	2 acres
Lila Ram	M	28	Harijan	landless
Bel Raj	M	32	Harijan	landless
Kamla	F	25	Harijan	landless
Ram Mehar	M	62	Ahir	3.5 acres
Sushila Devi	F	40	Ahir	3.5 acres
Krishna	F	30	Ahir	2 acres

There is no NGO or cooperative society in the village. All the developmental activities are done by the panchayats in which the Block Development Officer's role is central. Although a general meeting is called whenever an important decision regarding the welfare of the village has to be taken, but people generally do not participate, leaving the matter to be decided by the panchayat. It is very often the case that in the first meeting the quorum is not complete and hence, a second meeting has to be called. Then also the quorum is rarely complete and then finally, decisions are taken by whatever be the number of members that are present. [Singh, 1999: Kherki Daula (Gurgaon)]

Box 2.46
Composition and Functioning of Gram Panchayat Sikarpur

There is a separate panchayat for the village. Though there is reservation for the post of Sarpanch and other members for women and SC's in the whole state, but in the village there is no such reservation for the Sarpanch. The elections for panchayat were held on 12 March 2000. There is one Sarpanch and 10 other members from 10 wards of the village. The Sarpanch is 30 years old from Jat community. There are 3 female panchayat members out of which 2 belong to backward class Kumhar and one from Jat community. Out of 7 male panchayat members 4 belong to backward classes, 2 belong to Jat community and one from Scheduled Caste. Only four members of panchayat are holding land ranging from 1 to 5 acres and remaining six members are landless people, which shows the strengthening of democratic set up at grassroots level, i.e. in villages. Most of the members are in between 35 and 45 years of age.

Although the Panchayati Raj Institutions are working in the state since early sixties but before the new Haryana Panchayati Raj Act, 1994 came, there was no reservation for women. In the village panchayat there were 3 female members but they hardly visit the meeting of Panchayats. It is their husbands who enjoy all the respect and powers of their Panchayats.

Gram Panchayat is not functioning well, because, it is divided on political lines and many times it becomes very difficult to get a resolution passed and only few members show active participation in the developmental activities of the village.

The Panchayat is not financially sound as only Rs. 70,000 is generated through lease of Shamlat agricultural land and village pond. This amount is not sufficient for repairs and maintenance of various assets owned by the Gram Panchayat. The Panchayat also receives funds under DRDA for different developmental activities.

Apart from developmental functions a number of villagers approach the panchayat for help in case of old age pension, widow pension etc. The Panchayat also helps Social Welfare Department in smooth functioning of various activities of ICDS. Overall, one can say that the Panchayat is functioning as an important unit in the village but is not playing the desired role because of political reasons and lack of commitment on the part of its members towards social causes. [Agarwal, 2001: Sikarpur (Hisar)]

Box 2.47
Composition and Functioning of Gram Panchayat

The Mukhiya of the panchayat is a 56 year old male of the Sikligar caste which is a Scheduled Caste. This is not a reserved seat but since majority of the villagers are Sikligars, he is an active sarpanch who actively pursues the cause of the village. The composition of the panchayat is as follows:

Name	*Male/Female*	*Age*	*Caste*	*Land Ownership*
Shymo Devi	F	38	Brahmin	Yes
Ompal	M	32	Bairagi	Yes
Kala Devi	F	50	Valmiki	No
Vachitra Singh	M	35	Sikligar	No
Deep Kaur	F	53	Sikligar	No
Jagjeet Singh	M	37	Sikligar	No
Tahal Singh	M	51	Sikligar	Yes
Jeend Kaur	F	41	Sikligar	No

The meetings of the panchayat are held regularly and that of the panchayat sabha twice a year.

Although the Panchayati Raj institutions are working in the state since the sixties, there was no reservation for women or for the SC prior to the Haryana Panchayati Raj Act, 1994. In the village there are now 4 female members in the panchayat. However, they hardly ever attend the panchayat meetings. It is their husbands who tend to exercise the power in their behalf.

One of the weaknesses in the working of the panchayat is on account of the division of the panchayat along party lines. Many times it becomes difficult to get a resolution through. The panchayat is also divided on caste lines. The Sarpanch who is a Sikligar is busy getting schemes approved for his caste people as was evident in the selection of IAY list of beneficiaries. In fact the Sarpanch managed to bring a member of the SC Commission to the village and also got some grants approved by the Commission.

The income of the panchayat is not sufficient for repairs and maintenance of various assets owned by the Gram Panchayat. Of course, it receives funds from the DRDA under different development schemes. Apart from development functions, a number of villagers approach the panchayat for help in case of old age pension, widow pension etc. The panchayat also helps the Social Welfare Department in the smooth functioning of various activities of ICDS.

In short, one can say that although the panchayat is functioning as an important institution in the village, it is unable to play the desired role effectively because of political reasons and lack of commitment on the part of its members with regard to issues of public importance.

Village Development Committees

An important institution set up especially under the present government is the 'Vikas Samitis' or Village Development Committees. These committees are entrusted with the responsibilities of carrying out development works. The VDC is made up of three members from the panchayat, a lady member, a person from the Scheduled Caste and a former service personnel. The Sarpanch is the president of the committee. Funds for the works under the VDC are given under the HRDF (Haryana Rural Development Fund) and are announced by the Chief Minister in his "Sarkar Aapke Dwar Programme". Two of the members of the VDC are given the authority to withdraw the money. Technical assistance is provided by the Block Development and Panchayat Officer and the concerned SDO (Panchayati Raj). The same officers ensure audit of the funds. There were two works taken up by the VDC till date. There was the construction of the Shamshan Ghat at a cost of Rs. 30,000 and the pavement of the village ring road with bricks at a cost of Rs. 2,00,000. The quality of both the works was found to be satisfactory. [Yadav, 2002: Bibipur (Karnal)]

Box 2.48
Sources of Funds for Panchayat Bibipur

Source of Fund	*Amount collected during the financial year 2001-2002 in Rs.*
Auctioning of Panchayat land	75,500
House Tax	9,600
Sale of Material	25,000
Grant in Aid (State Government)	5,000

The Panchayat reserves the right to provide land from the Shamlat for developmental work if otherwise not available in the village. [Yadav, 2002: Bibipur (Karnal)]

Box 2.49
Panchayat Functioning in Guskani

The panchayat in the village is hijacked by the dominant caste of the village, i.e. the Jats. The Jats are numerically and economically the strongest segment in the village. The panchayat consists of 7 members out of which the Jats are 5. There are 2 female members who are also Jats. There is one person from the SC and one person from the BC. The role of the women and the weaker sections is virtually nil. The women are members of the panchayat in name only. For all practical purposes, the husbands of the female members are the real members. They are more active in all the panchayat meetings and forums. In fact the female members rarely participate in the meetings of the panchayat. Even if they do, they do so only after wearing a veil across their faces. As far as members of the weaker sections are concerned, they are mere rubber stamps. They cannot effectively articulate the interests of their community as they are too weak to do so.

As far as the general effectiveness of the panchayat is concerned, it is quite disappointing. Real power has not been conceded to the panchayats by the government. And in areas where they can be effective, they fail because of party politics and inability to take steps against the powerful. In the village I came across a situation where 8 acres of the panchayat land was encroached by the economically powerful persons and those quite close to the sarpanch and other panchayat members. Hence the panchayat would not initiate any action against them.

For panchayats to be really effective, there is a need for increased awareness among the people. For this, the most important thing is literacy and education. Issues like eradication of the caste system, increasing role and empowerment of women etc. are all rooted in increasing awareness levels of the people of the village. [Suresh, 1997: Guskani (Rohtak)]

CASE STUDIES

Case Study 1

A day in the life of a woman

Savitri Devi is a 45 year old lady from the SC colony in Ransika. She is mother of three children, two girls and one boy. The girls are 7 and 12 years old. The son is eight. Her husband Keshav is owner of a small agricultural holding. Less than two years ago Savitri's life was a mere tale of drudgery, the same as that of a woman in any other landless family. All that changed. She is now a member of the Self Help Group. The group has been in existence for just over a year and a half. There are 15 members in the group. They now have a saving of Rs. 20,000 and a NABARD direct bank linkage of Rs. 25,000. The group has taken 2 acres of land on lease in which they are cultivating fish. There is a perceptible level of empowerment that she exudes.

Savitri gets up at five in the morning and is off to the farm to work in the fields. After a short lunch she works right upto five in the evening. At six, she is back home. But her work for the day is not yet done. There is a meeting of her SHG to be attended. The meeting is at seven. Group accounts are taken stock of and savings for the day turned in. The Attendance Register, the Resolution Book and the Internal I, ending Registers are updated. A lot of this work is now done by Savitri and group members.

After the meeting, she gets back home and has her dinner. Sharp at half past eight she is at her Literacy Centre where her daughter, who is a matriculate, is the instructor. The class lasts an hour. It is only after this that Savitri gets time to relax at home.

Case Study 2

Social Status of a Dalit Family

Ravidas, his wife Gomti and two sons aged seven and nine years reside in the old SC quarters of Ransika. They belong to the *dhobi* caste. Both are deeply religious. Both are agricultural workers, though, to supplement his income Ravidas also runs a cycle repair shop in the lean season. Ravidas closely follows his sons' education. Although it is not accepted very overtly by the upper castes, it is evident that there is some distance between them and lower castes. The lower castes live in separate hamlet and do not mix a great deal with the upper ones. They have different sources of drinking water and different meeting places though both go to the same temple. There is also a marked difference between their economic status though there has been some improvement in the social status of the lower castes in the recent past.

Case Study 3

Employment Status of a Landless Agricultural Labourer

Ramsarup is from Ransika village. He is 35 years old. He is a Chamar by caste. He lives in the SC colony with his wife and two children. Both Ramsarup and his wife work as agricultural workers. His children, a son and a daughter aged 6 and 8 years respectively go to the local Primary School. The life of the village revolves around agriculture and so do the earnings of Ramsarup. The onset of the Kharif season in June brings backbreaking work for Ramsarup and his wife. Jointly they earn upto Rs. 180 per day in the peak of paddy transplantation: Ramsarup earning upto Rs. 100 per day. The process of transplantation is staggered and Ramsarup and his fellow labourers move from village to village in the soporific heat, working from six in the morning till five in the evening taking a break only for an hour for lunch. This work continues for a month and a half, from the beginning of June to the middle of July and by the end of it, Ramsarup has worked through a cluster of 15 villages. After this there is a lull. A new crop is being grown. Not much labour is required in this period. It is a lean period for Ramsarup. He has to scrounge for work. Wage rates dip. However, people prefer this period for hiring labour for various activities such as construction. Whenever they can find work Ramsarup makes up to Rs. 60 per day and his wife upto Rs. 40. In November, the crop is ready for harvesting. Ramsarup is once more in demand. Wage rates touch the transplantation time heights. By the end of November, harvesting is over. In December transplanting begins again and continues till the beginning of January. Ramsarup thus works for two months at a trot. Then the slack season hits him again. But Ramsarup doesn't need to wait too long. By the end of March it is harvesting time again. In a year Ramsarup's family can earn upto Rs. 30,000 if they are lucky but rarely less than Rs. 24,000. [Tayal, 2000: Ransika (Gurgaon)]

Case Study 4

A Study of the Poorest Person

It was difficult to identify the poorest person of the village. If the question was put to any person, he would start claiming himself to be the poorest one thinking that it would fetch some benefits from the government. However, after having stayed in the village for two days the situation became quite clear. There are two widow landless women in the village who were identified as the poorest persons of the village. Parvati, has a maturing son and he has started working as a labourer while Bhateri has three daughters only. Thus, we selected Bhateri for this study.

Bhateri, who belongs to a family of 4 brothers and 5 sisters, was married off to Kundan, a Kumhar by caste 17 years back. Her husband had no land but he worked as an agricultural labourer. He also had his traditional tools of carpenter and would earn some money by making bed posts, doors etc. for the residents of the village. However, just 4 years after their marriage, he fell ill and after 8 years of prolonged illness he died. He left behind himself, Bhateri, his wife and three daughters. Bhateri was left totally helpless.

Now, he does the job of filling drinking water in the pots at the local school. For this, she is paid Rs. 1800 per annum. The school pays this amount to her when the grant comes in the month of March/ April. Besides this, she gets widow pension from the government, which is Rs. 100 per month and is paid either every month or in two months. These are her only sources of regular income. Besides this, she works as construction labour/agricultural labour whenever the work is available. Two months back she married off her eldest daughter. For the wedding she had to spend Rs. 25,000 all of which she had to borrow. She borrowed Rs. 20,000 from local brahmin at an interest rate as high as 24 per cent. She also borrowed Rs. 5,000 from her own brother. Thus, she is already heavily indebted and she still has the burden of marrying off two more daughters.

She has not received any kind of help from the government till now. She says she would very much like to have a house of her own and wanted help under the IAY scheme, but the Panchayat has so far refused to help her out. [Misra, 1996: Kasumbhi (Bhiwani)]

CONCLUSIONS, RECOMMENDATIONS AND POLICY SUGGESTIONS MADE BY PROBATIONERS

These studies are full of impressions of young minds encountering the realities of village life. At the end of the study, they carry with them tentative conclusions regarding the usefulness of the study and about the prevailing realities. It is a fact that Haryana is forging ahead in urbanization and industrialization. The growth of centres like Panchkula, Faridabad and Gurgaon are pointers to the future development of the state. It is, therefore, natural for probationers to attach importance to these developments. However, Haryana continues to be dominated by villages. More than anything else it is agriculture and allied activities that constitute the backbone of economic and social life.

The important changes that are taking place are therefore in the power structure of rural life. The emergence of Panchayats with representation of weaker sections and women are leading to new interpretations of rural governance. The organisation of Self Help Groups is another innovation, which seems to promise empowerment. There is literacy, education and sanitation which continue to remain matters of concern. There are limitations of the wheat-paddy cycle that need to be broken. Suggestions on these and other related issues are contained in the narratives of the probationers that follow.

Box 2.50

Relevance of Poverty Alleviation Programmes and Their Study in Haryana

Haryana came into being only in the year 1966, as an independent state. Hitherto it had been merely a backward appendage of the state of Punjab. However, once having come into being the state has taken tremendous strides in the field of economic development especially agriculture. Haryana has been one of the pioneers in the field of modern

(Contd.)

Box 2.50 (Contd.)

agriculture and has been a harbinger of Green Revolution along with Punjab. The consequent prosperity has meant that household facilities such as cooking gas, channel television, vehicles (tractors, cars, etc.) have penetrated the village thereby increasing the disparity among the landless and landlords. This, however, is not to say that the condition of the poor has not improved in real terms. All the segments have gained from this overall prosperity, but quite expectedly more benefit has gone to those who own land. One more reason for this growth of demand for modem facilities is that many people from the village have either permanently migrated to nearby towns or they commute daily to these towns for work and when they visit their village, they try to provide their homes with such modern facilities.

Main source of light in the village is electricity. Out of the 54 houses surveyed, all of them are using electricity which includes households belonging to the SC also. In addition, some are using kerosene lantern/petromax also. Modern latrines and pit latrines are being used by more and more households but some still use open fields as place of defecation.

Poverty alleviation programmes such as IRDP, JRY, IAY, MWS etc. are not so relevant in the state of Haryana or Punjab as they may be in other states like UP, Bihar, MP, Andhra Pradesh, etc. This is so because the incidence of poverty is not as acute as it is in other states. Therefore, money, which is spent through such national schemes would be more efficaciously utilized if it were spent on larger projects that would have community as their focus rather than doling out aid to individuals. Most of the houses in the village belong to *pucca* or *kachha/pucca* category. The wage rate under JRY, EAS are so low as compared to the open market that nobody is willing to work under these schemes. Whenever some development work takes place under any of the above mentioned schemes, the labour has to be got from outside, as the villagers are generally not interested in the work because of the low wages. Therefore, the government officials too, have to devise ways and means to show in their records as to how the local labour has been used and how their payments are made. For example, what the government officials are doing is showing that the worker is paid for 2 days whereas he has worked for only one day.

(Contd.)

Box 2.50 (Contd.)

In the end one would like to make a suggestion to the course teams of future, that for states like Haryana and Punjab, instead of over-focusing on Poverty Alleviation Programmes, the survey or study should concern more with other developmental activities in the state or an area thereof. For example, two institutions have done commendable work in Haryana—the Haryana Urban Development Authority (HUDA) and the Haryana State Industrial Development Corporation (HSIDC). Such a study would be more relevant for an officer trainee who would be working in Haryana. [Singh, 1999: Kherki Daula (Gurgaon)

Box 2.51
Policy Suggestions

The villagers should be taught the importance of active participation in the meeting of Gram Sabha. Since now most of the funds are directed straight away to the Sarpanch, hence, it is the duty of the villagers to see that the developmental work is carried out properly and to restrain the Sarpanch from misusing his office for individual gains. The concept of democratic decentralization will only be successful through active participation. In this regard, since, VDCs, i.e. Village Development Committees, are responsible for execution of many developmental works in the villages, their training is needed for effective planning and efficient execution, so that, allocated resources can be used in an optimum manner. Even technical training to the members of VDCs is necessary to ensure better supervision of different work.

Regarding SHGs formation in the village under the SGSY Scheme for self-employment, all the banks, i.e. commercial, rural and co-operative, should play an important role in identification and execution of the scheme. Even the role of NGOs in this aspect cannot be ignored and they should also be involved in SHGs formation and supervision of different works. Even Anganwadi workers of ICDS need to be involved in motivation and monitoring of SHGs. SHGs are very necessary for generating self-employment in the villages and monitoring and recovery is also easy in this case. Even the chances of misuse of loans and subsidy is less in case of SHGs. It should be propagated in a big way by involving different agencies.

In the education sector, the adults should also be covered through provisions for adult education. The villagers should be taught about

(Contd.)

Box 2.51 (Contd.)

importance of education for girls also. Even a programme is needed for motivating the school teachers of the village so that they can perform their duty properly and help in nation building.

The villagers should also be taught the importance of sanitation for proper health as many water borne diseases can be taken care off by proper sanitation. They should also be discouraged from visiting the quacks for treatment. There is also need for augmenting their faith and confidence in government run sub-centres and PHCs.

The villagers must be explained at length that they must break the wheat-paddy cycle and diversify their products with better quality. The government is lifting wheat and paddy because of political reasons but the way the stocks are rotting in the godowns and even in the open market, the government may be reluctant in future to procure wheat and paddy. They should now diversify their crops and even more to allied sectors, i.e. animal husbandry, horticulture, floriculture, vegetables, food processing etc. The earlier they diversify their crops and activity better it would be for them. [Agarwal 2001: Sikarpur (Hisar)]

Box 2.52
Suggestions and Policy Recommendations

Functioning of Panchayats

Whereas the activities in the village suggest a high level of awareness among the villagers and the panchayat, due to the lack of institutional strength of the panchayat and accountability, this awareness instead of being channelised into productive energy is wasted on complaining. Most of the time the panchayat members have knowledge about their roles and the powers that they have for initiating works, however, they have little knowledge of how to operationalise the required works. They have to spend on the panchayat Secretary for record keeping and this allows a large loophole in the functioning of the panchayat, as it is generally alleged that the panchayat secretary or the Junior Engineer of the BDPO office engage labour and materials and take their commission. The sarpanch is either not aware or is a party to this kind of activity. Consequently the work executed is sometimes of inferior quality. This leads to an environment of distrust and inactivity. This is more true in the case of the VDC which is outside the purview

(Contd.)

Box 2.52 (Contd.)

of the normal system of panchayati raj in which there is a manner of removing the sarpanch and the dismissal of the panchayat under the Panchayat Act of 1994. The proper training and involvement of the people in the process of the panchayats is important for realizing the aim of taking democracy to the grassroots level. There is also a need for a proper grievance redressal mechanism to be put in place in the offices of the BDPO, the DDPO and the Deputy Commissioner.

Poverty Alleviation Programmes

The Self Help Groups despite their reaching the second stage are still not being run in the true spirit of the scheme, wherein they are expected to share the experience and also share the risk. Most of the times these groups are formed on *ad hoc* basis at the instance of the DRDA staff to have a speedier compliance report. This *adhocism* often leads to a failure of the group at a later stage when they are unable to complete their first or second grading. The groups do not share the experiences and the expertise gained in the activities. There are no regular meetings and the repayment is done at the risk of the individual. To counter this, firstly, the information base of the needy persons has to be strengthened. After the applications are received and the groups are formed, there has to be a coordinated effort by the DRDA, the commercial bands, the BDPO office and most importantly by the panchayat and the Gram Sabha.

The selection under IAY should be made more transparent and the houses need to be made on the basis of the individual preferences and the ground conditions in the area. Also, in places where there is a mass housing problem, instead of recommending individual cases, a comprehensive plan should be prepared so that the problem can be handled effectively. This would ensure a planned growth of housing along with fewer disgruntled elements in the society.

Education

The problem faced acutely by the teachers and the education system in the village was on account of the migratory nature of the population, especially the Sikligars, who leave the village along with their entire family. This leads to repeated breaks in the education of the children and consequent dropouts. Also there was a shortage of teachers because of the remoteness of the place. Many of the teachers were not found in the village. The one who were more regular was from the adjoining village. One of the teachers was on deputation to another primary school.

(Contd.)

Box 2.52 (Contd.)

There was lack of basic civic amenities in the school. The drinking water from the hand pump was not hygienic. The sanitary toilets in the school were being built under the Rural Sanitation Project. The mid-day meal scheme is not being run properly. The food grains are stored in the custody of the head teacher and are distributed to the children at the end of the month. Most of the time the father collects the foodgrain and sells it in the market. While the idea behind the scheme was to prevent dropouts and improve the nutritional status of the students by providing them a cooked mid-day meal, the implementation got derailed.

Health

The dependency of the people on private medical practitioners and quacks indicate the level of dissatisfaction with the existing government medical system. The wide network of PHCs and its sub-centres have to be strengthened. This would mean providing maintenance support for this infrastructure. The World Bank and European Commission have begun providing funds in this area. This could go a long way in bridging the gap. This is also an opportunity to come up with new ideas like setting up of regular mobile units which could go to the villages for regular check-ups. These units could provide good training to the doctors and also be effective in reaching out to the people. The immunization programme under the Pulse Polio campaign was very successful. This shows the effectiveness of involving the people and the effect that a campaign has when taken to the doorsteps of the people.

Agriculture

The agricultural sector has been witnessing regular progress in the areas of input management and introduction of technology. Modern agricultural equipments like combine harvesters and threshers are commonly seen. However, the area of finance and insurance remains to a large extent unaddressed despite various schemes like Kisan Credit Card. For example, during the summer months there are lots of fires in which standing crops are destroyed. There are no insurance scheme to cover such accidents and losses. Also the credit flow is too low to meet the requirements of the farmers. Most important expenditures are on social occasions. These lead the farmers into the clutches of the *Arhaties* or the middlemen in the *mandis* who practically act like money lenders.

(Contd.)

Box 2.52 (Contd.)

There is also a need to set up a cold storage system in the nearby towns so that farmers could diversify into cash crops and increase their incomes. The need for strengthening the agricultural extension system is also important. The role of social forestry and farm forestry needs to be highlighted. The soil in the area is sandy-clayey, quite suitable for cultivation of trees on the boundaries of the fields. [Yadav, 2002: Bibipur (Karnal)]

Box 2.53

Natural Resources/Common Resources and People's Needs, Problems and Solutions

From the data collected during the survey, it is clear that people are aware of their voting rights but people's participation is somewhat poor in development works and people are not much keen on the activities of panchayat. They feel their job is done once they have elected their representatives. In any case a large number of SC respondents felt that since the panchayat was heavily dominated by the Ahirs, their voice is rarely heard. In the village there is no concentrated effort of the villagers to develop and protect common resources for the benefit of the entire community. Most the common panchayat land is under illegal possession especially the so-called "*raaste*" or the common ways and path ways. The sarpanch's role in this is negligible, since the poor man is helpless as he cannot force the higher caste people to relent and vacate the encroached lands.

One of the felt needs of the people is to have a PHC in the village, because the nearest medical facility available is some 11 kms. away. This has been a long standing demand of the village but so far no action has been taken on it.

It has been more than thirty years since this village was electrified, still the quality of power supply as in the rest of rural Haryana is very poor. It needs to be mentioned, however, that this village is among the major defaulting villages in this region as regards the payment of electricity dues. Though electricity to rural areas is supplied at a very nominal rate yet the people have defaulted over a number of years and now the situation has come to a pass where some of the farmers' electricity bills run into tens of thousands of rupees and obviously there is a reluctance to pay up. How the state government gets the people to pay their dues is not just an administrative but a political

(Contd.)

Box 2.53 (Contd.)

problem and this problem has to be solved on an urgent basis as the Haryana State Electricity Board is in financial crisis due to the populist decisions of the successive state governments and the World Bank aided reform programme in the electricity sector will be derailed if the government cannot ensure compliance in this regard. [Misra, 1996: Kasumbhi (Bhiwani)]

Annexure A

Statement of Socio-Economic Surveys Conducted by IAS Probationers of the Haryana Cadre Between 1983 and 1994

District	*Year*	*Village*	*Probationer*
Bhiwani	1996	Kasumbhi	Shyamal Misra
Faridabad	1994	Silakhari	A.K. Gupta
Gurgaon	2000	Ransika	Deepak Tayal
Gurgaon	1999	Kherki Daula	Brijendra Singh
Hisar	2001	Sikarpur	Pankaj Agrawal
Karnal	2002	Bibipur	Nitin Yadav
Rohtak	1997	Guskani	D. Suresh (U.T. Cadre)
Sonipat	1999	Kakana Bhadri	Rakesh Gupta

NOTES

1. Director of Agriculture and Director of Land Records, Government of Haryana.
2. Derived from *Statistical Pocket Book of India (1992),* Government of India and *Statistical Handbook of Haryana (1991-92),* Government of Haryana.
3. Derived from Gupta, D.P., *Agricultural Development in Haryana* (1985).
4. *Statistical Pocket Book of India (1992),* Government of India.
5. *Agricultural Census (1985-86),* Government of India.
6. *Statistical Handbook of Haryana (1991-92),* Government of Haryana.

3

Himachal Pradesh

H.R. SHARMA and VIRENDER KUMAR

INTRODUCTION

The state of Himachal Pradesh came into existence as a part of C states on 15th April, 1948, consequent to the amalgamation of 30 Punjab and Shimla hill states into the Indian Union. Its total area was 27,168 square kilometres which subsequently increased to 28,335 square kilometres in 1954 with the merger of neighbouring Bilaspur state. The state's territorial area, however, increased substantially in 1966 when as a result of re-organisation of Punjab four more hilly districts, namely Shimla, Kangra, Kullu, and Lahaul & Spiti along with some more areas such as Nalagarah tehsil of Ambala district, some parts of Hoshiarpur district and Dalhausie of Gurdaspur district were merged with the state. The state attained full statehood on 25th January, 1971. Geographically, it is located between 30° 22′ 40″ to 33° 12′ 20″ north latitude and 75° 45′ 55″ to 79° 04′ 20″ east longitudes and share boundaries with Jammu & Kashmir in north, Punjab in the west, Haryana in the south and Uttar Pradesh in south-east. Its altitude ranges from 350 metres to 6975 metres above the mean sea level and is endowed with myriad of climatic niches. The area available for cultivation is 11 per cent of the total geographical area, out of which around 17 per cent is under irrigation. The small and marginal holdings (less than 2 hectares), account for about 85 per cent of the total holdings, and the average size of holdings is 1.16 hectares. Administratively, the state has been divided into twelve districts, 75 tehsils, 34 sub-tehsils and 72 community development blocks (Table 3.1).

Table 3.1: Administrative Profile of Himachal Pradesh—2001

Sl. No.	*Particulars*	*Nos.*
1.	No. of districts	12
2.	No. of Sub-divisions	52
3.	No. of Tehsils	75
4.	No. of Sub-tehsils	34
5.	No. of C D Blocks	75
6.	No. of Villages: Inhabited	16,997
	Uninhabited	2,391
	Total villages	19,388
7.	No. of Gram Panchayats	3,037
8.	No. of Assembly constituencies	68
9.	No. of Towns	57
10.	No. of Municipal Committees/Corporations	21
11.	No. of Nagar Panchayats	24
12.	No. of Cantonments	7

Source: Districts in Figures, 2002, H.P (Pamphlet), Department of Economics and Statistics, Government of Himachal Pradesh, Shimla.

Agro-climatically, the state has been divided into four zones keeping in view the altitude, rainfall, temperature, humidity and topography. The salient features of the four agro-climatic zones have been given in Table 3.2. As it may be seen from the table, while maximum geographical area of the state falls under high hills and temperate dry zone (Zone-IV), the highest percentage of cropped area is in the mid-hills and sub-humid zone (Zone-II). Likewise, the maximum precipitation is experienced in Zone-II which ranges from 1500 to 3000 mm per annum. The salient features of different zones have been briefly described below.

(i) Sub-montane and Low Hills Subtropical Zone (Zone-I)

The soils of this zone are productive, if fertilized. The textured of the soil varies from loamy to sandy loam. The average rainfall is 110 cm of which 80 per cent is received during July to September. The farming is rainfed as only 16.6 per cent of total area is under irrigation. The main crops are maize, rice and wheat but other crops like potato, ginger and sugarcane are also grown in some areas as cash crops. Citrus, mango and litchi are important fruit crops.

Table 3.2: Salient Features of Agro-Climatic Zones of Himachal Pradesh

Particulars	*Sub-montane Low Hills Zone (Zone-I)*	*Mid-hills High Humid Zone (Zone-II)*	*High Hills Temperate Wet Zone (Zone-III)*	*High Hills Temperate Dry Zone (Zone-IV)*
Geographical Area (000 ha)	913.2 (16.4)	1183.2 (21.3)	1280.9 (23.0)	2190.0 (39.0)
Total Cropped Area	355.1 (38.0)	383.4 (41.0)	171.8 (18.4)	24.0 (2.6)
Elevation	Below 650 metres (above mean sea level)	650-1800 metres (above mean sea level)	1800-2200 metres (above mean sea level)	2200 metres and above (above mean sea level)
Soil *p*H	Neutral, Coarse Texture	Acidic, Coarse Texture	Acidic in reaction shallow in depth and sloppy	Neutra! reaction Coarse Texture
Rainfall	About 1000 mm	1500-3000 mm	About 1000 mm	250 mm
Field Crops	Rice maize, wheat and pulses	Rice, maize, wheat, barley, pulses	Maize, potato and wheat, off-season vegetables	Barley, potato wheat and off-season vegetables
Fruits	Sub-tropical fruits	Apple, other temperate fruits, stone fruits, nuts and sub-tropical fruits, particularly mango and litchi	Apple, other temperate fruits and nuts	Nuts, dry fruits and apple
Percentage of irrigated area	16.6	17.5	7.8	40.6

Source: National Agricultural Research Project, Report of the ICAR Review Committee, Indian Council of Agricultural Research, Krishi Bhavan, New Delhi, July 1982, p. 47.

(ii) Mid-hills Sub-humid Zone (Zone-II)

The texture of the soils in Zone-II is loam to clay loam. These are deficient in nitrogen and phosphorus and have poor water and nutrient holding capacity. The area from Dharamshala to Jogindernagar in the foothills of Dhauladhar ranges receives rainfall as high as 3000 mm most of which comes between mid-June to mid-September. In the remaining areas, it is around 150 mm. While maize, rice, wheat, potato, pulses and oilseeds are major field crops, stone and citrus fruits are important fruit crops. The area under irrigation is only 17.5 per cent and *kuhls* (gravitational flow channels) are the important source of irrigation.

(iii) Mid-hills Temperate Dry Zone (Zone-III)

The soils of this zone are shallow in depth, acidic in reaction and silt loam to loam in texture. These are deficient in nitrogen and phosphorus. The average rainfall is 1000 mm most of which is received during the monsoon season. The zone is suitable for growing horticultural crops, particularly apple, plum and apricot. Recently, the cultivation of off-season vegetable crops like peas, cabbage, cauliflower and tomato has gained ground in some areas.

(iv) High Hills Temperate Dry Zone (Zone-IV)

The soils of the zone are mainly sandy loam, neutral to alkaline in reaction and have low fertility. This zone has the highest per cent of irrigated area (40.6 per cent). The important crops include potato, barley, buck wheat, peas and minor millets. The area is particularly suitable for growing off-season vegetables and seed production. In general, only one crop can be grown during the whole of the agricultural year because of heavy snowfall in winter from November to April. The details of the districts and tehsils falling under different agro-climatic zones are given in Table 3.3.

The economic development in general and agricultural development in particular, in the mountainous regions is circumscribed by the mountain specificities, namely, inaccessibility, marginality, fragility, niche and human adaptation mechanism created by unique vertical dimensions that distinguish them from the plains and other eco-systems. While the first three specificities contribute in varying degrees, among other things, to physical isolation, distance and high transportation costs, the latter two indicate positive features and the potential for agricultural development. The development strategy followed by the state over the years has explicitly taken into consideration the above-mentioned mountain specificities. The state has thus succeeded in transforming the living conditions of its people

Table 3.3: Districts and Tehsils in Different Agro-Climatic Zones

Agro-Climatic Zones	*Areas*	*Height Above Mean Sea Level (metres)*
Sub-montane low hills sub-tropical (Zone-I)	Una, Bilaspur and Hamirpur districts and parts of Sirmaur, Kangra, Solan and Chamba districts	Upto 650
Mid-hills sub-humid (Zone-II)	Palampur and Kangra tehsils of district Kangra, Rampur tehsil of Shimla district and parts of Mandi, Solan, Kullu, Chamba and Sirmaur districts	651-1800
High hills temperate wet (Zone-III)	Shimla district (except Rampur tehsil) parts of Kullu, Solan, Chamba, Mandi, Kangra and Sirmaur districts	1800-2200
High hills temperate dry (Zone-IV)	Kinnaur, Lahaul & Spiti districts and parts of Chamba district	Above 2200

Source: National Agricultural Research Project, Report of the ICAR Review Committee, Indian Council of Agricultural Research, Krishi Bhavan, New Delhi, July 1982, p. 51.

since its formation, when it was considered as one of the least developed regions in the country (Sharma, 1987)[1] . Commenting upon the socio-economic transformation and its impact of the quality of life, Dreze and Sen in their recent book write, 'Fifty years or so down the lane, living conditions in Himachal Pradesh seem to have been radically transformed for the better.' They further write, 'The experience of Himachal Pradesh illustrates an important feature of contemporary development patterns in India, namely, that examples of positive achievements are not confined to the well known case of Kerala' (Dreze and Sen, 2002: 102 and 110). The development strategy pursued in the state has come to be recognized as a model especially for other mountainous states not only in India but also in the whole of Hindukush Himalayan region.

Against this background, the present paper briefly discusses different aspects of socio-economic transformation in the state such as changes in the demographic profile, access to infrastructural facilities including health and education, agricultural development and crop diversification, land reforms and land distribution structure, rural farm and non-farm employment, factors that facilitated the process of socio-economic transformation, the emerging challenges and possible solutions and the important lessons that follow from development experience of the state.

Trends in Population

The population of the state has increased from 34,60,434 in 1971 to 60,70,305 in 2001, registering an annual compound growth rate of 1.90 per cent per annum (Table 3.4). The total population consisted of 30,80,781 males and 29,89,524 females; around 90 per cent of the population lives in rural areas. The sex ratio is 968 females per one thousand of males. The population of the state has registered a decadal growth rate of 23.04 per cent during the seventies, 20.79 per cent during the eighties and 17.39 during the nineties. The population

Table 3.4: Demographic Profile of Himachal Pradesh, 1971-2001

Sl. No.	*Particulars*	*Year*			
		1971	*1981*	*1991*	*2001*
1.	Total Population	3460434	4280818	5170877	6070305
	Male	1766957	2169931	2617467	3080781
	Female	1693477	2110887	2553410	2989524
2.	Rural Population	3218544	3954847	4721681	5475424
	Male	1628623	1988331	2372193	2749776
	Female	1589921	1966516	2349488	2725648
3.	Urban Population	241890	325971	449196	594881
	Male	138334	181600	245274	331005
	Female	103556	144371	203922	263876
4.	Sex Ratio (Females per 1000 males)	958	973	976	968
5.	Population Density (Persons/sq. km)	62	77	93	109
6.	Urbanisation (%)	7.0	7.61	8.69	9.79
7.	SC Population (Per cent of total population)	22.24	24.62	25.34	—
8.	ST Population (Per cent of total population)	4.09	4.61	4.22	—

Source: Statistical Outline of H.P. 1971 (pp. 18, 20, 21, 37, 39); 1985 (pp.8, 10-12, 22, 23, 25, 27); 1995 (pp. 6, 22 to 25) and 2002-03 (pp. 6, 20, 21, 39, 40), Directorate of Economics and Statistics, Government of Himachal Pradesh, Shimla.

density is 109 persons per square kilometre. Further, according to 1991 census, while the Scheduled Caste population accounted for around one-fourth of the total population, the per cent share of Scheduled Tribe Population was 4.22 per cent.

Access to Infrastructural Facilities

The extent of infrastructural development in the state has been brought out in Table 3.5. The table shows that the availability of basic amenities like hospital beds, safe drinking water and electricity is much higher in the state compared to the all-India average. The number of educational institutions, health centres and post offices per lakh of population is also much higher in the state. The road length per sq. km is, however, low mainly because of difficult mountain terrain and resultantly much higher cost of building roads.

The distance-wise availability of basic facilities like roads, bus stop, banks, post office, telegraph office, etc. to different villages has been brought by the data thrown up by the NSS 58th round. The per cent distribution of villages according to the distance-wise availability of different infrastructural facilities has been provided in Table 3.6 and Table 3.7. Table 3.6 shows that around four-fifths of the villages have got access to metalled road and more than three-fourths of the villages to the all weather road within a distance of five kilometres. Likewise, around ninety per cent of the villages have got access to post office and fifty per cent to fertilizer/pesticide shops again within a distance five kilometres. More than ninety per cent of the villages have also got access to fair price shop within the distance of five kilometres. The information about the access to education and health related facilities to different villages in terms of the distance has been provided in Table 3.7. As may be seen from the table, more than eighty per cent of the villages in the state have got access to the primary school within two kilometres, while for the remaining twenty per cent of the villages have got this facility at a distance of less than five kilometres. Likewise, more than ninety-five per cent of the villages have got middle school at a distance of less than five kilometres. So far health facilities were concerned, the table shows that while around ninety per cent of the villages have got access to dispensary within a distance of five kilometres, the access to primary health centre was available to more than fifty per cent of the villages within the distance of five kilometres.[2]

Table 3.5: Selected Indicators of Infrastructural Development: Himachal Pradesh *vis-à-vis* All-India Average

Sl. No.	*Indicator*	*Unit*	*Himachal Pradesh*	*All-India*
1.	Hospital beds per million persons, (1991-98*)	No.	1663	926
2.	Proportion of rural households having access to safe drinking water (1991)	%	77	64
3.	Proportion of households with electricity connection (1998-99)	%	94	60
4.	Road length per 100 sq. km. (1996)	km	44.30	73.00
5.	Telephone per 100 sq. km. (2000)	No.	5.20	8.70
6.	Telephone per 100 population (2000)	No.	4.30	2.90
7.	Proportion of ever married women aged 15-49 exposed to any media (1998-99)	%	84	60
8.	Primary health centres (1997-98)	No/lakh of pop.	5.00	—
9.	Primary schools (1997-98)	No/lakh of pop.	138.65	—
10.	Middle/high school (1997-98)	No/lakh of pop.	18.60	—
11.	Post offices (1997-98)	No/lakh of pop.	49.35	—
12.	Bank branches (1997-98)	No/lakh of pop.	12.75	7.70
13.	Agricultural credit societies (1996-97)	No/lakh of pop.	35.11	9.06
14.	Non-Agricultural credit societies (1996-97)	No/lakh of pop.	5.56	3.73

*Latest for the year for which the data are available within the period 1991-98.

Source: (i) Shariff and Ghosh (2000) and *Economic and Political Weekly* (2001).

(ii) Statistical Appendix in Dreze Jean and Amartya Sen (2002), *India: Development and Participation*, Oxford University Press, New Delhi.

(iii) Government of Himachal Pradesh (1999), *Statistical Outline of Himachal Pradesh*, Directorate of Economics and Statistics, Government of Himachal Pradesh, Shimla.

(iv) International Institute for Population Sciences (2002), *National Family Health Survey India, 1998-99, Himachal Pradesh*, Bombay.

(v) Himachal Pradesh, *Human Development Report*, 2001.

INDICATORS OF SOCIAL DEVELOPMENT

The indicators of social development in the state *vis-à-vis* all-India are given in Table 3.8. The table shows that despite difficult mountain terrain and associated constraints, the state has performed better in comparison to the all-India level. Most of the indicators such as infant mortality rate, total fertility rate, proportion of children who have been vaccinated, death rate, life expectancy, proportion of births attended by health professionals, and so on attest a better performance of the state as compared to the all-India average.

Table 3.6: Distribution of Villages by Distance from the Nearest General Facilities in Himachal Pradesh, 2002

(Per cent)

Sl. No.	*Facility*	*Within village*	*Less than 2 km*	*2 km to less than 5 km*	*5 km to less than 10 km*	*10 km or more*	*Total*
1.	Panchayat headquarters	22.50	47.70	21.30	4.80	3.7	100
2.	Tehsil headquarters	—	2.30	5.50	28.20	63.90	100
3.	District headquarters	—	3.00	—	1.80	97.90	100
4.	Railway station	—	1.40	1.80	2.60	94.20	100
5.	Bus stop	49.10	13.70	30.0	3.50	3.40	100
6.	Metalled road	39.70	12.30	27.40	15.00	5.60	100
7.	All weather road	49.60	13.60	13.60	2.90	20.30	100
8.	Post office	21.60	34.00	36.00	3.90	4.40	100
9.	Telegraph office/PCO/ e-mail	25.30	19.40	35.80	4.60	14.90	100
10.	Bank	5.30	12.50	39.40	15.70	27.10	100
11.	Veterinary hospital	18.00	20.00	44.50	11.20	6.20	100
12.	Fertiliser/pesticide shop	14.90	17.20	21.10	25.20	21.60	100
13.	Fair price shop	31.80	22.40	39.60	2.70	3.50	100
14.	Market/weekly market	20.10	9.80	19.10	12.70	38.40	100

Source: Report on Village Facilities, National Sample Survey, 58th Round, 2002, NSS Report No. 487, Table 1, p. 7.

Likewise, indicators related to the extent of female literacy, access to education for children of different income and social groups, share of expenditure on education including elementary education in the net state domestic product and per capita expenditure on education and health suggest better performance in comparison to the

Table 3.7: Distribution of Villages by Distance from the Nearest Education and Health Related Facilities in Himachal Pradesh, 2002

(Per cent)

Sl. No.	*Facility*	*Within village*	*Less than 2 km*	*2 km to less than 5 km*	*5 km to less than 10 km*	*10 km or more*	*Total*
Education							
1.	Pre-primary school	49.20	20.10	18.50	—	12.20	100
2.	Primary school	56.20	25.30	18.50	—	—	100
3.	Middle school	29.20	25.20	41.60	3.90	—	100
4.	Secondary school	16.00	20.80	46.40	10.50	6.30	100
5.	Higher secondary school/junior college	2.60	11.40	43.40	24.70	17.80	100
6.	College with degree course	—	2.30	3.30	14.10	80.60	100
7.	Industrial training institute	2.00	2.30	4.40	4.90	88.10	100
8.	Non-formal education centre (NEFC)	7.00	4.00	—	—	98.90	100
Health							
1.	Integrated child development service centre (anganwadi/balwadi)	51.50	14.20	32.90	1.40	—	100
2.	Sub-centre/dispensary	24.40	27.90	36.40	6.30	5.00	100
3.	Primary health centre	7.80	8.10	37.90	19.60	26.60	100
4.	Community health centre/government hospital	2.00	5.80	26.70	14.20	53.00	100
5.	Private hospital	2.00	3.00	9.10	10.90	79.50	100
6.	Private clinic/doctor	9.40	16.20	25.70	8.90	39.90	100
7.	Medicine shop	11.10	11.60	39.90	13.10	24.30	100

Source: Report on Village Facilities, National Sample Survey, 58th Round, 2002, NSS Report No. 487.

performance at the all-India level. As alluded to above, the state has also recorded a much lower decadal population growth (1991-2001), 17.53 per cent compared with 21.34 per cent at the all-India level.

INDICATORS OF ECONOMIC DEVELOPMENT

The easy availability of health, education and other infrastructural facilities has led to a substantial improvement in the living conditions of the people manifested, *inter alia,* in low incidence of poverty in all its manifestations like magnitude, depth and severity, high per capita household expenditure and its growth, daily real wage earnings

Table 3.8: Selected Indicators of Social Development in Himachal Pradesh *vis-à-vis* All-India Average

Sl. No.	*Indicator*	*Unit*	*Himachal Pradesh*	*All-India*
1.	Infant mortality rate (1997-99) (Per 1000 births)	NO.	63	71
2.	Total fertility rate (1996-98)	%	2.4	3.3
3.	Decadal population growth (1991 to 2001)	%	17.53	21.34
4.	Proportion of young children who have received	%	83	42
	All vaccinations		71	30
	At least one dose of vitamin A (1998-99)			
5.	Proportion of births attended by health professional, (1998-99)	%	40	42
6.	Proportion of mothers who know about ORS, (1998-99)	%	93.00	62.00
7.	Proportion of households using adequately iodised salt, (1998-99)	%	91	40
8.	Life expectancy at birth (1998-99)	Yrs		
	Female		65.2	61.8
	Male		64.6	60.4
9.	Death rate per 1000 (1997-99)	%	7.70	8.90
10.	Birth rate per 1000 (1997-99)	%	23.00	26.60
11.	Female male ratio, (2001)		970	933
12.	Proportion of child population (0-6) in total population (2001)	%		
	Male		13.34	15.47
	Female		12.32	15.36
	Person		12.84	15.42
13.	Proportion of women aged 20-24 married before 18 (1998-99)	%	11	50
14.	Proportion of currently married women who are practicing contraceptives, (1998-99)	%	68	48
15.	Literacy rate (2001) Female	%	68	54
	Male		86	76
	Persons		77	65
16.	Proportion of children attending school, (1998-99)	%		
	Female		97	74
	(6 to 14 yrs) Male		99	83
17.	Female school attendance in the 6-17 age group (1998-99)	%	93	66
18.	Proportion of children aged 6-14 who have been to school (1993-94)	%		
	By income group Low income		91.00	65.00
	Lower-middle income		96.00	75.00

(*Contd.*)

Table 3.8 (Contd.)

Sl. No.	*Indicator*		*Unit*	*Himachal Pradesh*	*All-India*
		Upper middle income		95.00	81.00
		High income		90.00	87.00
	By social groups	Caste Hindu		93.00	72.00
		Scheduled caste/tribe		88.00	62.00
		Muslims		80.00	62.00
	By gender	Female		90.00	65.00
		Male		96.00	77.00
19.	Share of expenditure in education and elementary education in NSDP (1995-96)		%	7.3	3.8
20.	Share of elementary education expenditure in NSDP (1995-96)		%	3.8	1.8
21.	Share of elementary education expenditure in total education expenditure, (1997-98)		%	52.1	47.4
22.	Growth rate of real per capita expenditure on elementary education (1990-91/ 1997-98)		%/yr.	3.3	1.4
23.	Per capita expenditure on education, (1997-98)		Rs.	995.92	—
24.	Per capita expenditure on health, (1997-98)		Rs.	294.95	—

Source: (i) Shariff and Ghosh (2000) and *Economic and Political Weekly* (2001).

(ii) Statistical Appendix in Dreze Jean and Amartya Sen (2002), *India: Development and Participation*, Oxford University Press, New Delhi.

(iii) Government of Himachal Pradesh (1999), *Statistical Outline of Himachal Pradesh*, Directorate of Economics and Statistics, Government of Himachal Pradesh, Shimla

(iv) International Institute for Population Sciences (2002), *National Family Health Survey India, 1998-99, Himachal Pradesh*, Bombay.

(v) Deaton Angus and Jean Dreze (2002), 'Poverty and Inequality in India: A Re-examination', *Economic and Political Weekly*, Vol. XXXVII, No. 36, pp. 3729-3748.

(vi) Chadha, G. K. and P.P. Sahu (2002), 'Post Reform Setbacks in Rural Employment: Issues that Need Further Scrutiny', *Economic and Political Weekly*, Vol. XXXVII, No. 21, pp. 1998-2026.

(vii). Sharma, H.R. (2001), 'Employment and Wage Earnings of Agricultural Labourers', *The Indian Journal of Labour Economics*, Vol. 44, No. 1, pp. 27-38.

(*Contd.*)

Table 3.8 (Contd.)

(viii) Himachal Pradesh, Human Development Report, 2001

(ix) Sharma, H.R. (2000), 'Agrarian Structure and Agricultural Development: Emerging Trends and Patterns', *Man and Development*, Vol. XXII, No. 2. pp. 22-41.

---

of agricultural labourers, and so on (Table 3.9). Further, in 1999-2000 while the state accounted for 0.1 per cent of total very poor households in the country, the share of very poor in total poor households in the state was 16.7 per cent. The high female labour force participation rates in the state appeared to have played an important role in influencing many other facets of social development such as high female literacy, low female death rates, low child mortality rate, and so on. Yet another set of economic indicators like the proportion of households having no cultivated land, proportion of agricultural labourers in total workers, proportion of asset poor households, Gini co-efficient of per capita consumer expenditure and Gini co-efficient of distribution of ownership and operational holdings point towards a relatively egalitarian economic structure compared with many other north Indian states. The relatively egalitarian economic structure of the society enabled people of all hues to participate in the transformation process thus fostering growth with equity and a process of widely shared economic development. In sum, the low incidence of poverty and the better availability of educational, health and other infrastructural facilities in the state stand in sharp contrast to the situation prevailing in other mountainous regions in India and abroad, including those of China where poverty, inequality and deprivations are endemic.[3] This also provides a contrast with the situation prevailing in the state during the fifties and the early sixties when it was widely, like many other regions in India, considered as an extremely backward state.

It, however, needs to be mentioned that all the regions/districts of the state do not have equal access to infrastructural facilities and are not equally developed. While some districts have performed better, others lag behind. The inter-district variations in different aspects of some indicators of socio-economic transformation like net state domestic product and its growth over time, and the availability of

Table 3.9: Selected Indicators of Economic Development in Himachal Pradesh *vis-à-vis* All-India Average

Sl. No.	*Indicator*	*Unit*	*Himachal Pradesh*	*All-India*
1.	Proportion of poor (1999-2000) Head Count Ratio	%	7.5	26.80
	Poverty gap Index		1.0	5.20
2.	Incidence of extremely poor, (1999-2000) Rural	%	0.00	0.8
3.	Incidence of very poor, (1999-2000) Rural	%	1.3	8.2
4.	Incidence of moderately poor, (1999-2000) Rural	%	6.2	18.3
5.	Average household expenditure per capita (1999-2000)	Rs./m	740	589
6.	Growth rate of real per capita state domestic product (1992-93 to 1998-99)	%/ yr.	4.6	4.4
7.	Annual growth of per capita expenditure (1993-94 to 1999-2000)	%	5.06	4.36
8.	Gini co-efficient of per capita consumer expenditure, (1999-2000)		0.10	0.18
9.	Proportion of rural households not owning any agricultural land (1992-93)	%	16	36
10.	Proportion of asset-poor households (1992-93)	%	7.0	40.0
11.	Gini co-efficient of ownership holdings, (1991-92)		0.60	0.71
12.	Gini co-efficient of operational holdings, (1991-2)		0.54	0.64
13.	Proportion of agricultural labourers in rural population (1991)	%	1.0	11.0
14.	Daily real wage earnings of agricultural labourers (1980-81=100) Male	Rs/D	10.82	7.62
	Female		8.85	5.42
15.	Proportion of population receiving subsidized foodgrains from the public distribution system (1993-94)	%	45	27
16.	Per capita consumption of foodgrains obtained through public distribution in rural areas (1993-94)	Kg/yr	31.8	30.0
17.	Growth rate of number of rural enterprises (1990-98)	%	2.63	2.27
18.	Growth rate of workers in rural enterprises (1990-98)	%	2.73	2.15
19.	Proportion of every married women (15 to 49 yrs) who have access to money (1998-99)	%	80	60

(Contd.)

Table 3.9 (Contd.)

Sl. No.	Indicator	Unit	Himachal Pradesh	All-India
20.	Rural workforce structure (1999-2000)	%		
	Agriculture Rural male		71.40	71.40
	Rural female		96.10	86.30
	Non-Agriculture Rural male		44.70	28.60
	Rural female		4.90	13.70
21.	Rural labour force participation rates (1999-2000)	%		
	Male		54.60	54.00
	Female		47.40	30.20
	Persons		50.90	42.30
22.	Rural workforce participation rates (1999-2000)	%		
	Male		98.20	98.30
	Female		99.40	99.00
	Persons		98.80	98.60

Source: (i) Shariff and Ghosh (2000) and *Economic and Political Weekly* (2001).

(ii) Statistical Appendix in Dreze Jean and Amartya Sen (2002), *India: Development and Participation*, Oxford University Press, New Delhi.

(iii) Government of Himachal Pradesh (1999), *Statistical Outline of Himachal Pradesh*, Directorate of Economics and Statistics, Government of Himachal Pradesh, Shimla.

(iv) International Institute for Population Sciences (2002), *National Family Health Survey India, 1998-99, Himachal Pradesh*, Bombay.

(v) Deaton Angus and Jean Dreze (2002), 'Poverty and Inequality in India: A Re-examination', *Economic and Political Weekly*, Vol. XXXVII, No. 36, pp. 3729-3748.

(vi) Chadha, G. K. and P.P. Sahu (2002), 'Post Reform Setbacks in Rural Employment: Issues that Need Further Scrutiny', *Economic and Political Weekly*, Vol. XXXVII, No. 21, pp. 1998-2026.

(vii) Sharma, H.R. (2001), 'Employment and Wage Earnings of Agricultural Labourers', *The Indian Journal of Labour Economics*, Vol. 44, No. 1, pp. 27-38.

(viii) Himachal Pradesh, Human Development Report, 2001

(ix) Sharma, H.R. (2000), 'Agrarian Structure and Agricultural Development: Emerging Trends and Patterns', *Man and Development*, Vol. XXII, No. 2. pp. 22-41.

basic infrastructural facilities have been brought out in Table 3.10. The table shows that regional variations, measured in terms of coefficient of variation, were more pronounced in the availability of basic infrastructural facilities like roads, schools, hospitals, primary agricultural and primary non-agricultural societies and area under non-food crops. This could be primarily attributed to difficult mountainous terrains in some districts like Lahaul & Spiti, Kinnaur and Chamba where the provision of these facilities is extremely difficult and costly.

Table 3.10: Inter-regional Variations in Levels of Socio-Economic Transformation in Himachal Pradesh: Some Selected Indicators

Sl. No.	*Indicators*	*Minimum*	*Maximum*	*Mean*	*SD*	*CV (per cent)*
1.	Net State domestic product (1999-2000, Rs. at Current prices)	12839	217927	92727.67	64427.72	69.48
2.	Growth rate of NSDP (1993-94/1999-2000)	8.60	16.83	12.75	2.56	20.09
3.	Per capita income, (1999-2000, Rs. at Current prices)	12479	38906	20368.58	8223.18	40.37
4.	Per cent of Poor (1998-99)	19.06	61.72	29.06	11.58	39.58
5.	Per cent of workers in non-farm sector (1991)	13.30	39.30	27.37	9.08	33.20
6.	Public sector employment (1997-98)	2329	65957	19668	17476.57	88.85
7.	Per cent area under non-foodgrains (1997-98)	1.15	38.46	16.31	13.07	80.11
8.	Road length/100 sq. km. (1997-98)	0.08	99.37	54.92	36.98	67.33

(Contd.)

Table 3.10 (Contd.)

Sl. No.	*Indicators*	*Minim.*	*Maxim*	*Mean*	*SD*	*CV (per cent)*
9.	Banks/lakh of population (1997-98)	10.69	24.24	14.37	4.40	30.64
10.	Schools/100 sq. km (2000)	1.85	61.44	35.33	20.46	57.91
11.	Hospitals/100 sq. km (2000)	0.30	9.21	5.09	2.94	57.76
12.	Telephones/100 persons (2002)	2.92	9.28	5.92	1.84	31.11
13.	Primary agricultural credit societies/100 sq. km (2001)	0.38	13.90	4.27	4.23	98.84
14.	Primary non-agricultural credit societies/100 sq. km (2001)	0.20	3.93	1.81	1.15	63.43
15.	Literacy, Males, (2001, per cent)	77.22	90.86	85.73	4.04	4.73
16.	Literacy, Females, (2001, per cent)	49.70	76.41	66.43	7.81	11.76

Source: Computed by the authors on the basis of district level data collected from various publications of Directorate of Economics and Statistics, Government of Himachal Pradesh.

Again, the high coefficient of variations in the area under non-foodgrains could be largely explained in terms of climatic variations across the districts. For example, the districts, which have temperate climate are particularly suitable to the growth of high value cash crops like off-season vegetables and temperate fruits like apple and, therefore, account for a higher per cent of area under non-foodgrains.

GROWTH OF STATE DOMESTIC PRODUCT

Consistent with the overall pattern of structural changes associated with the process of economic development, the contribution of agriculture to the net state domestic product declined continuously; from around 35 per cent in 1980-81 to 19.52 per cent in 1999-2000

(Table 3.11). The contribution of primary sector as a whole during the period plummeted from around one-half to around one-fourth. Consequently, the contribution of secondary and tertiary sectors increased respectively from 20.10 per cent and 31.82 per cent in 1980-81 to 31.99 per cent and 42.52 per cent in 1999-2000. Further, while in secondary sector the contribution of manufacturing registered significant increase from 2.26 per cent to 11.23 per cent, in the tertiary sector, the increase was more pronounced in per cent share of community and personal services (from 14.33 per cent to 22.26 per cent). Table 3.12 shows that during the twenty years period since 1980-81, the net state domestic product originating in agriculture and animal husbandry recorded a growth rate of 1.91 per cent per annum. The secondary sector registered a growth rate of 8.51 per cent whereas the tertiary sector experienced a growth rate of 6.37 per cent

Table 3.11: Sectoral Distribution of Net State Domestic Product (NSDP) in Himachal Pradesh: 1980-81 to 2000-01

Sl. No.	*Sectors*	*1980-81*	*1985-86*	*1990-91*	*1995-96*	*2000-01*
1.	Primary Sector	48.08	43.54	40.24	32.14	25.49
	(i) Agriculture and Animal Husbandry	34.95	34.97	31.77	24.37	19.52
	(ii) Forestry	12.10	6.90	6.62	6.54	4.67
	(iii) Fishing	0.27	0.30	0.36	0.29	0.20
	(iv) Mining & Quarrying	0.76	1.37	1.49	0.94	1.10
2.	Secondary Sector	20.10	21.76	22.37	31.55	31.99
	(i) Manufacturing	2.26	3.99	6.05	10.04	11.23
	(ii) Construction	18.22	15.29	12.90	15.54	15.54
	(iii) Electricity, Gas and Water supply	-0.39	2.48	3.42	5.97	5.22
3.	Tertiary Sector	31.82	34.70	37.39	36.31	42.52
	(i) Transport	1.79	2.03	1.24	1.55	2.41
	(ii) Trade	7.67	8.29	8.83	8.99	8.76
	(iii) Finance and Insurance	8.03	8.86	9.45	9.10	9.09
	(iv) Community and Personnel Services	14.33	15.52	17.87	16.67	22.26
4.	All Sectors	100	100	100	100	100
5.	Net State Domestic Product (NSDP), at 1993-94 prices (Rs. in lakh)	251720	287526	391891	492052	667155
6.	Per capita NSDP (Rs.)	5933	6160	7632	8801	10942

Source: Directorate of Economics and Statistics, Government of Himachal Pradesh, Shimla.

Table 3.12: Sectoral Compound Growth Rates of NSDP in Himachal Pradesh: 1980-81 to 2000-01

Sl. No.	*Sectors*	*1980-81 to 1990-91*	*1991-92 to 2000-01*	*1980-81 to 2000-01*
1.	Primary Sector	2.35	1.10	1.90*
	(i) Agriculture and Animal Husbandry	3.46	0.75	1.91*
	(ii) Forestry	-3.92	1.05	1.59
	(iii) Fishing	7.03*	-1.76	4.30*
	(iv) Mining & Quarrying	16.79*	11.92*	5.22
2.	Secondary Sector	5.85*	10.64*	8.51*
	(i) Manufacturing	14.83*	13.77*	14.24*
	(ii) Construction	2.39	7.66*	5.48*
	(iii) Electricity, Gas and Water supply	14.92	15.24	13.46*
3.	Tertiary Sector	6.84*	7.58*	6.37*
	(i) Transport, Storage and Communication	1.55	12.40*	5.20*
	(ii) Trade, Hotel and Restaurant	5.38*	5.78*	6.06*
	(iii) Finance and Real Estate	6.56*	4.81*	5.70*
	(iv) Community and Personal Services	8.11*	9.39*	7.07*
4.	All Sectors	4.65*	6.33*	5.25*

* Denotes significance at 0.05 level of probability.
Source: Computed by the authors.

per annum. And while in the former manufacturing sector recorded a growth rate as high as 14.24 per cent, in the latter the highest growth during the period occurred in electricity, gas and water supply. The overall growth rate of state economy was 5.25 per cent per annum. Between the two periods, the growth rate in the primary sector was higher during the eighties compared to the nineties in comparison to the secondary and tertiary sector where the growth rates were higher during the nineties. The state's per capita state domestic product has always remained above the all-India average state domestic product except for one-two years in 1984-85 to 1986-87 when it dipped below all-India average.

LAND USE PATTERN

According to 'Village Papers', i.e. the reporting area, for which revenue papers exist in the state, was 2930.9 thousand hectares in 1972-73 and increased to 4531.8 thousand hectares in 1999-2000. Thus, the unreported area in comparison to geographical area from the viewpoint of land use has declined from 47 per cent of the total geographical area in 1972-73 to only 19 per cent in 1999-2000. The per cent changes in land use pattern for the state and at four points of time, i.e. 1972-73, 1980-81, 1990-91 and 1999-2000 are given in Table 3.13. The table invites the following comments. The area under forests increased from around 22 per cent in 1972-73 to 24 per cent in 1999-2000. While the area put to non-agricultural uses remained constant at around 5-6 per cent, the area under barren land registered more than four-fold increase from 4.43 per cent to 19 per cent during the period. The area under culturable waste, (the land that can be brought under plough), however, decreased from 4.33 per cent to 2.63 per cent. There has also been no change in the area under miscellaneous trees that remained constant at 1.5 per cent. In terms of growth rates (Table 3.14), for the total period of thirty years, while the barren land

Table 3.13: Trends in Land Use Pattern under Different Categories in Himachal Pradesh, 1972-73 to 1999-2000

(Per cent)

Type of Land Use	*1972-73*	*1980-81*	*1990-91*	*1999-00*
1. Forests	21.75	27.03	30.85	24.14
2. Area Not Available for Cultivation				
(i) Barren	4.43	4.74	5.46	18.91
(ii) Non-Agricultural uses	6.49	5.42	5.74	6.67
Total	10.92	10.16	11.20	25.58
3. Other uncultivated land excluding Current Fallows				
(i) Culturable waste	4.33	7.49	3.72	2.63
(ii) Permanent pastures	40.64	33.03	33.72	32.47
(iii) Miscellaneous Tree Crops	1.50	1.32	1.43	1.42
Total	46.47	41.84	38.87	36.52
4. Fallow Lands				
(i) Current Fallows	1.69	1.39	1.33	1.24
(ii) Other Fallows	0.11	0.42	0.46	0.35
Total	1.80	1.81	1.79	1.59
5. Net Sown area	19.06	19.17	17.31	12.17
6. Total	100.00	100.00	100.00	100.00
	(2930.9)	(2985.2)	(3367.6)	(4531.8)

Note: Figures in parentheses give total geographical area according to village papers on the basis of which percentages have been calculated.

Source: Annual Season and Crop Reports (for the corresponding years), Directorate of Land Records, Government of Himachal Pradesh, Shimla.

Table 3.14: Compound Growth Rates of Land Use under Different Categories in Himachal Pradesh, 1972-73 to 1999-2000

(per cent per annum)

Type of Land Use	I	II	III
1. Forests	3.21*	1.39*	2.36
2. Area Not Available for Cultivation			
(i) Barren	1.87*	12.73	4.96*
(ii) Non-Agricultural uses	-0.85	1.15	0.70
Total	0.33	8.24	3.15
3. Other uncultivated land excluding Current Fallows			
(i) Culturable waste	1.98	-1.39*	-1.31
(ii) Permanent pastures	-0.46	1.30	0.53
(iii) Miscellaneous Tree Crops	-0.94	5.99	1.90
Total	-0.18	1.26	-0.06
4. Fallow Lands			
(i) Current Fallows	-1.66	2.45*	0.19
(ii) Other Fallows	16.70*	3.24*	8.92*
Total	0.59	2.67*	1.59*
5. Net Sown area	0.53*	-0.41*	0.06

Note: * Denotes significance at 0.05 per cent level of probability
I = 1972-73 to 1980-81; II = 1980-81 to 1990-91; III = 1972-73 to 1999-2000

Sources: Computed by the authors on the basis of data from Annual Season and Crop Reports (for the period 1972-73 to 1999-2000), Directorate of Land Records, Government of Himachal Pradesh, Shimla.

recorded a compound growth rate of around 5 per cent per annum, the area under other fallows increased at a rate of around 9 per cent per annum. Between two periods, the compound growth rate of forests was higher in the first period whereas the growth rate of barren land was extremely high (12.73 per cent) albeit statistically insignificant in the second period. The area under other fallows also recorded a very high statistically significant growth rate (16.70 per cent) during the first period.

AREA, PRODUCTION AND PRODUCTIVITY OF MAJOR CROPS

Table 3.15 tells the story of changing levels of area, production and productivity of major crops in the state since 1972-73. It may be seen from the table that among cereal crops, there was an increase in the

Table 3.15: Area, Production and Yield of Major Crops, 1972-73 to 1999-2000

Sl. No.	Crops	*Area (ha) in Triennium Ending*			*Production (tonnes) in Triennium Ending*			*Yield (kg/ha) in Triennium Ending*		
		1974-75	*1986-87*	*1999-00*	*1974-75*	*1986-87*	*1999-00*	*1974-75*	*1986-87*	*1999-00*
1.	Rice	96058	93823	82841	101657	82726	119269	1058	882	1440
2.	Maize	261976	303505	304248	452261	551900	654797	1726	1818	2152
3.	Wheat	315740	378268	375883	330228	404299	568624	1046	1069	1513
4.	Barley	41594	33275	26782	48783	33306	33862	1173	1001	1264
5.	Other Cereals*	53047	27683	16251	32121	45954	10118	606	456	623
6.	All Cereals	768414	836554	806005	965069	1118184	1386669	1256	1337	1720
7.	Pulses	72926	44916	34112	27778	10439	24601	398	232	721
8.	Foodgrains	838289	881470	840117	999717	1128623	1411271	1193	1280	1680
9.	Sugarcane	3643	2932	3267	6116	3394	15394	1679	1157	4712
10.	Potato	14915	14576	14359	57905	48099	152833	3882	3300	10644
11.	Ginger	2018	2218	1799	1047	1159	2779	519	522	1544
12.	Oilseeds	23095	21853	19241	9695	4476	10093	420	205	525

*Includes ragi and other common millets

Source: Annual Season and Crop Reports (1972,73, 1973-74, 1974-75, 1984-85, 1985-86, 1986-87, 1997-98, 1998-99 and 1999-2000), Directorate of Land Records, Government of Himachal Pradesh, Shimla.

area under most of the crops except rice, barley and other cereals. The area under pulses nosedived from about 72 thousand hectares in the triennium ending 1974-75 to 27 thousand hectares in the triennium ending 1999-2000. Among the non-foodgrain crops, while the area under potato stayed practically unchanged, that under sugarcane, ginger and oilseeds declined by varying degrees. The production of foodgrains during the period increased from 9.99 lakh tonnes to 14.11 lakh tonnes. The production of non-foodgrain crops also increased by varying degrees; the maximum surge was witnessed in potato production, from about 57 thousand tonnes to 1.52 lakh tonnes. The yield levels of different crops did also increase during the period. For example, the yield of rice increased from 10.58 q/ha in the triennium ending 1974-75 to 14.40 q/ha in the triennium ending 1999-2000, that of maize from 17.26 q/ha to 21.52 q/ha and wheat from 10.46 q/ha to 15.13 q/ha. The yield levels of non-foodgrain crops like sugarcane, potato, ginger and oilseeds too experienced significant increases.

In terms of compound growth rates, there was an overall decline in the growth rates of area under different crops except that under wheat and maize (Table 3.16). The maximum decline occurred in case of pulses, other cereals and barley. There was no neat pattern in growth rates in the yield levels of different crops in two periods. The foodgrains production increased at the rate of 1.55 per cent per annum. Among different foodgrain crops, production of wheat recorded the highest growth (2.56 per cent per annum), followed by maize (1.68 per cent). Among the non-foodgrain crops, the production of sugarcane and potato recorded higher growth rates, though these were statistically insignificant. Further, the growth rates of production in most of the crops were higher in the second period (1985-86 to 1999-2000) compared with the first period (1972-73 to 1984-85). The growth rate of yield was the highest in case of wheat (1.93 per cent) during the overall period among the cereals.

The state has also made significant strides in horticultural development and has come to be known as 'apple state of India'; in 1999-2000, the horticultural sector in the state contributed around 16 per cent of the gross value of output originating in agriculture. Table 3.17 shows that while area under fruit crops increased from 26,307 hectares in the triennium ending 1967-68 to around 2 lakh hectares in the triennium ending 1999-2000, fruit production increased from 48 thousand tonnes to 2.72 lakh tonnes. The yield levels, however,

Table 3.16: Compound Growth Rates of Area, Production and Yield of Major Crops in Himachal Pradesh, 1972-73 to 1999-2000

Sl. No.	Crops	Area			Production			Yield		
		I	II	III	I	II	III	I	II	III
1.	Rice	-0.39	-1.00*	-0.72*	-2.51	3.45*	0.12	-2.12	4.50*	0.84
2.	Maize	1.30*	-0.04*	0.73	1.36	2.08	1.68	0.06	2.12*	0.95*
3.	Wheat	1.68*	-0.03	0.61*	1.47	1.78	2.56*	-0.20	1.82	1.93*
4.	Barley	-1.65*	-1.66*	-1.98*	-3.06*	-0.46	-1.44*	-1.43*	1.21	0.55
5.	Other Cereals	-2.82*	-4.46*	-4.41*	-7.25*	-0.12	-5.17*	-2.55*	4.55	-0.79
6.	All Cereals	0.82*	-0.32*	0.21	0.85	1.87	1.63*	0.03	2.19*	1.42*
7.	Pulses	-4.83*	-2.28*	-3.16*	-10.01*	10.17*	-2.40	-5.44*	12.73*	0.78
8.	Foodgrains	0.44*	-0.41*	-0.001	0.60	1.96	1.55*	0.16	2.38*	1.54*
9.	Sugarcane	-1.78	2.03	-1.15	-6.14*	20.44*	1.95	-4.44	18.05*	3.13
10.	Potato	-0.51	-1.16	-0.30	-3.95	6.52	4.31	-3.46	7.78	4.63*
11.	Ginger	-0.81	-2.04	-1.98*	-0.84	12.72	0.13	-0.03	15.06*	2.15
12.	Oilseeds	-0.13	-0.99	-0.33	-6.57*	7.69*	-0.02	-6.45*	8.78*	0.32

Note:
1. * Denotes significance at 0.05 level of probability
2. I = 1972-73 to 1984-85; II = 1985-86 to 1999-00 and III = 1972-73 to 1999-2000

Source: Computed by the authors.

Table 3.17: Trends in Area, Production and Yield of Fruits in Himachal Pradesh, 1965-66 to 1999-2000

Triennium Ending	*Area (ha)*			*Production (tonnes)*			*Yield (tonnes\ha)*		
	Apple	*Others*	*Total*	*Apple*	*Others*	*Total*	*Apple*	*Others*	*Total*
1967-68	15148 (57.48)	11159 (42.42)	26307 (100)	307482 (63.41)	17744 (35.59)	48492 (100)	2.03	1.59	1.84
1977-78	36895 (53.49)	32085 (46.51)	68980 (100)	150282 (84.87)	26800 (15.31)	177082 (100)	4.07	0.83	2.57
1987-88	52805 (39.03)	82464 (60.97)	135269 (100)	264405 (86.51)	41242 (13.49)	305647 (100)	5.01	0.50	2.26
1999-2000	84772 (41.23)	120841 (58.77)	205613 (100)	225679 (82.89)	46585 (17.11)	272264 (100)	2.66	0.38	1.32

Note: Figures in parentheses are percentages.

Source: Horticultural Development in Himachal Pradesh: Facts and Figures at a Glance, (1975-76,1976-77, 1977-78, 1997-98, 1998-99 and 1999-2000), Directorate of Horticulture, Government of Himachal Pradesh, Shimla.

fluctuated and had declined in recent years, *inter alia*, because of erratic weather and mounting incidence of diseases and insect pests. Further, among the horticultural crops, apple continued to be the most important fruit crop accounting for around two-fifths of the total area and more than four-fifths of total fruit production. Table 3.18 shows that during the period 1965-66 to 1999-2000, while the area under all fruits registered a growth rate of 6.46 per cent per annum, the fruit production increased at a rate of 4.94 per cent per annum. The growth rate of yield of all fruits during the same period was, however, negative. Nevertheless, the yield of apple registered a growth rate as high as 11.89 per cent per annum. Between the two time periods, the yield levels of apple and other fruits registered negative growth rate during the second period, i.e. from 1981-82 to 1999-2000. It may, however, be mentioned that post 1980 period has not been so good for apple production. The major setback came in the early eighties when the scab disease took a heavy toll. And subsequently, the apple production has fluctuated due to the frequent outbreaks of diseases and erratic weather conditions, especially at the time of fruit setting.[4]

Table 3.18: Compound Growth Rates in Area, Production and Yield of Fruits in Himachal Pradesh, 1965-66 to 1999-2000

Particulars	*Area (ha)*			*Production (tonnes)*			*Yield (tonnes\ha)*		
	I	*II*	*III*	*I*	*II*	*III*	*I*	*II*	*III*
Apple	7.59*	4.06*	4.73*	10.45*	3.11	7.47*	2.76	-2.99*	11.89*
Other Fruits	10.89*	4.27*	8.13*	-2.05*	0.93	1.17	-11.50*	-3.27*	-5.91*
Total Fruits	9.07*	4.12*	6.46*	7.36	0.95	4.94*	-1.43*	-3.13*	-1.41*

Note: * Denotes significance at 0.05 level of probability
I = 1965-66 to 1980-81; II = 1981-82 to 1999-00; III = 1965-66 to 1999-2000

Source: Computed by authors.

CROP DIVERSIFICATION

The agriculture in the state has, over the years, has undergone the process of diversification towards high value crops, thanks to the availability of bewildering micro climatic niches. The process of crop diversification that began with the introduction of apple in the late fifties and the early sixties has gained momentum recently with the introduction of off-season vegetable and other cash crops like peas, cabbage, cauliflower, beans, capsicum, tomato, garlic and so on. At the state level, an idea of the extent of agricultural diversification at the state level can be had by looking into the changing contribution of crop production, horticulture and livestock towards the gross value of output originating in agriculture. The data given in Table 3.19 show that, fluctuations notwithstanding, during 1993-94 and 2000-01, crop production contributed nearly half of the total value of output originating in agriculture. Further, while the contribution of livestock sector remained stagnant at around 35.36 per cent, that of horticultural crops fluctuated sharply, ranging from as high as 17.35 per cent to as

Table 3.19: Share of Crop Production, Horticulture and Livestock in the Gross Value of Output Originating in Agriculture, 1993-94 to 2000-01 at 1993-94 Prices

Year	*Crop Production*	*Horticulture*	*Livestock*	*Total*	*Gross Value of Output Originating in Agriculture (Rs. in lakhs)*
1993-94	47.80	14.51	37.69	100	155407
1994-95	54.35	8.27	37.38	100	157031
1995-96	50.74	13.28	35.98	100	166409
1996-97	49.36	14.71	35.93	100	171372
1997-98	52.39	11.44	36.17	100	175474
1998-99	47.48	17.35	35.17	100	180856
1999-00	57.05	4.62	38.33	100	167735
2000-01	48.30	15.99	35.71	100	184314

Source: Directorate of Economics and Statistics, Government of Himachal Pradesh, Shimla.

low as 4.62 per cent. Yet another way to understand temporal changes in the process of agricultural diversification is to study the changes in the cropping pattern. In this context, Table 3.20 shows that among foodgrain crops the share of area under rice declined steadily while that under maize and wheat registered a small but persistent increase. Among the non-foodgrains, the area under apple, other fruits, potato and other vegetables increased over the period by varying degrees. It, however, needs to be underlined that state level averages, especially in the context of Himachal Pradesh where there are marked variations in the agro-climatic conditions among different districts and even among different areas in the same district, do not reveal much about the extent of crop diversification. For example, two tribal districts

(Lahaul & Spiti and Kinnaur) and most of the areas of Shimla, Kullu and Chamba and some areas of Sirmaur, Solan and Mandi that fall in the temperate region (Zone III) did have a considerable potential to grow temperate fruits and vegetables. It is, therefore, essential to examine changes in the area under different crops at a much more disaggregated level, preferably at a block level. However, due to data constraints, we look at the temporal changes in per cent share of area under foodgrain and non-foodgrain crops at the district level. It may be mentioned that non-foodgrain crops in the state mostly include off-season vegetable and horticultural crops. The requisite information has been brought out in Table 3.21. The table shows that while there has been a significant increase in the extent of crop diversification in terms of per cent share of area under non-foodgrain crops in four districts, namely Kullu, Shimla, Kinnaur, and Lahaul & Spiti, the increase was less pronounced in three others (Solan, Sirmaur and Chamba). Further, in all these districts, the process of crop diversification had gathered momentum in recent periods, especially

Table 3.20: Temporal Changes in Cropping Pattern in Himachal Pradesh, 1972-73 to 1999-2000

(Per cent to total cropped area)

Sl. No.	*Crops*	*1972-73*	*1977-78*	*1982-83*	*1987-88*	*1992-93*	*1999-2000*
1.	Rice	10.54	10.90	9.45	9.25	8.42	8.38
2.	Maize	28.16	29.11	30.10	30.78	31.91	31.35
3.	Wheat	34.27	34.30	39.24	38.50	38.93	38.73
4.	Barley	4.55	4.04	3.94	3.23	2.79	2.71
5.	Other Cereals*	5.90	4.13	3.40	2.85	2.08	1.60
6.	Pulses	7.76	8.66	4.48	4.52	4.22	3.40
7.	Sugarcane	0.39	0.45	0.35	0.31	0.24	0.32
8.	Apple	1.27	1.57	2.08	2.62	3.56	4.25
9.	Other fruits	0.52	0.60	0.92	1.06	1.22	1.78
10.	Potato	1.56	1.56	1.39	1.53	1.46	1.50
11.	Other Vegetables	0.54	0.61	0.83	1.32	1.15	2.12
12.	Ginger	0.24	0.27	0.20	0.21	0.17	0.21
13.	Oilseeds	2.58	2.33	2.43	2.38	2.25	1.97
14.	Others	1.72	1.47	1.19	1.44	1.60	1.68

* Includes ragi and other common millets

Source: Annual Season and Crop Reports (1972-73, 1977-78, 1982-83, 1987-88, 1992-93 and 1999-2000), Directorate of Land Records, Government of Himachal Pradesh, Shimla.

after 1987-88. In remaining four districts (Kangra, Bilaspur, Hamirpur and Una), which mostly fall in sub-tropical region, the per cent share of area under foodgrain and non-foodgrain crops stayed practically unchanged.

Table 3.21: Temporal Changes in the Area under Non-Foodgrain Crops across Districts in Himachal Pradesh: 1972-73 to 1999-2000
(Per cent to total cropped area)

District	*1972-73*	*1977-78*	*1982-83*	*1987-88*	*1992-93*	*1999-00*
Bilaspur	3.01	3.11	3.30	3.15	3.24	3.33
Chamba	6.36	6.87	7.49	8.02	7.46	9.75
Hamirpur	1.38	1.42	1.28	1.19	1.15	1.21
Kangra	11.21	9.57	9.34	9.53	11.04	9.91
Kinnaur	8.09	10.08	14.45	22.00	25.77	37.43
Kullu	6.83	9.08	11.90	12.20	16.96	21.33
Lahaul & Spiti	24.70	39.13	46.97	59.31	63.73	72.43
Mandi	5.89	6.69	6.80	7.90	7.10	9.11
Shimla	17.16	17.62	20.76	26.74	33.14	43.73
Sirmaur	9.99	12.52	10.75	13.13	12.72	15.46
Solan	9.73	8.30	8.25	10.93	10.19	12.52
Una	7.79	7.77	7.83	8.55	8.83	8.87
H.P.	8.81	8.86	9.38	10.87	11.65	13.82

Source: Annual Season and Crop Reports (1972-73, 1977-78, 1982-83, 1987-88, 1992-93 and 1999-2000), Directorate of Land Records, Government of Himachal Pradesh, Shimla.

The process of diversification towards high value crops has made significant impact on the level of income and employment of the households. The results of a study, based on primary data gathered from sample households in different areas that had attained different levels of crop diversification show that the net returns over different farm management costs from high value crops like peas, cabbage, cauliflower, etc. were much higher compared to those from traditional crops (Table 3.22)[5]. Not only that in many cases, especially in apple cultivation, the individuals did leave their jobs in the service sector to look after their orchards at home.[6]

LAND REFORM MEASURES

The state of Himachal Pradesh has enacted and implemented a number of land reform measures following the guidelines of the Central

Table 3.22: Net Returns from High Value Crops *vis-à-vis* Cereal Crops

Theog Block (District Shimla) (*Rs.ha*)

Sl. No.	Returns over	Potato	Peas	Cabbage	Cauliflower	Tomato	Beans	Capsicum	Wheat	Maize
1.	Cost A_1 (Rs.)	64646	56028	120821	83032	49160	33759	64269	-3140	264
2.	Cost A_2 (Rs.)	64646	56028	120821	83032	49160	33759	64269	-3140	264
3.	Cost B_1 (Rs.)	63907	54248	119131	81749	49155	33537	63427	-3751	-395
4.	Cost B_2 (Rs.)	61469	52309	116007	77237	46921	32202	60139	-4846	-1472
5.	Cost C_1 (Rs.)	53845	42862	105225	67327	36855	28133	43471	-8546	-7748
6.	Cost C_2 (Rs.)	51407	42257	102100	63151	34621	18797	40810	-9640	-8525
7.	Returns per quintal over cost C_2 (Rs)	350	559	450	478	385	355	544	-102	-22

Sangrah Block (District Sirmaur)

Sl. No.	Returns over	Potato	Peas	Garlic	Ginger	Colocasia	Wheat	Maize	Barley
1.	Cost A_1 (Rs.)	57776	60201	197467	66918	34137	3448	7936	1335
2.	Cost A_2 (Rs.)	57776	60201	197467	66918	34137	3448	7936	1335
3.	Cost B_1 (Rs.)	56561	59159	196805	66750	34116	2999	7006	714
4.	Cost B_2 (Rs.)	52803	57719	184288	65764	32956	2384	6117	435
5.	Cost C_1 (Rs.)	45118	47857	177663	57184	26976	-1501	-311	-4314
6.	Cost C_2 (Rs.)	41359	46274	173262	53772	22103	-2116	-1201	-5034
7.	Returns per quintal over cost C_2 (Rs.)	202	578	1773	773	242	-132	-32	-291

(*Contd.*)

Table 3.22 (Contd.)

Seraj Block (District Mandi)

Sl. No.	*Returns Over*	*Potato*	*Peas*	*Cabbage*	*Cauliflower*	*Tomato*	*Wheat*	*Barley*	*Maize*
1.	Cost A_1 (Rs.)	45738	51182	121511	83446	95924	5666	4722	5418
2.	Cost A_2 (Rs.)	45738	51182	121511	83446	95924	5666	4722	5418
3.	Cost B_1 (Rs.)	45463	51081	121367	83419	95901	5533	4606	5284
4.	Cost B_2 (Rs.)	42865	49725	119918	80860	94095	4552	3890	4464
5.	Cost C_1 (Rs.)	33806	43658	106418	65239	73312	-1518	-1939	-3562
6.	Cost C_2 (Rs.)	33682	42313	104968	62680	71506	-2499	-1987	-4333
7.	Net returns per quintal over cost C_2 (Rs)	234	604	505	464	429	-102	-93	-158

Source: Sharma, H.R., R.K. Sharma, S.K. Chauhan and Virender Kumar (2004), *Mountain Agriculture in Transition: A Study of Processes, Determinants and Implications Using Micro Evidence from Himachal Pradesh*, Department of Agricultural Economics, H.P. Agricultural University, Palampur (H.P.), pp. 104-108.

Government to reform agrarian relations by ensuring land to the tiller and reducing glaring inequalities in the distribution of landholdings. In fact, over the years, the land reform measures enacted and implemented in the state have aimed at: (a) conferring ownership rights on the tenant cultivators; (b) reducing inequalities in respect of distribution of landholdings; (c) encouraging consolidation of holdings to solve the problem of fragmentation of land; (d) revision and updating of land records; and (e) allotting wasteland/village common land to landless and other eligible persons under Nautor Rules, 1968 and Utilisation of Surplus Areas Scheme, 1975 (Economic Review, 1997:19). The Himachal Pradesh Abolition of Big Landed Estates and Land Reform Act was enacted way back in 1953. However, with passing of Punjab Re-organisation Act, 1966, certain areas of erstwhile Punjab were merged with Himachal Pradesh. This led to the enactment of Himachal Pradesh (Transferred Territory) Tenants Protection of Rights Act in 1971. Again, to incorporate the guidelines evolved by the Chief Ministers' Conference in 1972 and also to plug the loopholes in the existing land ceiling legislations, the land legislation Act was amended and H.P. Ceiling of Landholding Act, 1972 and Himachal Pradesh Tenancy and Land Reform Act, 1972 were enacted. To eradicate the phenomenon of landlessness and to augment the pool of surplus land, the Government of Himachal Pradesh enacted H.P. Village Common Land Vesting and Utilisation Act, 1974. The Act placed *shamlat* (common) land at the disposal of the government for allotment to the landless and other eligible households.

Unlike other states, the progress of the implementation of land reform measures in Himchal Pradesh has been fairly good. For example, in respect of tenancy laws, out of 4.34 lakh occupancy tenants, about 3.96 lakh tenants have already been conferred proprietary rights. Among different revenue divisions, there were 2,35,472 non-occupancy tenants in Kangra division out of which 2,17,332 have been conferred proprietary rights so far. The remaining tenants fall under the category of tenants of protected categories of landowners like widow, minor, army personnel, disabled and infirm persons. As one village study reported, though the land has not been transferred to the names of such tenants, the land was in their possession, they are cultivating it without any interference from their landlords and were not paying any rent. Thus they were the *de facto* owners of land, though *de jure* they belonged to the category of tenants, euphemistically called 'bookish tenants' (Rajneesh, 1999). Likewise, in Mandi division, there were 1,07,107 non-occupancy tenants out of which 95,621 have been conferred proprietary rights. In Shimla division, 30,078 tenants have been conferred proprietary rights out of 31,477 non-occupancy tenants. In a similar vein, nearly one lakh landless agricultural labourers have been allotted land acquired under ceiling laws and H.P. Village Common Land Vesting and Utilisation Act, 1974. Regarding the implementation of Land Ceiling Laws, 3.17 lakh acres of land was declared surplus out of which 3.05 lakh acres were actually taken into possession. The land distributed to the beneficiaries amounted to 0.04 lakh acres and 3.12 lakh acres was not distributed as the land was barren and not fit for cultivation. The land under litigation was 0.07 lakh acres. There are very few landless households in the state who are left without allotment of land. As far as the beneficiaries of land allotment were concerned, 0.04 lakh belonged to Scheduled Caste, 0.003 to the Scheduled Tribe and 0.02 to other castes. The amount of land allotted to these categories of households was 0.03 lakh acres, 0.002 lakh acres and 0.01 lakh acres, respectively. As a result of the distribution of surplus and common land, the incidence of landless households is very low; according to National Sample Survey Data, the landless households were 10.46 per cent in 1991-92. It, however, needs to be underlined that the allotment of land was a one time affair and the factors like unrelenting population pressure coupled with lack of non-farm employment opportunities and consequent subdivision of holdings might have pushed some of the land allottees to the army of landless households. So far consolidation of holdings is concerned, out of total 49 lakh hectares of land identified for consolidation of holdings, 21.93 stood consolidated upto March 1996. The conferment of ownership rights on the tenants and the distribution of surplus land among the eligible households, especially to those belonging to Scheduled Caste, has also been brought out by different village studies in the state (Panda, 1999). The distribution of surplus land among the eligible households including those belonging to Scheduled Caste has made a significant impact on the socio-economic status of the land allottees. For example, besides social empowerment of beneficiaries in terms of increase in their social prestige in the aftermath of the distribution of surplus land, the results of an empirical study, presented in Table 3.23, show that there has been a significant impact of the land allotment on levels of income and employment of the beneficiaries, both Scheduled Caste and non-Scheduled Caste households, leading to a substantial decline in the incidence of poverty in all its manifestations like magnitude, depth and severity[7]. The increase in the income from the allotted land could still be increased further if the land allottees are provided easy access to inputs like seeds, fertilizers and credit.

Table 3.23: Levels of Income, Employment and Poverty Before and After Land Allotment

Particulars	*Before Land Allotment*		*After Land Allotment*	
	Scheduled Caste	*Non-Scheduled Caste*	*Scheduled Caste*	*Non-Scheduled Caste*
Agricultural Income (Rs./ household)	249	371	6913	8674
Employment (Days/ha)	—	—	189	220
Poverty (Per cent)				
Head Count Ratio	55.97	35.37	17.14	9.00
Poverty Gap	22.30	10.22	6.01	2.08
FGT	8.77	4.83	2.35	0.75

Source: Sharma, H.R., R.K. Sharma and Virender Kumar (2000), *Distribution of Surplus Land among Landless Households and its Impact on Income, Employment and Poverty: A Study of Himachal Pradesh*, Research Report No. 15, pp. 105-108, Department of Agricultural Economics, H.P. Agricultural University Palampur (H.P.).

LAND DISTRIBUTION STRUCTURE

The above-mentioned land reform measures did impact on the land distribution structure in the state; these measures halted the process of increasing land concentration. Nevertheless, it would be instructive to understand the changes in the land distribution structure over the period in the state. There are two data sets, thrown up by the different quinquennial rounds of agricultural censuses and landholdings surveys of National Sample Surveys (NSS) that are available to study the changes in the land distribution structure. However, as is well known, the data thrown up by agricultural censuses after re-tabulating the existing revenue records cannot be put to scientific uses because of highly unsatisfactory state of revenue records in most of the states, especially related to tenancy. One is, therefore, left with NSS data to understand the changes in the land distribution structure and tenancy relations. In the following section, we look into the changes in the distribution of landholdings in general as also among different social groups and magnitude and terms of tenancy in the state during 1981-82 and 1991-92 using data emanating from 37th and 48th NSS rounds.

The data given in Table 3.24 show that the concentration of both the ownership and operational holdings in the state in the eighties became more skewed both by the values of Gini co-efficients and the per cent share of land owned and operated by the households/holdings at the top 20 per cent, 10 per cent, 5 per cent and 1 per cent. So far the distribution of landholdings among different categories of households was concerned, the information given in Table 3.25 shows that between 1981-82 and 1991-92 the incidence of landlessness increased from 7.77 per cent to 10.46 per cent. The proportion of marginal households and the proportion of land owned by them also increased significantly. The proportion of large households owning more than four hectares of land and the area owned by them also declined. Likewise, the huge proliferation in numerical proportion

Table 3.24: Concentration of Landholdings in Himachal Pradesh, 1981-82 to 1991-92

Year	*Gini co-efficient*	*Share of Bottom*		*Share of Middle*		*Share of Top*			
		40%	*50%*	*40 to 80%*	*50 to 80%*	*20%*	*10%*	*5%*	*1%*
Ownership Holdings									
1981-82	0.5524	7.35	12.86	34.46	29.13	58.01	39.26	25.58	7.99
1991-92	0.6020	6.42	10.98	30.18	25.62	63.40	46.30	31.87	11.72
Operational Holdings									
1981-82	0.4683	12.56	17.99	35.36	29.93	52.08	34.37	22.60	6.61
1991-92	0.5379	9.47	14.61	31.77	26.63	58.76	41.15	28.15	11.72

Source:
1. Report on Some Aspects of Landholdings; 37th Round 1981-82, NSS Report No. 330.
2. Report on Some Aspects of Landholdings; 37th Round 1981-82, NSS Report No. 331.
3. Report on Some Aspects of Household Ownership Landholdings (1); 48th Round, 1991-92 NSS Report No. 399.
4. Report on Some Aspects of Operational Holdings (1); 48th Round, 1991-92, NSS Report No. 407.

Table 3.25: Distribution of Landholdings among Different Categories of Households/Holdings in Himachal Pradesh, 1981-82 to 1991-92

(*Per cent*)

Year	*Landless*	*Marginal Upto (1.00ha)*		*Small (1.01-2.00)*		*Medium (2.01-4.00)*		*Large (Above 4.01 ha)*		*All*	
		H	*A*	*H*	*A*	*H*	*A*	*H*	*A*	*H*	*A*
Ownership Holdings											
1981-82	7.77	54.24	20.95	19.36	23.07	12.37	26.04	6.26	29.94	100	100
1991-92	10.46	68.73	34.97	11.54	20.35	6.43	21.58	2.84	23.10		
Operational Holdings											
1981-82	—	54.23	20.69	25.17	25.94	14.89	28.59	5.71	24.78	100	100
1991-92	—	80.17	41.43	12.30	22.50	6.00	21.38	1.53	14.69		

Note: H stands for holdings (no.) and A stands for area.

Source: 1. Report on Some Aspects of Landholdings; 37th Round, 1981-82, NSS Report No. 330.

2. Report on Some Aspects of Landholdings; 37th Round 1981-82, NSS Report No. 331.

3. Report on Some Aspects of Household Ownership Landholdings (1); 48th Round, 1991-92, NSS Report No. 399.

4. Report on Some Aspects of Operational Holdings (1); 48th Round, 1991-92, NSS Report No. 407.

of marginal holdings was accompanied by an equally significant increase in the proportion of land operated by them.

Table 3.26 presents the respective share of different social groups namely Scheduled Caste, Scheduled Tribe and non-Scheduled Caste and Tribe in the total population and total land. The table shows that during the eighties while the proportion of Scheduled Caste population increased marginally, that of Scheduled Tribe declined. On the other hand, the proportion of land owned by them recorded marginal increase in case of Scheduled Caste and significant decline in case of Scheduled Tribe. There was also a marginal increase in the proportion of landless households among Scheduled Castes. It was, however, important to note that the per cent of landless household among the Scheduled Castes was significantly lower compared to such households both among Scheduled Tribe and non-Scheduled Caste and Tribe. This could largely be attributed to the allotment of surplus and common land to these households under the land distribution programme.

Table 3.26: Share in Population and Land of Different Social Groups in Himchal Pradesh, 1981-82 to 1991-92

(Per cent)

Social Groups	Year	Population	Land	Landless Households
Scheduled Caste	1982	24.62	13.86	6.06
	1992	25.34	14.76	7.09
Scheduled Tribe	1982	4.61	6.75	—
	1992	4.22	2.07	10.00
Non-Scheduled Cast and Scheduled Tribe	1982	70.77	79.39	8.73
	1992	70.44	83.17	11.65

Source: 1. Report on Some Aspects of Landholdings; 37th Round 1981-82, NSS Report No. 330.
2. Population Census, 1981 and 1991.

Further, there was also a significant decline in the levels of land concentration among Scheduled Caste households. As may be seen from Table 3.27, the value of Gini co-efficient and the proportion of area owned by the households at different levels of hierarchy at the top declined significantly in 1991-92 compared with the 1981-82. The land concentration, however, increased both among the Scheduled Tribe and non-Scheduled Caste and Tribe households; it was evident from increase in the value of Gini co-efficient and the per cent share of land owned by the households at the top of the land ownership hierarchy of both the groups. The changes in the distribution of land among different categories of households like marginal, small, medium and large, (Table 3.28) show that the small increase in the per cent of marginal households among Scheduled Caste was associated with huge increase in the proportion of land owned by them. There was also a large decrease in both in the proportion of large households and land owned by them. More or less similar pattern was discernible among the households belonging to scheduled tribe category.

Regarding changes in different aspects of tenancy relations, the information provided in Table 3.29 shows that during 1981-82 and 1991-92, there has been an increase in the incidence of tenancy both in terms of decline in the per cent of entirely owned holdings and increase in the per cent of entirely leased-in holdings. The per cent of

Table 3.27: Concentration of Landholdings among Different Social Groups in Himachal Pradesh, 1981-82 to 1991-92

Social Groups/Year	*Gini-co-efficient*	*Share of Bottom*		*Share of Middle*		*Share of Top*			
		40%	*50%*	*40 to 80%*	*50 to 80%*	*20%*	*10%*	*5%*	*1%*
Scheduled Caste									
1981-82	0.6356	3.27	8.58	45.40	40.10	51.32	53.88	38.17	9.19
1991-92	0.4879	12.10	18.12	44.16	38.14	43.74	35.41	22.97	7.77
Scheduled Tribe									
1981-82	0.3277	39.37	43.06	14.70	10.95	45.93	28.41	16.42	3.71
1991-92	0.5341	7.44	13.95	34.55	28.05	58.00	39.97	23.92	8.54
Non-Scheduled Caste and Tribe									
1981-82	0.5038	9.95	15.58	37.79	32.16	52.27	36.37	24.27	7.53
1991-92	0.6087	5.59	10.10	31.59	27.08	62.82	45.31	31.74	11.58

Source: 1. Report on Some Aspects of Landholdings; 37th Round 1981-82, NSS Report No. 330.
3. Report on Some Aspects of Household Ownership Landholdings (1); 48th Round, 1991-92 NSS Report No. 399.

Table 3.28: Distribution of Landholdings among Different Categories of Households belonging to Different Social Groups in Himachal Pradesh, 1981-82 to 1991-92

(*Per cent*)

Social Groups/Year	*Landless*	*Marginal Upto (1.00 ha)*		*Small (1.01-2.00)*		*Medium (2.01-4.00)*		*Large (Above 4.01 ha)*		*All*	
		H	*A*	*H*	*A*	*H*	*A*	*H*	*A*	*H*	*A*
Scheduled Caste											
1981-82	6.06	81.18	44.06	5.95	11.99	1.29	5.89	4.98	38.06	100	100
1991-92	7.09	84.95	67.42	5.46	16.29	2.09	11.25	0.41	5.04	100	100
Scheduled Tribe											
1981-82	—	18.03	4.10	53.22	43.42	17.60	21.38	11.15	31.10	100	100
1991-92	10.00	65.78	38.46	15.26	24.36	7.37	25.64	1.59	11.54	100	100
Non-Scheduled Caste and Tribe											
1981-82	8.73	45.37	18.34	22.79	23.28	16.63	29.95	6.48	28.43	100	100
1991-92	11.65	63.07	29.14	13.60	20.97	7.95	23.30	3.73	26.59	100	100

Source: 1. Report on Some Aspects of Landholdings; 37th Round 1981-82, NSS Report No. 330.
2. Report on Some Aspects of Household Ownership Landholdings (1); 48th Round, 1991-92 NSS Report No. 399.

Table 3.29: Incidence of Tenancy in Himachal Pradesh, 1981-82 to 1991-92

(*Per cent*)

Year	Entirely Owned Holdings	Mixed Holdings	Entirely Leased-in Holdings	Neither Owned Nor leased-in Holdings	Owned Area	Leased-in Area	Neither Owned Nor Leased-in Area
1981-82	87.24	12.27	0.49	—	94.6	3.2	2.2
1991-92	84.08	3.8	5.01	0.71	92.18	4.83	2.99

Source: 1. Report on Some Aspects of Landholdings; 37th Round 1981-82, NSS Report No. 331.
2. Report on Some Aspects of Operational Holdings (1); 48th Round, 1991-92, NSS Report No. 407.

Table 3.30: Terms of Tenancy in Himachal Pradesh, 1981-82 to 1991-92

(*Per cent*)

Year	Holdings				Area			
	Fixed Money	Fixed Produce	Share Tenancy	Other Terms	Fixed Money	Fixed Produce	Share Tenancy	Other Terms
1981-82	1.83	1.88	2.32	3.22	0.24	0.52	1.06	1.38
1991-92	1.36	0.9	1.08	5.72	0.66	0.43	0.52	3.21

Source: 1. Report on Some Aspects of Landholdings; 37th Round 1981-82, NSS Report No. 331.
2. Report on Some Aspects of Operational Holdings (1); 48th Round, 1991-92, NSS Report No. 407.

operated area leased-in also increased, though marginally. The terms of tenancy also changed (Table 3.30); while there was a marginal decrease in the per cent of holdings leasing-in under fixed money, fixed produce and share tenancy, there was a significant change both in per cent of holdings leasing-in and area leased-in under other terms, which among other things include usufructuary mortgage, from relatives, etc. Table 3.31 further shows that towards the close of the nineties, around two-thirds of the total holdings and operated area leased-in were accounted for by the other terms. It, however, needs to be underlined that there are empirical studies to show that tenancy relations have undergone qualitative changes and no longer entails semi-feudal exploitation of the tenants because of their precarious economic position. The incidence of interlocking of land-labour market was, however, reported by some studies (Panda, 1999). Under interlocking of markets, the tenant does not pay rent but agree to perform labour services whenever required by the landlords. The interlocked transaction is one in which two or more independent exchanges are simultaneously agreed upon and an employer and employee enter into several transactions at the same time in wage hiring, land renting, production and consumption credit, and so on (Bardhan, 1980; Basu, 1983; Bell and Srinivasan, 1989). In the literature on rural development, while Marxists view the pervasiveness of these interlocked transactions as a source of exploitation and surplus appropriation (Bhaduri, 1984; Bhardwaj, 1974), the neo-classicals explain their existence in terms of market imperfections manifested in high transaction cost, asymmetry information, moral hazards, adverse selection, and so on (Braverman and Stiglitz, 1982).

FARM AND NON-FARM EMPLOYMENT

As is well known, the growth of non-farm employment opportunities in the rural areas is essential to lessen the pressure on agriculture and provide new avenues of employment to increasing workforce. It would, therefore, be useful to analyse the changing importance of farm and non-farm employment in the state. The changes in the proportion of usual status workers, i.e. male, female and persons, employed in farm and non-farm sectors, based on data emanating from different quinquinnial NSS surveys on employment and unemployment, have been brought out in Table 3.32. The table shows

Table 3.31: Distribution of Area Leased-in by Terms of Tenancy in Himachal Pradesh, 1981-82 to 1991-92

(*Per cent*)

Year	Holdings				Area			
	Fixed Money	Fixed Produce	Share Tenancy	Other Terms	Fixed Money	Fixed Produce	Share Tenancy	Other Terms
1981-82	7.43	16.21	33.11	43.25	7.28	16.5	33.01	43.21
1991-92	14.99	9.91	11.94	63.16	13.64	8.98	10.87	66.51

Source: 1. Report on Some Aspects of Landholdings; 37th Round 1981-82, NSS Report No. 331.
2. Report on Some Aspects of Operational Holdings (1); 48th Round, 1991-92, NSS Report No. 407.

that the usual status workers employed in agriculture decreased from 87.05 per cent during the early1980s to around 75 per cent towards the close of the 1990s. As a result, the percentage of workers employed in the non-farm sector increased to around 25 per cent. Further, while crop production and livestock were the two major sectors employing most of the workers in agriculture, construction activities followed by services, trade, transport, storage and communication were important non-farm sectors. The changes in the distribution of male workers among major sectors over time show that the share of male workers in agriculture declined significantly from 77 per cent in 1983 to 55.26 per cent in 1999-2000. In the non-farm sectors, the workers employed in construction activities registered a significant increase from 5.77 per cent in 1983 to 11.94 per cent in 1993-94 and further to 16.16 per cent in 1999-2000. The service sector, including community and personal services, was another important sector, wherein the proportion of male workers employed increased from 6.57 per cent in 1983 to 8.33 per cent in 1993-94 and marginally to 8.85 per cent in 1999-2000. Transportation, and storage and trade were the other two important sectors employing 2.16 per cent and 2.91 per cent of the total male workers, respectively. Further, while the percentage share of workers employed in trade increased during the first period (1983 to 1993-94), the percentage of those employed in transport, storage and communication increased during the second period (1993-94 and 1999-2000). So far the employment of usual status female workers is concerned, agriculture continued to employ more than 95 per cent of the total female workers. In the agriculture sector, the female workers employed in the livestock sector recorded a huge increase, from 11.31 per cent in 1993-94 to 24.19 in 1999-2000. In the non-farm sectors, community and social service was the only important sector employing women. The proportion of female workers employed in the service sector increased marginally from 1.07 per cent in 1983 to 1.53 per cent in 1993-94 and further to 2.42 per cent in 1999-2000. In all the other sectors, the proportion of female workers employed was less than one per cent except in agro-based manufacturing where it was around one per cent. The very high proportion of female workers in the agricultural sector can be understood in terms of very high incidence of the service sector in the state. The male workers employed in the service sector including the services are generally posted in areas far from their villages, leaving the management of agriculture and other household affairs to females.

Table 3.32: Distribution of Usual Status Rural Workers among Major Sectors by Sex in Himachal Pradesh 1983 to 1999-2000

(*Per cent*)

Production Sector	1983			1993-94			1999-2000		
	Male	Female	Persons	Male	Female	Persons	Male	Female	Persons
Agriculture	77.00	97.48	87.05	65.77	95.55	80.23	55.26	95.14	74.85
Crop Production	72.82	85.25	78.92	60.74	82.30	71.21	47.99	68.74	58.18
Plantation	1.49	0.16	0.84	2.57	1.90	2.25	2.73	2.11	2.42
Livestock	2.45	12.04	7.15	2.01	11.31	6.53	4.16	24.19	13.99
Forestry and Logging	0.20	—	0.10	0.44	0.05	0.25	0.35	0.03	0.19
Fisheries	—	0.03	0.02	—	—	—	0.05	0.00	0.02
Mining	0.47	0.00	0.24	0.22	0.03	0.13	0.03	0.00	0.01
Manufacturing									
(a) Agro-based	3.58	0.82	2.21	3.58	1.55	2.59	3.29	1.04	2.19
(b) Others	1.91	0.23	1.09	1.71	0.11	0.94	4.54	0.05	2.33
Utilities	0.54	0.00	0.28	1.30	0.19	0.76	1.83	0.11	0.99
Construction	5.77	0.20	3.03	11.94	0.39	6.33	16.16	0.44	8.44
Trade	1.80	0.05	0.94	5.17	0.64	2.97	5.10	0.63	2.91
(a) Wholesale	—	0.00	0.00	0.31	0.14	0.23	0.08	0.00	0.04
(b) Retail	1.80	0.05	0.94	4.86	0.50	2.74	4.02	0.64	2.87
Transport, Storage and Communication	1.09	0.00	0.56	1.61	0.00	0.83	4.15	0.10	2.16
Finance, Insurance and Real Estate	0.34	0.00	0.17	0.37	0.00	0.19	0.79	0.06	0.43
Services, Community Social and Personal Services	6.57	1.07	3.91	8.33	1.53	5.03	8.85	2.42	5.69
Agriculture	77.00	97.48	87.05	65.77	95.55	80.23	55.26	95.14	74.85
Non-Agriculture	22.07	2.37	12.43	34.23	4.45	19.77	44.74	4.86	25.15
All Sectors	99.07	99.85	99.48	100.00	100.00	100.00	100.00	100.00	100.00

Note: Persons include both male and female workers.

Source 1. Government of India, *SARVEKSHANA*, Vol. XIV, No. 172, *October-December* 1990;

2. 1993-94 and 1999-2000 data are extracted from household level data on CD-ROM supplied by NSSO, Government of India.

The annual compound growth rates of usual status workers employed in different sectors, both agriculture and non-agriculture, have been presented in Table 3.33. The table shows that the growth rates of employment in the state for rural males, females and persons declined significantly both in the farm and non-farm sectors during the post-reform period. For example, while the growth rate of usual status persons in the agricultural sector registered a negative growth rate (-1.39), in the non-agricultural sector, it declined from 7.30 per cent to 4.45 per cent. Not only that, other sectors including crop production, and forestry and logging in the agricultural sector and mining, agro-based manufacturing, and wholesale and retail trade in the non-agricultural sector recorded negative growth rates. More importantly, female workers appear to have been affected more adversely as compared to their male counterparts; it was evident from the fact that the growth rate of usual status female workers employment was negative in most of the sectors with the notable exceptions of livestock and plantation in the agricultural sector and services, retail trade and construction in the non-agricultural sector.

The changing relative importance of different sectors in employing rural workers can be better understood by analysing the per cent distribution of incremental workers. The results are provided in Table 3.34. The table shows that during the first period, i.e. between 1983 and 1993-94, more than half the incremental workers were absorbed in agriculture; crop production, livestock and plantation were the important sub-sectors in agriculture. In the non-farm sectors, construction activities employed around 17 per cent of the incremental workers followed by the service sector with 8.72 per cent. There was, however, a huge difference in the proportion of absorption of incremental male and female workers. For example, while agriculture absorbed around 30 per cent of the incremental male workers, as high as 88 per cent of the incremental female workers got absorbed in agriculture. In the non-farm sector, the construction, retail trade and service sectors, respectively absorbed 29.81 per cent, 13.77 per cent and 13.30 per cent of the total incremental usual status male workers. These sectors also played an important role in absorbing the incremental female workers. Regarding the second period (1993/94 to 1999-2000), there was a net decrease in the workers employed in the agricultural sector; however, a significant proportion of the incremental workers was absorbed in the livestock sub-sector. In the non-farm sectors, manufacturing other than agro-based,

Table 3.33: Annual Compound Growth Rate of Employment for Usual Status Rural Workers by Sex and Major Sectors in Himachal Pradesh: 1983/1999-2000

(*Per cent per annum*)

	Male		*Female*		*Persons*	
Production Sector	*1983 to 1993-94*	*1993-94 to 1999-00*	*1983 to 1993-94*	*1993-94 to 1999-00*	*1983 to 1993-94*	*1993-94 to 1999-00*
Agriculture	1.22	-2.96	2.38	-0.23	1.85	-1.39
Crop Production	0.99	-3.95	2.23	-3.11	1.64	-3.49
Plantation	8.24	0.86	29.82	1.60	12.51	1.15
Livestock	0.85	12.71	1.96	13.34	1.77	13.23
Forestry and Logging	10.81	-4.13	—	-5.08	11.73	-4.21
Mining	-4.54	-29.63	—	—	-3.45	-31.02
Manufacturing	2.39	6.64	7.16	-6.85	3.23	4.40
(a) Agro-based	2.75	-1.48	8.99	-6.52	4.08	-2.73
(b) Others	1.70	17.49	-4.27	-12.33	1.25	16.61
Utilities	11.71	5.79	—	-9.13	13.02	4.54
Construction	10.12	5.06	9.37	1.95	10.10	4.98
Trade	13.61	0.34	30.85	-0.41	14.47	-0.35
(a) Wholesale	—	-20.19	—	—	—	-24.58
(b) Retail	11.54	-0.62	27.17	3.04	12.35	-0.23
Transport Storage and Communication	6.64	16.96	—	—	6.64	17.35
Finance, Insurance and Real Estate	3.53	13.40	—	—	3.53	14.56
Services, Community Social and Per-sonal Services	5.10	0.91	6.14	7.74	5.24	2.00
Non-Agriculture	7.14	4.45	8.93	1.29	7.30	4.15
All Sectors	2.84	-0.11	2.59	-0.16	2.72	-0.13

Note: 1. Persons include both male and female workers.
2. Because the information on the workers employed in the fisheries sector for 1993-94 is not available; the growth rates could not be calculated.

Source: 1. Government of India, *SARVEKSHANA*, Vol. XIV, No. 172, October-December 1990;
2. 1993-94 and 1999-2000 data are extracted from household level data on CD-ROM supplied by NSSO, Government of India.

construction, retail trade, transportation, storage and communication, service and real estate employed a significant proportion of the incremental workers. So far the absorption pattern of incremental

Table 3.34: Distribution of Incremental Usual Status Rural Workers among Major Sectors by Sex: 1983 to 1999-2000

Production Sector	*1983 to 1993-94*			*1993-94 to 1999-2000*		
	Male	*Female*	*Persons*	*Male*	*Female*	*Persons*
Agriculture	30.83	88.79	56.71	-1704.09	-138.32	-827.81
Crop Production	23.43	72.30	45.25	-2049.53	-1529.31	-1758.67
Plantation	5.70	7.54	6.52	21.29	20.49	20.85
Livestock	0.68	8.86	4.33	332.09	1364.20	909.97
Agricultural Services	-0.12	—	-0.07	—	7.63	4.27
Forestry and logging	1.14	0.19	0.72	-15.51	-1.33	-7.57
Fisheries	—	-0.10	-0.04	7.58	—	3.34
Mining	-0.54	0.13	-0.24	-29.90	-3.42	-15.08
Manufacturing						
(a) Agro-based	3.48	3.91	3.67	-47.94	-55.55	-52.21
(b) Others	1.09	-0.27	0.48	438.64	-6.55	189.49
Utilities	3.50	0.82	2.31	81.90	-9.11	30.96
Construction	29.81	1.01	16.95	645.76	5.19	287.26
Trade						
(a) Wholesale	1.21	0.60	0.94	-35.79	-15.32	-24.34
(b) Retail	13.77	1.97	8.50	19.24	13.64	16.11
Transport Storage and Communication	3.10	—	1.72	394.18	10.33	179.36
Finance, Insurance and Real Estate	0.44	—	0.24	65.07	6.08	32.06
Services, Community Social and Personal Services	13.30	3.02	8.72	72.93	93.04	84.21
Total	100.00	100.00	100.00	100.00	100.00	100.00

Note: Persons include both male and female workers.

Source: 1. Government of India, *SARVEKSHANA*, Vol. XIV, No. 172, October-Deceber 1990;

2. 1993-94 and 1999-2000 data are extracted from household level data on CDROM supplied by NSSO, Government of India.

male and female workers was concerned, construction, retail trade, transport, storage and communication, finance and real estate, and service were the important sectors that employed most of the additional female workers. In comparison, varying proportions of incremental male workers were absorbed in most of the non-farm sectors except agro-based manufacturing and wholesale trade wherein the number of workers actually employed decreased.

FACILITATING FACTORS

As seen above, the state of Himachal Pradesh has undergone a high degree of socio-economic transformation manifested in better access to basic amenities of life and ultimately in the improvement in the quality of life of population in terms of a number of economic indicators compared with the all-India average. It may, however, be mentioned that the state of Himachal Pradesh continues to be an agrarian state and, therefore, much of its socio-economic transformation is largely driven by the spread of the cultivation of high value crops in the state, especially in districts that enjoy favourable agro-climatic conditions. This has generated both backward and forward linkages that have spawned a number of non-farm activities in other sectors of the economy. For example, it has led to mushrooming of activities in trade and business; numerous shops have come up to supply chemicals and other inputs, post-harvest material like packing boxes, transportation facilities, nursery plants, and so on. Many people in these areas have bought tractors, pick up vans and trucks, and are engaged in a number of activities like supplying construction material, transporting fruits and vegetables, etc. The most important effect has, however, been on the construction activities culminating into a big surge in demand for carpenters, masons, and unskilled labour apart from increase in demand for construction material like cement, iron and steel and bricks. This has made a significant dent on wages and employment of the local labourers, both skilled and unskilled. The cultivation of high value cash crops in the state has also helped sustaining agro-forestry in the neighbouring states of Punjab and Haryana that has become an important source of timber for packing boxes. The economic and ecological impacts of the cultivation of apple and other high value cash crops have been well documented by now (Chand, 1998; Sharma, 1996, Sharma *et al.*, 2002).

Against this background and also from the policy perspective, it is important to understand and throw bare the factors that triggered the whole process of agricultural development and crop diversification in the state. These factors operated both at the micro and macro level. While the factors at the macro level created enabling environment for agricultural development and crop diversification to get underway, those at the household level induced the farmers to make use of the enabling environment by switching over to the cultivation of high value and more remunerative crops which, among other things, depended on landholdings, availability of labour, credit, marketing and so on. The present section discusses some of the important macro factors that facilitated the process of agricultural development and diversification.

First, the adoption of development strategy incorporating mountain specificities has been the single most important contributory factor in facilitating the whole process of agricultural development and crop diversification in the state. The planners accorded very high priority to create basic infrastructural facilities, *ab initio*. Table 3.35 shows that transport and communication, power and social services including education and health, accounted for more than half of the total plan outlay in the first three five year plans. These heavy allocations created a reasonably good network of roads, schools and hospitals. This led to the enhancement of 'social opportunities' and created enabling conditions for a process of widely shared growth, both across regions and sections of society. The roads connected the interiors with the main towns thus breaking the barriers of inaccessibility and isolation and fostering the process of crop diversification. More recently, the widespread expansion of telephone facilities in interiors including tribal areas has given further impetus to the ongoing process of crop diversification. The hypothesis that breaking of inaccessibility barrier triggers the whole process of crop diversification has been supported by the results of the regression equation, given below, fitted to a cross-section of data for twelve districts. The regression coefficients associated with the road length per hundred hectares of net sown area and the number of telephones per hundred of persons were positive and statistically significant as well.

$$Y = -14.58 + \underset{(4.96)}{0.24^{*}} X_1 + \underset{(2.07)}{3.59^{**}} X_2 \; R^{-2} = 0.76 \text{ and } N = 12$$

Where Y is per cent of total cropped area under non-foodgrain crops; X_1 is road length per hundred hectares of the net sown area and X_2 is the number of telephones per 100 persons.

The figures in parentheses are 't' values
* and ** denote significance at 0.01 and 0.05 levels of probability, respectively

Second, a network of institutions was created that facilitated the process of crop diversification. The Himachal Pradesh Horticultural Produce Marketing and Processing Corporation (HPMC) was set up in 1971 with the assistance of World Bank to provide post-harvest infrastructural facilities such as link roads, cold storage, grading and packing facilities. A network of R & D institutions had been created to evolve new technologies and provide technical know-how and extension back up to the farmers. In addition to an Agricultural University, a separate University of Horticulture and Forestry was established in 1985 to provide technical and extension back up to the growing horticultural sector. The Central Government also established research institutions/centres in the state to strengthen the R & D infrastructure; Central Potato Research Institute at Shimla, National Institute of Mushroom Research at Solan, IARI Regional Research Station for Vegetable Research at Katrain (Kullu) and Institute of Himalayan Bio-resources Technology at Palampur are the notable examples. These research institutions/centres provided much needed technical back-up to the cultivation of high value cash crops by evolving suitable technologies in terms of breeding high yielding varieties and advising the farmers about varieties suited to the agro-climatic conditions of their respective areas, their agronomic practices and crop protection measures. Some of the high yielding varieties evolved by the R & D institutions/centres located in the state during the eighties like Arkel (early peas), Azad P-1 (Main season peas), Kufri Jyoti (Potato), Pusa Snow Ball K-1 (Cauliflower), Golden Acre (Cabbage), Contender (French bean) and California wonder (Capsicum) gave a big boost to cultivation of high value cash crops in the state. These varieties have been widely adopted by the farmers of the state. The readily available technical know-how in these institutions and its transfer to the farmers through their network of regional research stations and government line departments played an important role in accelerating the process of crop diversification.

Table 3.35: Pattern of Resource Allocation in Different Five Year Plans: First Five Year Plan to Ninth Five Year Plan

(Per cent)

Sectors	*First Plan 1951-56*	*Second Plan 1956-61*	*Third Plan 1961-66*	*Annual Plan 1966-69*	*Fourth Plan 1969-74*	*Fifth Plan 1974-79*	*Sixth Plan 1980-85*	*Seventh Plan 1985-90*	*Eighth Plan 1992-97*	*Ninth Plan 1997-02*
1. Agriculture & Allied Services	17.56	22.90	28.43	27.74	30.76	22.49	22.61	25.70	20.72	19.22
2. Irrigation	9.78	3.22	2.69	4.85	2.91	5.10	6.21	7.09	4.78	4.54
3. Power	5.87	14.52	7.05	19.56	15.23	25.11	24.94	25.22	20.21	18.23
4. Industry	1.95	3.23	3.62	4.27	4.14	3.66	3.22	2.53	3.02	2.63
5. Transport & communication	44.66	31.16	34.08	28.65	29.90	23.04	21.91	15.67	13.23	10.78
6. Social Services	19.96	23.16	22.63	14.25	16.69	18.14	19.33	20.19	29.90	36.95
of which: Education	8.86	7.74	7.98	5.82	7.01	5.19	3.17	6.21	11.36	14.33
Health	6.37	5.41	6.12	3.37	4.09	3.13	2.89	2.50	4.84	5.57
Others	4.73	10.01	8.53	5.06	5.69	9.82	13.27	11.48	13.70	17.04
7. Miscellaneous	0.22	1.81	1.50	0.68	0.37	2.46	2.50	3.60	8.14	7.65
8. Total	100.00	100.00	100.00	100.00	100.00	100.00	100.00	100.00	100.00	100.00
9. Plan Outlay (Rs. lakhs)	564.40	1,472.53	2.793	4,022	10,140	23,895	56,000	1,05,000	2,50,200	5,70,000
10. Per capita per annum investment (Rs.)	4.00	11.00	21.00	40.00	61.20	100.50	287.80	544.59	1353.60	2205.03

Source: (i) Statistical Outline of Himachal Pradesh, 1971, 1976, 1981, 1989, 1994 and 1999, Directorate of Economics and Statistics, Government of Himachal Pradesh, Shimla.

(ii) Annual Season and Crop Report, 1997-98, Himachal Pradesh, Directorate of Land Records, Government of Himachal Pradesh, Shimla.

The implementation of New Policy on Seed Development (NPSD) by the Government of India since October 1988 further made the import of good quality seeds much easier and hastened the spread of the cultivation of high value cash crops. In addition, the support prices for different fruit crops have been introduced to insulate farmers from fluctuations in the market prices. In more recent times, the market intervention scheme has been launched under which the prices of different fruit crops are fixed according to their grade and quality, and if prices happen to fall below these levels, the state government purchases the produce at fixed prices. These state initiatives are yet other hallmarks of the development strategy that has been implemented over the years.

Third, rapid spread of the cultivation of high value cash crops has also been on account of very high level of market consciousness among the farmers. A number of factors have contributed towards this development. The farmers in Shimla, Solan and Kullu districts have been traditionally growing cash crop like potato, and have always remained in touch with markets outside the state. They have acquired a spirit of entrepreneurship and innovativeness and are always ready to experiment with new crops/enterprises that promise high economic returns. In retrospect, for instance, when potato ceased to be a cash crop in the fifties and the early sixties due to dwindling yields and falling demand, they switched over to fruit cultivation mainly apple, and subsequently to off-season vegetables. Likewise, in recent times, when apple production is fluctuating and becoming uncertain because of erratic weather, farmers in some areas have started switching over to high value cash crops like garlic and off-season vegetables and even to more risky crops like floriculture (Sharma, 1996).[8]

Fourth, the availability of huge market at Delhi and in other cities in the neighbouring states of Punjab and Haryana has been yet another important contributory factor encouraging the cultivation of fruits and off-season vegetables in the state. It needs to be mentioned here that practically from all the far-off parts of the state, the distance to Delhi can be covered in less than twenty-four hours. This puts the state in an advantageous position compared to other mountainous regions including Jammu & Kashmir and north-eastern states where lack of nearby markets has been one of the most limiting factors in the cultivation of high value cash crops. In fact, accessibility of the mountain areas to final markets is a common theme underlying all success stories of crop diversification, especially towards off-season vegetables, in whole of the Hindu kush Himalayan region (Nagpal, 1999).

Fifth, the emergence of relatively efficient marketing system is also an important factor that has contributed towards the adoption and popularization of high value cash crops. In areas where the cultivation of off-season vegetables is 15-20 years old, the local youths have formed some sort of informal groups to market their produce. In some other areas a different marketing system has got evolved that is relatively less efficient. Under this, the growers sell their produce to traders at a price much lower than that prevailing in the market. However, the formation of informal groups by the local youth has also started taking place in these areas. The state marketing board also played an important role in facilitating the marketing of high value cash crops. It has opened marketing yards and established regulated markets where the small and marginal growers can sell their produce. There are around 45 regulated markets including marketing yards in the state, and more than thirty are located in the off-season vegetable producing districts.

Sixth, the emergence of self-help institutions like fruit growers' associations/cooperatives in some of the producing regions is yet another factor that has played an important role in promoting the cultivation of high value cash crops. These institutions help farmers, particularly the small and marginal, in different ways like procuring inputs and also in marketing their produce. The Lahaul Potato Growers Cooperative Society, the Fruit Growers' Associations in Kullu and Shimla districts are notable examples of such cooperative endeavours by the farmers.[9]

EMERGING CONCERNS

The process of socio-economic transformation in the state is beset with a number of problems that are bound to affect its pace and pattern. While there are some common problems being confronted by most of the states, others are specifically related to the sectors and activities that have so far remained the niche areas for the state. Some of these problems are discussed below:

First, the employment in the public sector, that has contributed, in varying degrees, towards the whole process of transformation, particularly in low hill districts like Hamirpur, Kangra, Una, Bilaspur, has already reached a saturation stage. In fact, as one commentator puts it, 'HP now has a dubious distinction of possessing the highest proportion of employees supported by any state government in the country. Salary, interest payments, and pensions put together constitute over a third of the state domestic product' (Sanan, 2004: 976). There thus remains a very little scope for providing jobs in the public sector. The process of liberalization and privatization also does not offer much hope so far the creation of jobs in the private sector in the state is concerned. Due to mountain terrain coupled with lack of modern industrial infrastructural facilities and raw material, not much private investment including foreign direct investment is forthcoming in the state. It is evident from the fact that between August 1991 and March 2002, the industrial investment approved in the state amounted to Rs. 9428 crore (0.88 per cent) compared to Rs. 10,76,327 crore for the whole country (*EPW,* 2002). As a result, the problem of unemployment, especially educated unemployment, has assumed serious proportions and is bound to worsen in times to come.

Second, the liberal financial assistance from the Central Government that facilitated transformation has also started shrinking. The plan assistance has declined, especially since the beginning of the nineties, which is partly attributed to the changes in the norms on the recommendations of the Ninth Finance Commission. The decline in the Central assistance coupled with mounting expenditure has led to a huge gap in the revenue and expenditure obliging the state to resort to market borrowing. As a result, debt burden has increased from Rs. 311.32 crore in 1990-91 to Rs. 1121.85 crore in 1999-2000; the total interest payment has increased to Rs. 770.63 crore accounting for nearly one-fifth of the total revenue expenditure of the state. The fiscal and revenue deficits as a percentage of state domestic product have reached very high levels. The decreasing financial assistance coupled with lack of internal sources of revenue has led to the financial unsustainability jeopardizing the whole process of rural development.[10]

Third, the state, like other mountainous states, also does not have strong industrial base partly because of mountainous terrain and partly because of its relative neglect in successive five year plans; the plan outlay for industrial sector has remained around three per cent from the First Five Year Plan to Ninth Five Year Plan (Table 3.35). The backward and forward linkages arising from the cultivation of high value cash crops have also not spurred the growth of industrial sector; especially small-scale agro-processing and other industries. The benefits have mostly spilled over to the neighbouring states like Punjab and Haryana. For example, the cultivation of high value cash crops has given a big boost to the construction activities. However, most of the construction material like bricks, iron and steel, etc. is being imported from the neighbouring states of Punjab and Haryana. As a matter of fact, a number of factories supplying bricks, iron and steel and other construction material have come up in areas of neighbouring states that border the state.

Fourth, areas/activities in which the state has traditionally enjoyed comparative advantage also face serious problems. For example, the cultivation of high value cash crops, especially horticultural crops, is showing increasing symptoms of unsustainability due to dwindling soil fertility, erratic weather conditions and the emergence of numerous insects, pests and diseases like scab, canker, red-mite, pre-mature leaf fall, and so on. The problem is being compounded due to the availability of spurious inputs, especially agro-chemicals. Consequently, there are sharp fluctuations in year-to-year production. The mono-cropping has led to the loss of micronutrients and deterioration in the overall soil health. The high incidence of diseases has led to an excessive use of agro-chemicals, which increased from 81 metric tonnes in 1985-86 to 192.5 metric tonnes in 1998-99. This has not only resulted in high production cost but has also affected the environment and bio-diversity adversely.

Fifth, the new outward looking open trade linked strategy and the launching of WTO has posed competition from cheaper imports that have affected the production of hops, sericulture, honey and rabbit wool adversely.[11] The problem is likely to become more serious in times to come, particularly for horticultural crops. The problem of procuring reliable seeds, quality plant materials and chemicals has become more serious in the post liberalization regime. There is a mushroom growth of numerous private companies supplying seeds and plant material without any accountability. The emerging Intellectual Property Rights regime shall make it more and more difficult to acquire good quality seeds and plant material. The multinational companies acquiring Intellectual Property Rights, more especially in the field of hybrid seeds, would oblige the farmers to buy these seeds at a very high price. The liberalized regime that facilitates the entry of multinationals and other private companies, who supply seeds, chemicals and other inputs, has posed new challenges to public sector R&D institutions and other public sector agencies. The role of these institutions and government line departments in supplying different inputs has diminished significantly in recent years.

Sixth, the shifting/erosion of micro niches/comparative advantages hitherto enjoyed by the state due to fast technological developments outside the producing regions has posed a new problem, unheard some years back. In an era of fast changing technological developments, the hilly regions, and for that matter any region, cannot take its comparative advantage as given for ever. The experience shows that the comparative advantages are now acquired through technology and new innovations. There are instances to show that many areas in the hills have lost their comparative advantage due to technological changes outside. This has already happened in case of production of many crops like mushrooms, herbs, off-season vegetables, seed potato, etc. that are grown on a large scale in the plains using poly house technologies. The process is likely to get accentuated with the intensification of the process of globalisation/liberalization, which is bound to bring in new technologies, infrastructural and support system (Jodha, 2000; Sharma, 1999).

Seventh, while in case of infrastructural facilities related to education and health the quality of the services leave much to be desired, the physical infrastructural facilities are increasingly proving to be inadequate to cope with the mounting pressure. For example, in a recently concluded micro study in three different high value cash crops growing regions of the state on the problems and constraints in sustaining the cultivation of high cash crops, a preponderant majority of the farmers growing high value crops reported the problem of inadequate transportation facilities, lack of value addition facilities, lack of quality packing material and inadequate marketing infrastructural facilities as the major problems encountered by them (Sharma *et al.*, 2002).

LOOKING AHEAD: SOME POLICY OPTIONS

Some of the policy measures listed below shall go a long way in sustaining the process of socio-economic transformation including the ongoing process of crop diversification in the state.

First, in the non-farm sector, the state should promote the rural small scale cottage industries like handicraft in Kullu and Chamba districts through making suitable policy interventions. In the changed economic dispensations, the possibility of the market for these products in other countries should be explored. Further, the state should take advantage of its dust free environment for the development of electronic goods and precision equipment industries. The promotion of eco-tourism in its earnest sense should enable the state to harness immense potential of its salubrious climate and picturesque valleys. Likewise, hydro-electricity potential needs to be exploited at the earliest to raise revenue. These measures shall help in not only enhancing the state's revenue but also in boosting the employment opportunities available to the local people on a more enduring basis.

Second, so far the agricultural sector is concerned, continuous technological improvements in terms of evolving high yielding disease resistance varieties of high value cash crops including fruit crops, especially apple, is *sine qua non* for promoting the economic viability and ecological sustainability of the cultivation of high value crops. The apple production in the state is showing wide fluctuations in recent years thanks primarily to erratic weather conditions and very high incidence of diseases. It is, however, pertinent to mention that nearly one-fifth of the bearing apple plantations in the state are over-aged which pulls down the overall productivity. These plantations need to be replaced by new dwarf, spur bearing and high yielding plantations. The most important policy support has, therefore, to be in terms of enhanced investment on R & D for evolving new technologies to not only retain but also strengthen the comparative advantage currently enjoyed by the state.

Third, the market infrastructural facilities for high value cash crops need to be further expanded and improved upon. The crops like floriculture and other off-season vegetables require quick refrigerated transport and storage facilities. The effective intervention is, therefore, required to improve upon the provision of efficient infrastructural facilities like metalloid roads, efficient means of transportation, market infrastructure like purchase centres, grading facilities, packaging, cold storage, etc. The far-flung inaccessible areas, particularly in districts like Kinnaur and Lahaul & Spiti, should be linked with road heads, may be through ropeways. The regulatory mechanism for ensuring proper quality of seeds, chemicals etc. is absolutely essential in the changed economic dispensations. The government should intervene by establishing appropriate regulatory mechanism and laying down the rules of the game to safeguard the interests of the farmers.

Fourth, the facilities for proper grading and standardization to improve upon the quality of product and improvement in the post harvest technology to minimize post-harvest losses are very essential to compete in the changed economic regime. Measures for value addition by encouraging the processing of raw produce cost effectively need to be undertaken. The encouragement of private companies to set up small-scale agro-processing plants for value addition is an important initiative required to be taken. In this regard, the possibility of encouraging contract farming in ways that ensures both the technology and other inputs and the market to small and marginal producers at comparable terms and conditions also needs to be explored. In this context, the government can help by bringing small and marginal farmers and agri-business together and building complementary institutions for contract enforcement.

Fifth, the hill farmers also need to be educated about the immediate threats they face and opportunities that are available to them in the changed economic dispensations. More important is to impart technical know how by arranging short duration training camps to enable them to adopt new high value cash crops like floriculture, medicinal plants and herbs and other production options like mushrooms, bee-keeping, poultry, etc. The liberalized regime also calls for continuous vigil on the quantity of imports of fruits like apple and other products and imposing/raising the tariffs on imports, of course within the tariff bindings, to protect the domestic growers from undue foreign competition.

CONCLUSIONS AND LESSONS LEARNED

To conclude, the state of Himachal Pradesh has succeeded in effecting significant improvements in the living conditions of its people during the last four decades; it is evident from a number of indicators related to literacy, health and other infrastructural facilities and quality of life. The state has recorded a fairly high growth rate in its state domestic product and the per capita state domestic product has remained above all-India average barring two-three years in the mid eighties. The state's agriculture has also recorded a fairly high growth during the past three decades. The foodgrains production increased from 9.99 lakh tonnes in the triennium ending 1974-75 to around 15 lakh tonnes in the triennium ending 1999-2000. The yield levels of different crops had also increased over the period by varying degrees. It has got diversified towards high value crops over the years; the story actually began with the introduction of apple in the fifties and the sixties which now include many other crops such as peas, cabbage, cauliflower, garlic and so on, especially in districts/areas enjoying favourable (temperate) agro-climatic conditions.

Regarding changes in the farm and non-employment, the evidence from NSS data shows that the usual status workers employed in agriculture decreased from 87.05 per cent during the early1980s to around 75 per cent towards the close of the 1990s. The structure of rural non-farm employment shows that construction and service sectors were the two important sectors accounting for more than half the workers employed in non-farm sector. Trade, transportation, storage and communication, and agro-based manufacturing were the other important sectors, with each of them employing around 2 to 3 per cent of the total usual status workers. Further, while the employment of male workers in different non-farm activities improved significantly during the post-reform period that of female workers remained practically unchanged. In the non-farm sectors, varying proportions of incremental workers got absorbed in all the non-farm sectors except wholesale trade and agro-based manufacturing. In the ultimate analysis, however, given the state's mountainous terrain, varied agro-climatic conditions and general lack of industrial development because of poor industrial infrastructure, agriculture has been and shall continue to remain a very important source of livelihoods in the times to come.

An in-depth analysis of the factors that facilitated the process of socio-economic transformation in the state shows that the adoption of mountain specificities sensitive development strategy has been the single most important contributory factor. The agricultural diversification from cereal crops to high value cash crops, especially in temperate and sub-temperate regions has, played an important role in triggering the process of socio-economic transformation. The factors such as political patronage, committed state intervention in terms of the provision of infrastructural facilities and easing of inaccessibility constraints, the technological and extension back-up from R & D institutions and supporting departments, the availability of huge market at Delhi and in other neighbouring states, among other things, played an important role in hastening the process of agricultural diversification.

All is, however, not well. The state's agriculture that has remained a driving force for the overall development of the state faces number of problems. The threat from erratic weather for the last couple of years looms large and is endangering the sustainability of high value cash crops. The erosion of natural production niches hitherto enjoyed by the state, because of, *inter alia,* fast technological changes taking place outside the production regions and the ongoing process of globalization is posing new problems. The problem of spurious seeds and chemicals, especially in the aftermath of liberalization and globalization, has assumed serious proportions. The financial health of the state is extremely precarious as was evident from very high fiscal and revenue deficits as per cent of state domestic product. The public sector that has hitherto remained an important source of employment has already reached a saturation stage and the problem of educated en-employment has assumed serious proportion.

The policy initiatives are required to address emerging concerns. The measures such as establishing some regulatory mechanism to ensure quality inputs, improving upon the quantity and quality of existing infrastructural facilities including physical, institutional and social, paying attention to proper grading and standardization and post-harvest technology to minimize losses and add value and enhancing investment on R&D for evolving new technologies shall go a long way in promoting economic viability and ecological sustainability of high value cash crop agriculture. Likewise, in the non-agricultural sector, initiatives such as paying attention to cottage and small industries, promoting electronic goods and precision equipment industries to take advantage of dust free environment, promoting eco-tourism to harness immense potential of its salubrious climate and picturesque valleys and harnessing the hydro-electricity potential are some of the policy initiatives that shall help in not only enhancing the state's revenue but also in boosting the employment opportunities available to the local people on a much more enduring basis.

In the end, the development experience of Himachal Pradesh throws up some important lessons. First, committed state intervention and adoption of development strategies incorporating regional specificities is an essential prerequisite for creating basic conditions for development process to get underway. Second, the creation of basic infrastructural facilities like transport, health, education, etc. is essential for harnessing of local niches and spurring widespread development across all regions. Third, the responsive and entrepreneurial farming communities, their initiatives to innovate, experiment and adopt new production options and form self-help institutions to solve problems in production and marketing is yet another important lesson that emerges from the experience of the process of agricultural development and crop diversification in the state. Fourth, rural transformation process facilitated by high value cash crop agriculture requires continuous technological upgradation. This assumes more importance in an era of fast changing technologies and liberalized economic regime when the comparative advantage of a region cannot be taken as given for ever. Fifth, the development of local resource based industries, especially rural industries, is essential to impart internal strength and resilience to the whole development process, enhance income and employment opportunities, augment revenue and improve upon long term financial sustainability of the state.

ACKNOWLEDGEMENTS

While preparing this paper, the authors have drawn extensively on their past works published in different professional journals. The list of the papers has been given in the references. In the process of writing those papers, they did receive useful comments and suggestions from several persons to whom they remain indebted. They are especially grateful to G.K. Chadha, T.S. Papola, S.S. Johl, Ramesh Chand, D.N. Rao, Mruthyanjaya and D.K. Sharma. The responsibility of all errors and omissions, however, stay with authors alone.

NOTES

1. The state was extremely backward in the fifties. The basic facilities (roads, schools, hospitals, banks, etc.) were almost non-existent. For details, see Sharma, 1987, chap. 2, pp. 19-44.

2. It has, however, argued that the quality of the infrastructural particularly related to educational facilities leave much to be desired. For example, the pass percentage has usually remained less than 50 per cent at class 10 and even lower than at the senior secondary level. *See* Sanan, 2004, pp. 975-978.
3. The poverty levels in the mountainous states of India for 2000 are given below in brackets with each state: Assam (36.89), Arunachal Pradesh (33.47), Nagaland (32.67), Manipur (28.54), Mizoram (19.47), Jammu & Kashmir (3.48), Nagaland (32.67), Sikkim (36.53), Tripura (34.49), Himachal Pradesh (7.63), Jammu & Kashmir (3.48). The poverty levels show that among different states, the incidence of poverty is the lowest in Himachal Pradesh except Jammu & Kashmir. For details see, Papola, 2004, pp. 93-117.
4. The horticultural sector in the state is currently at the cross roads because of the threats it faces from the ongoing process of globalisation, technological and climatic changes. See Sharma *et al.*, 2003.
5. Different Farm Management Cost Concepts have been defined below:
   (i) Cost A1 = Include value of hired human labour (permanent and casual); value of bullock labour (owned and hired), expenditure on Machinery (owned and hired); expenditure on seed (owned and hired); expenditure on fertilizers and manures (owned and purchased); expenditure on insecticides and pesticides; irrigation charges; canal water charges; land revenue and other taxes; depreciation on farm buildings and equipments; interest on working capital and miscellaneous charges.
   (ii) Cost A2 = A1 + rent paid for leased-in land.
   (iii) Cost B1 = Cost A1+ imputed interest on owned fixed capital (excluding land).
   (iv) Cost B2 = Cost A2 + imputed rental value of owned land (less land revenue) imputed interest on owned fixed capital (excluding land).
   (v) Cost C1 = Cost B1 + imputed value of family labour.
   (vi) Cost C2 = Cost B2 + imputed value of family labour.
   (vii) Cost D = Cost C2 + 10 per cent of Cost C2.
6. The mountain regions are generally known to be thriving on the so-called money order economy because of large-scale male migration from these regions. However, in those areas of the state where high value cash crop cultivation has made much headway, the process of reverse migration has taken place; many males who had migrated to other places have left their jobs to take care of their orchards at home.

7. In the literature, there are different methods to measure the incidence of poverty, each having its own merits and demerits. For instance, if one is interested to find out the number of people below poverty line, the most commonly employed method is head-count ratio. This measure is just a head count of the people whose income/expenditure falls below the required level. Notationally, the measure is HCR = HC/n, where HC is the number of people below the poverty line and n is the total population. However, as is well known, an obvious limitation of head count ratio is that it does not tell anything about the extent to which individual income/expenditure actually falls below the poverty line. One way to take this into account is to use a measure of average income shortfall from the poverty line. The measure that takes this aspect into account is Poverty Gap Ratio (PGR). It is defined as the ratio of average income needed to lift all poor people above the poverty line. In notational terms, the measure is written as under: PGR = $\Sigma_{yi<p}(p\text{-}y_i)_{/nm,}$ where y_i is the income of households blow poverty line, p_i is the poverty line, n is the number of people below the poverty line and m is the poverty line. It, however, needs to be mentioned that these two measures do not take into account some other important aspects of poverty. For example, neither of the measures mentioned above, satisfies the principle of weak axiom that states that a transfer of income of an individual below the poverty line to anyone less poor, while keeping the set of poor unchanged, must raise the incidence of poverty. The most popular measure that takes into consideration the distributional underpinnings of poverty is the class of measures proposed by Foster, Greer and Thorbecke (1984). The measure proposed by them incorporates the distributional sensitivity by raising the poverty gap to a power. For any power á, a class of poverty measure given by Foster, Greer and Thorbecke can be stated as under: $p_\alpha = 1/n\ \Sigma_{yi<p}$ $(p\text{-}y_i/p)^\alpha$.The change in the values of á has interesting implications. For instance when $\alpha = 0$, the measure P_0 is just head count ratio, when $\alpha = 1$ it becomes poverty gap ratio. And as the value of α increases beyond 1, the poverty gap starts acquiring larger weights and the measure becomes increasingly sensitive to the gaps between individual's income and the poverty line. Thus, FGT measure states that when there is no inequality in the distribution of income, the poverty can be measured by head count ratio but in the presence of inequality, it raises the poverty. In the present case, we had taken a poverty line of Rs. 20,000 per annum for a family of five members.
8. For an historical account of the introduction of different cash crops like potato, tea, etc. in different districts like Kullu, see Singh, 1998.

9. Dreze and Sen have attributed the rapid economic and social transformation of Himachal Pradesh to three important enabling factors:

   (i) well directed public intervention in support of social opportunities;

   (ii) active agency of women; and

   (iii) local democracy and social cooperation.

   For details see, Dreze and Sen 2002, pp. 105-110 and 179-184.

10. For details about the magnitude of financial crisis, see Himachal Pradesh: Human Development Report, 2001, Chapter XIV.

11. In the post-liberalization period, the products like raw silk and silk products and honey are being imported from China, Korea, and Australia are sold at a much lower price. This year, the price of mulberry cocoon has fallen by as much as Rs. 100 per kg. Likewise, the price of hops has declined from Rs. 35 per kg in 1995-96 to Rs. 10 in 1999-2000. As a result, the area under hops in the Lahaul valley has declined from 120 hectares in 1991-92 to 40 hectares in 2000-01.This did affect the income and employment of local producers adversely.

REFERENCES

Bardhan, Pranab (1980): 'Interlocking Factor Markets and Agrarian Development: A Review of Issues', *Oxford Economic Papers*, Vol. 32, Nos. 1-2, pp. 82-97.

Basu, Kaushik (1983): 'The Emergence of Isolation and Interlinkage in Rural Markets', *Oxford Economic Papers*, Vol. 35, No. 2, pp. 262-280.

Bell, Clive and Srinivasan, T.N. (1989): 'Interlinked Transactions in Rural Markets: An Empirical Study of Andhra Pradesh, Bihar and Punjab', *Oxford Bulletin of Economics and Statistics*, Vol. 51, No. 1, pp. 73-83.

Bhaduri, Amit (1984): *Economic Structure of Backward Agriculture*, Macmillan India Ltd., New Delhi.

Bhardwaj, Krishna (1974): *Production Conditions in Indian Agriculture*, Cambridge University Press.

Braverman, A. and Stiglitz, J.E. (1982): 'Sharecropping and Interlinking of Agrarian Markets', *American Economic Review,* Vol. 72, No. 4, pp. 695-715.

Chadha, G.K., Sucharita Sen and H.R. Sharma (2004): *Land Resources in Indian Agriculture: Policy, Use and Future Strategic Choices*, Academic Foundation, New Delhi.

Chand, Ramesh (1998): *Agricultural Diversification and Development of Mountain Regions*, M.D. Publications, New Delhi.

Dreze Jean and Amartya Sen (2002): *India: Development and Participation*, Oxford University Press, New Delhi.

Economic and Political Weekly (2001): 'Current Statistics', Volume XXXVI, No. 25, p. 2212.

Foster, J., J. Greer and E. Thorebecke (1984): 'A Class of Decomposable Poverty Measures', *Econometrica*, Vol. 52, No. 3, pp. 571-576.

Jodha, N.S. (2000): 'Globalisation and Fragile Mountain Environment: Policy Challenges and Choice', *Mountain Research and Development*, Vol. 20, No. 4.

Nagpal, Shantanu (1999): 'Food Security in Hindukush Himalaya', *Economic and Political Weekly*, Vol. XXXIV, No. 38, pp. 2717-2720.

Panda, Subhasish (1999): 'The Survey of Rural India: Case Study of a Village Khala-Kiar', Report Submitted to Lal Bahadur Shastri National Academy of Administration, Mussoorie, India.

Papola, T.S. (2004): 'Poverty in Mountain Areas: Nature, Causes and Alleviation Strategy', in *Poverty Alleviation in Mountain Areas of China* (Eds) N.S. Jodha, Binayak Bhadra, Narendra Raj Khanal and Jurgen Richter, Inweent gGmbH, Capacity Building International, Germany, pp. 93-117.

Sanan, Deepak (2004): 'Delivering Basic Public Services in Himachal Pradesh: Is the Success Sustainable?' *Economic and Political Weekly*, Vol. XXXIX, No. 9, pp. 975-978.

Shariff, Abusaleh and P. K. Ghosh (2000): 'Indian Education Scene and the Public Gap', *Economic and Political Weekly*, Vol. XXXV, No. 16, pp. 1396-1406.

Sharma, H.R. (1992). 'Agrarian Relations in India since Independence', *Journal of Indian School of Political Economy*, 4 (1):201-62.

Sharma, H.R. (1994). 'Distribution of Landholdings in Rural India, 1953-54 to 1981-82: Implications for Land Reforms', *Economic and Political Weekly*, 29 (13): A12-A25.

Sharma, H.R. (1995). *Agrarian Relations in India: Patterns and Implications*, New Delhi; Har Anand Publications.

Sharma, H.R. (1996): *Mountain Agricultural Development Processes and Sustainability: Micro Level Evidence from Himachal Pradesh, Indian Himalayas*, Discussion Paper Series No. MFS 96/2, ICIMOD, Kathmandu, Nepal.

Sharma, H.R. (1997). 'Land Reforms: Status and Opportunity', in Desai M. Bhupat (ed.): *Agricultural Development Paradigm for Ninth Plan under New Economic Environment*, pp. 712-39. Delhi: Oxford & IBH.

Sharma, H.R. (1998). 'Distribution of Landholdings in Rural India: A Comparative Study of Scheduled Castes, Tribes and Non Scheduled Caste and Tribes', *Artha Vijnana,* 50 (2):196-226.

Sharma, H.R. (1999): 'Issues and Options for Horticulture Based Marginal Farms and Lands', Paper Presented at Planning Meeting on Investigating Issues and Options for Improving Livelihoods of Marginal Mountain Farms, ICIMOD, Kathmandu, Nepal.

Sharma, H.R. (2004): 'Agricultural Development and Crop Diversification in Himachal Pradesh: Understanding the Patterns, Processes, Determinants and Lessons', *Indian Journal of Agricultural Economics*, Forthcoming.

Sharma, H.R. 2000, 'Tenancy Relations in Rural India: A Temporal and Cross-sectional Analysis'. *Indian Journal of Agricultural Economics*, 55 (3):295-307.

Sharma, H.R., R.K. Sharma and Virender Kumar (2000): *Distribution of Surplus Land among Landless Households and its Impact on Income, Employment and Poverty: A Study of Himachal Pradesh*, Research Report No. 15, Department of Agricultural Economics, H.P. Agricultural University Palampur (H.P.).

Sharma, H.R., R.K. Sharma, S.K. Chauhan and Virender Kumar (2004): *Mountain Agriculture in Transition: A Study of Processes, Determinants and Implications Using Micro Evidence from Himachal Pradesh*, Department of Agricultural Economics, H.P. Agricultural University, Palampur (H.P.).

Sharma, H.R., Virender Kumar and R.K. Sharma (1999): 'Rural Non Farm Employment in Himachal Pradesh, 1971-1991: A District Level Study', *The Indian Journal of Labour Economics,* Vol.40, No. 2, pp. 251-263.

Sharma, L.R. (1987): *The Economy of Himachal Pradesh: Growth and Structure*, Mittal Publications, Delhi.

Singh, Chetan (1998): *Natural Premises: Ecology and Peasant Life in Western Himalayas, 1800-1950,* Oxford University Press, New Delhi.

4

Madhya Pradesh

S.N. CHAUDHARY

THE REGION

Madhya Pradesh is one of the largest states in the country. It is surrounded by five states, namely Andhra Pradesh, Bihar (Now Jharkhand), U.P., Rajasthan, Gujarat and Maharashtra. After Independence, hundreds of princely states were merged to form the boundaries of the present state of Madhya Pradesh. Thus, undivided Madhya Pradesh came into being on November 1, 1956, with the merger of Bhopal, Madhya Bharat and Vindhya Pradesh provinces, Mahakaushal region of the former M.P. province, and the Sironj sub-division of Rajasthan. Bhopal was made the capital of this newly constituted state. The state of Chhattisgarh was carved out of the parent state of M.P. on November 1, 2000. The population of Madhya Pradesh is just over 60 million, which is 7.8 per cent of the total population of India. It is the seventh most populous Indian state. The sex ratio (i.e., number of females per thousand males) has improved from 912 in 1991 to 920 in the 2001 Census. However, there are regional and communitywise variations. The Growth Rate (1981-1991) for urban and rural population was 44.98 per cent and 22.11 per cent respectively, as against the all India figures of 36.19 per cent and 19.17 per cent respectively. The Growth Rate during 1991 and 2001 was 24.34 per cent for Madhya Pradesh as against 21.34 per cent for India. There are 48 districts in the state. Some of the special features, which are administrative and demographic, are given in Table 4.1. All the 48 districts may be grouped under different regions. These are: Malwa Region formed of Dhar, Indore, Jhabua, Barwani, Dewas, Mandsaur, Neemuch, Ratlam, Sajapur, Ujjain, Khandwa, Burhanpur, Khargon, and Harda. The Mahakaushal Region consists of areas of Betul, Hosangabad, Balaghat, Chhindwara, Jabalpur, Katni, Mandla, Dindori, Narsinghpur and Seoni. The Chambal Region comprises Bhind, Morena, Sheopur, Datia, Guna, Ashoknagar, Gwalior, and Shivpuri. The Bundelkhand Region comprises Chhatarpur, Damoh, Panna, Sagar and Tikamgarh. The Vindhya Region has areas of Rewa, Satna, Sahdol, Anuppur, Umariya, and Sidhi; while the region of Ex-Bhopal dynasty consists of Bhopal, Raisen, Rajgarh, Vidisha, and Sehore.

HEALTH AND EDUCATION

Life expectancy at birth is one of the most comprehensive indicators of health status. The best available estimates for the state of life expectancy are from the Sample Registration Scheme (SRS) of the Registrar General of India. The latest SRS estimated life expectancy at Birth in Madhya Pradesh is 55.2 years for the period 1992-96, which has a significant increase from 47.2 years and 49.0 years during 1970-75 and 1976-80 respectively. This, however, is still behind the national estimate of 60.7 years. The gap between national and state life expectancy rates has been increasing over the years, to a current difference of 5.5 years (a difference of 9 per cent). There are also differences in life expectancy between rural and urban areas, pegged at 53.7 years and 63 years respectively. The level of deprivation in the state seems even more when compared to that of the state of Kerala (a significant difference of 18 years), where life expectancy was estimated at 73 years as against 55 years for Madhya Pradesh during the period 1992-96. The crude birth rate in the state was high as compared to the prevailing national rate according to the Sample Registration System 1999. The death rate is still one of the highest in the country.

Table 4.2 shows that the birth rate, death rate and infant mortality rate (IMR) in the state have decreased over the time. In 2001, the crude birth rate, crude death rate and infant mortality rate for India were 24.28, 8.78 and 63.19 respectively (*Source*: 2001 CIA India Fact Book). In spite of the many health care programmes in Madhya

Table 4.1: Madhya Pradesh at a Glance

Population	6,03,85,118 (Census, 2001)
Male	3,14,56,873 (52.09%)
Female	2,89,28,245 (47.91%)
Scheduled Tribes	96,82,000 (19.94%)
Scheduled Castes	74,78,000 (15.40%)
Area (in sq. kms.)	308,000
Revenue Divisions	9
Districts	48
Tehsils	272
Development Blocks	313
Decennial Growth Rate	24.26
Gram Panchayats	21,999
Literacy rate	64.11%
Male	76.80%
Female	50.28%
Density of Population	196 per sq. km.
Male-Female Ratio	1000:933
Total Villages	55393
Inhabited Villages	52143
Tribal Blocks	89
Towns (2001)	394
Municipalities	86
Nagar Panchayat	237
Police Thana	934
Lok Sabha Seat	29
Rajya Sabha Seat	12
Vidhan Sabha Seats	230
Total Working population (in thousands)	25794
Main working population (in thousands)	19103
Marginal working population (in thousands)	6691
Cultivators (in thousands)	11038
Agricultural labours (in thousands)	7401
Workers in household industries (in thousands)	1033
Other workers (in thousands)	6322
Non-working population (in thousands)	34554
Post office (2004-05)	8345
Letter Box (2004-05)	40962 (Approx)
Telephone Kendra (2004-05)	2789
Doordarshan transmiter (2004-05)	78
Doordarshan Studio (2004-05)	03
Radio Station (2004-05)	16

Source: NIC site, GOMP. Give full details of the reference.

Table 4.2: Crude Birth and Death Rates for Madhya Pradesh

Year	*Crude Birth Rate*	*Crude Death Rate*	*IMR*
1971-1975	38.5	17.1	145
1976-1980	38.0	16.0	143
1981-1985	38.2	14.9	129
1986-1990	36.6	13.3	117
1991-1995	34.4	12.4	105
1996-2000	31.5	10.8	93
2000	31.4	10.5	87
2001	30.8	10.0	86

Source: The State of Population, MPHDR, 2003.

Pradesh, the number of infants and children dying prematurely is still very high. The Word Health Chart depicts India's IMR in relation to the rest of the world (Vietnam has a lower infant mortality compared to India despite lower per capita income (www.whc.ki.se). Madhya Pradesh has one of the highest IMR rates in comparison to those prevailing in other states. The IMR for Madhya Pradesh has been estimated at 88 in 2000 by Sample Registration Survey (SRS) as compared to the national average of 68 (UNICEF, 2000). The rural IMR was 94 and urban 54 in 2001 in Madhya Pradesh. The IMR trend for undivided Madhya Pradesh and India is shown in Table 4.3. Mortality of infants (early neo-natal, neo-natal and infant mortality) shows some decline in post neo-natal mortality rates. However, there is no decline in neo-natal rates but an increase, which is a grave concern. The child mortality rates are nearly twice the national average as per NFHS-2, 1998-99. Deaths due to complications in pregnancy and childbirth (or maternal deaths) are among the leading causes of death in women in the reproductive age group in Madhya Pradesh. Evidence from various rural surveys suggests that maternal deaths account for more than 2 per cent of total deaths and about 4 per cent of total female deaths (Department of Economics and Statistics, GOMP, 1996). SRS estimates for 1997 suggest that about 498 women die of complications associated with pregnancy, delivery and in the post-partum period for every 100,000 live births. However, there are regional and district-wise variations. The maternal mortality ratio was the third highest in the country. Major causes of maternal mortality are given in Table 4.3. The National Family Health Survey (NFHS-2) 1998, shows that only

22.4 per cent childern received the full schedule of immunization in the state, indicating that nearly 80 per cent of children are potentially vulnerable to preventable diseases. The National Sample Survey (NSS) data show a decreasing trend in immunization with increasing age of the child.

Table 4.3: Trends of Infant and child death (neonatal, post-neonatal, infant) per 1000 life birth in undivided Madhya Pradesh and India

Survey and Year	*Neonatal Mortality*	*Post Neonatal Mortality*	*Infant Mortality*	*Child Mortality*	*Under 5 Mortality*
NFHS 1 MP:1988-92	53.2	32	85.2	49.3	130.3
NFHS 2 MP:1994-98	54.9	31.2	86.1	56.4	137.6
NFHS 2 India	43.4	24.2	67.6	29.3	94.9
SRS 1992	63.9	39.7	104	—	—
SRS 1997	64.0	30.4	94	—	—

Source: NFHS-1 and various volumes of SRSs.

Table 4.4: Causes of Maternal Deaths

	(In per cent)
Haemorrhage	29
Anaemia	19
Puerperal Sepsis	16
Obstruction	10
Hypertensive Disease	8
Unsafe Abortion	9

Source: Department of Economics and Statistics, GOMP, 1996.

Cases of water born diseases as well as the cases of death are very common and alarming in the state, except asthma, the percentage of persons suffering from T.B., Jaundice and Malaria is quite high. In Jhabua village, as reported by Shobhit Jain (2000), Malaria, Diarrhoea and T.B. are common diseases.

The percentage of infant mortality, maternal mortality, death due to disease is high in M.P. in comparison to the all India scenario. There are multiple historical and contextual factors responsible for this. Poverty and lack of institutional support to the people living in

Table 4.5: Cases of Water Borne Diseases

Diseases	Cases		Death	
	1989	*1993*	*1989*	*1993*
Gastro-enteritis	47172	31826	168	1021
Dysentery	212551	38568	199	178
Cholera	36	56	01	01
Jaundice	3690	2083	71	107
Meningitis	4569	803	507	N.A

Source: Third Environmental Status Report (1996 EPCO, Bhopal, p. 272).

Table 4.6: Percentage of Persons Suffering from

	Asthma	*T.B*	*Jaundice during past 12 months*	*Malaria during past 3 months*
M.P	2.273	0.602	1.927	10.015
India	2.468	0.544	1.361	3.697

Source: M.P. Third Human Development Report, 2002:58.

rural and tribal areas and their over dependence on tradition and cultural practices and health management mechanisms are the broader reasons. However, a trend in favour of villagers, especially tribals' dependence on institutional arrangements is under way. Broadly these efforts are of seven types, that is, (i) policies prepared by government, such as, ensuring geographic and economic access to primary and secondary quality health care and family welfare services to all people of M.P within a span of five to seven years; (ii) prevention of disaster, to the extent possible, and preparedness for disaster management as and when required; (iii) reducing the MMR to 220 by 2011 from the level of 498 (1997 level); (iv) reducing the IMR to 62 by 2011 from the level of 97 (1997 level); (v) total fertility rate to reach replacement level fertility (i.e. a TFR of 2.1) by the year 2011; (vi) stabilize the prevalence of HIV/AIDS at low level, and (vii) address problems related to mental health and initiate action to create information base and preventive intervention for improved mental health in the state. The strategies to achieve these objectives were: schemes and programmes run by government schemes run by NGOs (both national and international), and private health practioners. Since its inception the Government of M.P. have taken number of efforts to establish, strengthen and popularize medical/health education and services in both rural and urban areas. Health schemes such as Swasth Jeewan Sewa Guarantee Yojana, Rogi Kalyan Samiti, Jan Swasthya Rakshak Scheme, Dai Training Programme, and State Illness Assistance Fund Scheme.

The state formulated a Women's Policy in 1995, becoming the second state in the country to recognize empowerment of women as key element in changing unequal social structures. The overall goals of the policy are to ensure the survival and protection of female life, fullest participation of women in civil society, strengthening their role in decision making, and enabling them to take advantage of developmental efforts in all fields.

But this is the macro perspective. If we look at the situation at the village level the picture is mixed. Shobhit Jain (*op. cit.*) reported from Jhabua village that there is a Village Health Committee but hardly any meeting takes place. However, the Gram Swastha Register is properly maintained. This register carries information related to birth, death, conception and marriage. PHC camps are there but villagers have no knowledge about it. Villagers know about condom but they rarely use it. Jain reported that for the meaningful functioning of Anganwadi Kendras it is necessary that health check up of pregnant women and malnourshied children are carried out and the severe malnourished children provided referral services. On the basis of above analysis it is clear that health status of rural population is by and large not upto the mark in Madhya Pradesh. Of course, the number of societal interventions have increased, now people's participation based strategies have been introduced since 1991 but due to variety of inter-connected reasons significant achievement is yet to be attained. This calls for formulation of area, target group and culture specific curative mechanisms with the participation and cooperation of all the concerned change agents.

In order to delink from the trauma of sick state symbol attempts, particularly in the field of education, have been made in Madhya Pradesh during last several years. This is reflected from the increasing number of interventions by the state from the primary education level onwards. Towards the end of 2005 M.P. had 81,335 primary schools and 12 Universities.

We have districtwise data on number of such educational institutions. The data show that highest number of Primary Schools is in Jhabua (3690), and lowest in Burhanpur (532), but in spite of that Jhabua has the lowest level of literacy (36.9%) in the state. Perhaps this state of affairs is due to highest seasonal out-migration, non-realization of importance of education, highest number of people under debt, highest levels of poverty and so on. As a result of all these constraints the district is forced to face the challenge of non-enrollment and dropout in a more serious manner in comparison to other districts.

Table 4.7: Categorywise Government run number of Educational Institutions (2005)

Sl. No.	*Name*	*Number*
1.	Primary Schools	81335
2.	Middle Schools	24293
3.	High/Higher Secondary Schools	8504
4.	Colleges	391
5.	Technical Institutes	127
6.	Universities	12

Source: Statistical Summary of M.P. (2006), Directorate of Economics and Statistics, Bhopal, GOMP.

In order to promote primary education and ensure maximum enrollment especially in the remote rural and tribal areas, number of steps have been taken during last several years. Important among these are: The Education Guarantee Scheme (1997); Incentives to Girl Students; SC/ST Students Griha Yojana; Padhna Badhna Andolan; and Sarva Shiksha Abhiyan.

Table 4.8: Social Composition of EGS Students

1.	Of the total children enrolled	44% are STs
2.	Of the total children enrolled	16% are SCs
3.	Of the total children enrolled	32% are OBCs
4.	ST/SC/OBC children comprise	92% of the total
5.	Of the total enrolled	47% are girl students
6.	Demographic Location	42% schools are in tribal areas

Source: The Bhopal Document (2002): Bhopal: GOMP, p.117.

The Education Guarantee Scheme (EGS) was launched in 1997. It ensures that every child has access to elementary level school education within a habitation not extending beyond a mile. It is named as Rajiv Gandhi Shiksha Mission. According to the philosophy of decentralization any village or a collection of households with a minimum of 25 children can demand an EGS school facility where no school exists, and the state government provides the same within a short span of 90 days. By July 2001, 23,854 schools were established, 28,435 teachers were appointed and 11,30,219 children were enrolled. It is observed that most of the students enrolled under EGS are from the marginalized sections.

Numbers of steps are in progress to promote the education of girls from SC/ST households. The state government awards Rs. 500 to each girl student who passes 5th standard and joins class 6th as a regular student. In the financial year 2000-01 a sum of Rs. 541.95 lakh was sanctioned to benefit about 1,06,800 SC/ST girl students. SC/ST Students' Griha Yojana provides for the payment of rent by the government for hiring a room to five or more students who fail to get admission into welfare hostels. During the year 2000-01, 800 such homes were taken to accommodate around 3,650 students. Padhna Badhan Andolan scheme was crafted in 2000 to revitalize the literacy movement in the state. It had eight strategies to achieve its objectives. These were: to involve non-literates to come together and form Padhna Badhan Samitis. Local educated persons be made their teachers (*Guruji*); all students should be registered with the nearest Panchayat or Jan Shiksha Kendra (Cluster Resource Centre) along with the name of the proposed *Guruji;* Government should verify the literacy status of the *Guruji* and provide training and teaching-learning material to him. During the literacy programme three basic literacy primers of the NLM would be taught and in addition to the three literacy Primers of NLM, a fourth Primer (*Chautha* Primer) was developed by the Rajiv Gandhi Mission on Human Rights such as land rights, gender rights, forest rights, labour rights, and development rights. The idea was that as the PBA Samiti transacts the Fourth Primer it repositions itself as a Self-Help Group and then form a thrift and credit society. The Government was to monitor, hold hands, and undertake a 100 per cent external evaluation of the learners. Based on the number of people who cleared the examination the *Guruji* would be given a *Gurudakshina* of Rs. 100 per learner to which the community was also free to add. The outcome of this intervention seems praiseworthy. The Andolan could, form 2,17,000 Samitis and enrol 5.18 million students. There was no restriction on who could be a *Guruji* and even grassroots level functionaries like *Gurujis* of EGS schools, erstwhile TLC volunteers could also become *Gurujis* of the 'Padhan Badhan Andolan'. The final evaluation was scheduled between 7-9 December and out of the 51.83 lakh people enrolled 32 lakh had completed the Third Primer (another 19.41 lakh had completed the second Primer) and took the examination. 29.85 lakh cleared the examination which was conducted openly with invitation advertised in newspapers requesting the public to witness the event. Results of external evaluation by expert panel approved by NLM are close to those of the 100 per cent state level evaluations corroborating the results of this one-year campaign. (Third Human Development Report: 34)

Sarva Shiksha Abhiyan (SSA) is one of the recent responses (2001) by the government to deal with the problem of non-enrollment, stagnation, and school dropouts among children living in remote rural and tribal areas. It was introduced to ensure that all the children between the age group of 6 to 14 attend school and receive quality elementary education within a fixed period. Specific objectives of SSA are that all children in School Education Guarantee Centre, Alternate schools should be back to School Camps by 2003 and they should complete five years of primary schooling by 2007. By 2010 all children should complete eight years of elementary schooling. The scheme focuses on elementary education of satisfactory quality which is relevant for life. SSA aims at bridging all gender and social gaps at the primary stage by 2007 and at elementary education level by 2010. It aims to achieve universal education by 2010. To actualize these objectives during 2001, Rs. 1600 crore were sanctioned by the Central Government which increased upto Rs. 7156 crore in 2005-06. Two per cent education cess was levied from 2004 to provide additional finances for elementary education. Critical examination of SSA in the light of the objectives mentioned above shows that the enrollment rate among both boys and girls have increased, due to mid-day meal the retention rate have also increased, gap between the sexes and social groups have also decreased. However, doubt is raised about the quality of the education imparted to children. This is clear from a finding of the study done by Chaudhary and Chaudhary (2007), which is on 15 schools of Sehore district. It states that all the 15 schools visited were upto the mark from infrastructure and basic facility point of view. Most of the teachers are from the upper castes. Most of the students are from the OBCs and from poor background. Mid-day meal was functioning in an excellent manner. SSA had positively impacted students in terms of their enrollment, health and presence in the classroom. But the level of knowledge of the interviewed students (150 from all the 15 schools) was a frustrating experience. More than 51 per cent respondents even did not know the name of the capital of Madhya Pradesh. Around 74 per cent of 4th and 5th standard students do not know the name of our Prime Minister. Hence, in terms of quality the situation is critical.

There is popularization of college education in Madhya Pradesh today. The increasing number of both government and private colleges in the entire 48 districts is an example. Also no matter where the colleges are located everywhere the students are opting for professional or job oriented courses. In many of these technical colleges, camps are held and direct appointments are made. This development has spread a ray of hope in favour of education and employment among the middle class youths.

Table 4.9: No. of Government Run Educational Institutions

Sl. No.	*Region Name*	*Pre-Primary/ Primary Schools*	*Middle Schools*	*High School/ Higher Secondary*	*Colleges*
1.	Mahakaushal	17056	5235	1881	68
2.	Bhopal	11279	3486	1240	46
3.	Malwa	22819	6562	2294	83
4.	Vindhya	12447	3178	1381	41
5.	Bhundelkhand	8134	2723	714	36
6.	Chambal	11279	3486	1240	46
	Total	83014	24670	8750	320

Source: Statistical Summary of M.P. (2006), Directorate of Economics and Statistics, Bhopal: GOMP.

AGRARIAN RELATIONS

According to Gupta (2005) the foray of the Britishers during the colonial period was delayed in Madhya Pradesh because of different reasons. Absence of productive forces was one among these which was also supported by existence of number of princely states. However, once established British administration resorted to massive economic exploitation of its large forest resources. Exploitation of forest resources was further followed by massive exploitation of mineral resources. In the field of agriculture it was felt by the "Raj" that the local population was not competent enough to initiate farm activities in a commercial manner and pay revenue to the administration. As stated by Rahul (unpublished) other social groups like Marathas from Maharashtra, Kunbis and Patidars from Gujarat and Jats from Rajasthan were encouraged to come and settle on tribal lands. According to Roy (2002) broadly there were two types of land revenue system during those days in this region, one with intermediaries between the tenant and the state and the other operated directly between the state and the tenant. As British entry was late in this area, the introduction of the tenurial system with a colonial imprint was delayed. However, once it happened numerous types of tenurial relations were introduced in Madhya Pradesh. Roy (*op. cit.*) further said that in spite of different ends of tenurial arrangements, the basic position of the tenant-cultivator during the colonial period remained pitiable. As Madhya Pradesh was thinly populated and unable to generate surplus, the land owning class was not interested in the productive collection of rents like in the permanent settlement areas. Hence, there was no real basis for rent and there was, in effect, a system of *ryotwari* being practiced with a direct relation prevailing between the state and the peasants. This explains why there was no massive dislocation on land and it was really indebtedness resulting from lack of proper production in land which contributed to indebtedness. Further, unlike in the permanent settlement areas there was no substantive large-scale peasant movement in M.P. for land reform issues either during the pre- or post-independence period. Roy further asserted that the poor peasants in the state escaped the large scale violence not because of the benevolence of the landed gentry of the region, but more because the mode of production was relatively free of exploitative elements as were found in the permanent settlement areas. As and when the occasion arose the landowners of the region thrived in reinventing the semi-feudal ties with the poor peasantry.

Zamindari Abolition, Land Reforms and Land Ceiling Acts

Madhya Pradesh had an intermediary system like other Indian provinces which was abolished by the Zamindari Abolition Act (No. 13 of 1951) and the Abolition of the Jagir Act, 1951. To bring uniformity in the land revenue system, the Madhya Pradesh Land Revenue Code, 1959 was enacted. It came into force on October 2,

1959. The M.P. Land Revenue Code incorporated almost all the important features of land reforms, that is, uniformity of tenures, protection of tenants against arbitrary ejection, and conferment of rights of *bhumiswamis* to tillers. The Code recognized only the class of tenure holders, namely *bhumiswamis*. It also protected the rights of sub-tenants who were given occupancy rights. With the abolition of intermediaries, the estates owned by these people were vested with the government. These included tanks, ponds, water channels, wastelands, community land, village forest, and mines. However, as in other states, abolition of *zamindari* system did not bring equity in the land distribution of Madhya Pradesh. In fact, intermediaries were conferred *bhumiswami* rights. As a result, a new land owning class emerged which evicted poor tenants in the name of personal cultivation. The purpose of land reform was thus defeated. After evaluating the failure of the *zamindari* system in providing equitable land distribution, the Planning Commission suggested that all states should enact agricultural ceiling acts to fix ceiling limits by 1958. However, the Madhya Pradesh Ceiling on Agricultural Holdings Act could be passed only in 1960, and came into force in November 1961. The Act stipulated that a person could hold 10.12 standard ha. of land in irrigated areas, 20.24 in partially irrigated areas, and 30.35 ha. in non-irrigated areas. There was a provision that allowed allotment of surplus land to joint farming societies formed by agricultural labourers, landless persons and displaced tenants.

Certain categories of landholdings that were exempted under this Act, including tea or coffee plantations, sugarcane farms, landholdings for cattle breeding, dairy farming, wool raising, efficiently managed and mechanized farms on which heavy investments or major structural improvements had been made, orchards/groves up to the size of 12.14 ha., landholdings of industrial or commercial undertakings and institutions for educational purposes. As a result, hundreds of landlords continued to possess thousands of acres of land under the category of mechanized farms, while in reality a major part of their land lay idle, for long periods. The government machinery did not verify whether a mechanized farm was in existence or not. Businessmen acquired ceiling free land for industrial purposes and converted the land into flourishing farms. The Ceiling Act of 1960 could not stop the illegal transfer of surplus land by landlords. Almost all the big landholders could evade the ceiling limit either by transferring land to their relatives or to fictitious adopted sons, or even to servants. There were even bizarre cases where a husband and wife divorced in the eyes of law to keep the surplus land under two holdings, but continued to live together as husband and wife for practical purposes. Therefore, the Ceiling Act, 1960 remained in the statute book instead of becoming a force of bringing dynamic change in the land distribution of Madhya Pradesh. Those who were supposed to implement the Act were from the big landholding class and they naturally did not take any serious initiative to implement it. Majority of the political leaders concealed their surplus land by indulging in clandestine transfers of land. For instance, when G.N. Singh became the Chief Minister of the state (1967-69), he transferred all his land (about 524 acres) to his sons and relatives to become a landless person. Landholding Act of 1960 was also frustrated by Dilip Singh Judav, a Gupta family of Durg; Vidya Charan Shukla, and V. Chandrakar from newly created Chhattisgarh state. Similarly, a large number of MLAs and MPs exercised indirect control over thousands of acres of land transferred in the name of their relatives, many of whom did not even stay in the state. Some political leaders sold off their land and turned 'socialists'. The real tiller, however, remained a 'subsisting cultivator' (*Mainstream*, May 6, 1972: 17).

The Ceiling Act did not touch upon *benami* landholdings. Taking advantage of non-availability of up-to-date land records in the revenue department, many landlords maintained vast tracts of land scattered in different villages. Another striking feature of the Ceiling Act of 1960 was that it did not cover land allotted on lease. There were instances where hundreds of acres of fertile land given to individuals on lease by erstwhile princely states remained exempt from ceiling limits. The ceiling also exempted government land given on lease. As a result of these flaws, the stated purposes of promulgating the Act were not realized. Inequitable land distribution continued in Madhya Pradesh, defeating the very purpose of the Ceiling Act, 1960 *(Mainstream,* August 21, 1971: 11). A research project taken up by the Planning Commission in 1965 to examine the enactment of land reform initiatives and legal and administrative impediments in the implementation of such legislation revealed that after passing of the M.P. Land Revenue Code in 1959 and the Agricultural Ceiling Act in 1960, the records maintained by the revenue department were inconsistent, inaccurate and contained errors. The study also candidly commented that '*patwaris*', in collusion with big landlords, did not report excess surplus land retained by the big landlords. As a result, there had been massive non-reporting of tenancy cases to the state government. Besides, there were inconsistencies in the estimates of surplus land, acquisition of surplus land and distribution of surplus land *(Kurukeshetra,* October issue, 1986: 5963).

Though political leadership scuttled the process of land reforms through deceitful means, it could not bury the popular demand for land reforms. Bowing to mass sentiment, the ruling Congress Party promised the people of Madhya Pradesh during the general elections in 1972 that if it was vcted to power, it would launch a vigorous land reform campaign by amending the existing ceiling Act. However, after the elections when the Congress government took initiatives to reduce the size of holdings and to amend the Agricultural Ceiling Act, 1960; the *kulak* lobby (mainly comprising big landlords) within the Congress Party resisted the initiative with might. The then Chief Minister, P.C. Sethi, however, took a firm stand and the Madhya Pradesh Ceiling on Agricultural Holdings Act was revised in line with national guidelines by the Amendment Act of 1972 which incorporated strict definition of family as a unit of five members, that is husband, wife and their minor children. It specified that the maximum land that could be held by an individual was 10 acres; a family of five could possess up to 15 acres and 18 acres could be held by a family of more than five members. The amendment removed all the exemptions given in the Ceiling Act. Exemptions were granted only to religious and charitable trusts, Wafq bodies and orchards. However, this amendment Act also had a significant number of flaws. It had retrospective effect only from January 1, 1972. Numerous fictitious transfers of land, which had taken place for a year or more when the big landlords got inkling that there was a move to curtail the ceiling limit, were regularized. Several thousand acres of land had been sold and resold many times, gifted or turned into property of some sort of religious trusts during that time (*Mainstream*, May 6, 1972, 17-19). In order to deal with the flows of Amendment Act of 1972 the Madhya Pradesh Assembly passed the new Madhya Pradesh Ceiling on Agricultural Holding Act in 1974. The new Act specified that the maximum land that could be held by a family was 10 acres for two crops of irrigated land and up to 54 acres in respect of dry land. All private and public companies, societies registered under the M.P. Societies Act and Cooperative Societies Act were exempted from the Act. Similar exemptions were given to the traders and industrialists who use their property for trade, industry and commerce purposes. Therefore, the Act of 1974 also failed to bring about any major change in the land reform process in Madhya Pradesh. This is evident from the findings of a study by the Lal Bahadur Shastri Academy of Administration on land reforms in M.P. in the late 1980s. The study found that big landowners belonging to upper castes (two-thirds of the landowners in M.P. belong to upper castes and one-fifth to OBC) had not been covered by the ceiling limit. Absentee landlords continued to control vast tracts of land in villages. At the state level, 69.1 per cent of the owners of surplus land had land in their village of residence and 30.9 per cent of them had land located away form their village of residence. According to one observation, "In Sirsod village of Gwalior 68.77 acres of un-irrigated land was allotted to 24 allottees on 30 June, 1978. They received nearly three acres of land each. Many of the allottees started selling their land from 1980 onwards. No land development was taken up for the help of the allottees. It may be mentioned here that 342.76 ha. of land were unfit for cultivation in this district, which constitutes 65 per cent of the land taken possession of by the government. Similarly, in district Satna, 422.72 ha of land were declared surplus, which was not fit for cultivation" (Jha, 2002:119). Another startling finding of the study was that there were 2,753 cases pending at the state level, which constituted only 0.64 per cent of the total 2,40,397 of land ceiling cases instituted in the state until September 1989. Around 80 per cent of the land ceiling cases were instituted between 1971 and 1975, 12 per cent between 1976 and 1980, and only 8 per cent of the cases were instituted before 1965. This implies that:

- Implementation of the Ceiling Act of 1960 had been a miserable failure.
- No cases have been instituted after 1980 indicating administrative apathy.
- A greater degree of both administrative and political will were exhibited between 1971 and 1980 in identifying and instituting land ceiling cases.

The study attributed these aspects to a combination of factors like administrative indifference, lack of political will and use of the legal system for delaying the acquisition of surplus land. Majority (73%) of land ceiling cases were disposed of by courts in less than five years; 8.9 per cent of the cases took 5 to 10 years and 17.90 per cent of the cases have lingered beyond 10 years. The cases lingering for longer time invariably involve large landowners, who have taken recourse to appeals, revision and writs. The major proportion (38.30%) of cases were pending at the level of the competent authority (25.82% of the cases were pending in courts; 19.59 per cent of cases were pending in civil courts and 16.29 per cent of cases were pending in the high court and the Supreme Court). Thus, though the amendment had envisaged expedition of the judicial process and quick disposal of cases, a large number of cases were pending (LBSNAA, 2002: 107-115).

There were considerable gaps between estimates of surplus land and actually acquired land and between acquired land and distributed land. In some cases big landlords had given up their rights on some portion of their lands or donated the land as part of the Bhoodan movement. But in reality the land transfer was done only on paper. The government issued entitlement of these lands to the landless poor without verifying the status of the lands. As a result, poor beneficiaries did not get possession of the land. Land which was declared surplus was not distributed, as can be seen from the observations of the Report of the Commissioner, Land Records, Gwalior upto November 1991, 22,124.28 acres of surplus land were not taken possession of by the government. Upto 1994, 1,39,642 lakh hectares of land, which was only 0.63 per cent of the operated area, had been declared as surplus land. The government could take possession of 1,13,798 lakh hectares and it could actually distribute only 74,951 lakh hectares, or around 50 per cent of the declared surplus land. This shows apathy on the part of the M.P. government relating to reducing the gap between words and deeds.

Social Movements

So far as role of social movements in land reform is concerned, no serious effort has been made in M.P. during the last 50 years or so apart from a few *ad hoc* protests except the **Narmada Bachao Andolan,** but most of these movements were addressed to issues of natural resources like forest, water, minerals and so on. For example, in Malwa district of Jhabua in 1975, a tribal protest took place for regularization of encroached forest lands under the leadership of non-tribal Mama Baleshwar Dayal (Rawal, 1975). However, the struggle for land run under the leadership of Chhattisgarh Mukti Morcha (CMM) and its leader late Shankar Guha Niyogi made some headway in this context. This fight against Mahant of Nadia Math of Rajnandgaon for the misuse of 350 acres of land by him is important but it is also reported that landowners employed private armies to diffuse such tensions (Singh, 2002). In the same order the role of *Sarvodaya* movement in land reform is not very significant in M.P. Most of the land acquired and distributed under this scheme is rocky, barren and waste in nature. Therefore, even after receiving land under this scheme the beneficiaries did not improve their life chances.

Apathy on the part of government has continued later also. This is clear from two examples such as, upto 31st March, 1998, government acquired 3,06,150 acres of land but it could distribute only 60.63 per cent of it, and till the same year it could get 4.10 lakh acres of land under *bhoodan* scheme but it could distribute only 2.60 lakh acres of land among the landless. As a result of this as said by Sail (2002: 60) concentration of ownership holdings and operational holdings in the state has not witnessed any major change despite claims made by political leaders and the government. It can be seen that 41.6 per cent of the landowners in the state have more than 100 acres of land, although the land ceiling in rural areas is 18 acres for irrigated land. Inequality in landholding size in terms of different categories of landholders is presented in Table 4.10.

In spite of relatively low density of population the problem of landlessness is acute in the state. The number of landless households is highest in Sagar (100155) and lowest in Indore (1535). This is clear from Table 4.11. SCs and STs constitute bulk of the population in the undivided Madhya Pradesh. Even after creation of Chhattisgarh as a separate state in M.P. they constitute 16 and 20 per cent population respectively for the Scheduled Castes and Scheduled Tribes. According to Sharma (2000:15) only 12.6 per cent of SCs in the state has land which constitutes only 8.1 per cent of the total landholdings in the state. Around 15 per cent of the SCs work as agricultural or non-agricultural labourers. The same is the situation with tribes, only 24.7 per cent of them have landholdings which constitute 25.2 per cent of the total landholdings. About 27.4 per cent of the tribes work as agricultural and non-agriculture labourers. Further, of the total rural labour force 43.6 per cent are SCs and 32.1 per cent are STs and

Table 4.10: Per cent Distribution of the Number of Holdings and Area Operated, M.P. 1961-1991

Year	Marginal		Small		Semi Medium		Medium		Large		Average size (ha.)
	No	Area	No	Area	No	Area	No	Area	No	Area	
1961-62	21.72	2.90	19.34	7.12	25.78	18.46	25.31	38.56	7.85	32.96	4.10
1971-72	26.11	3.40	20.29	8.86	25.77	21.15	21.64	37.99	6.19	28.58	3.92
1981-82	32.80	4.24	19.13	8.17	21.39	17.65	19.89	35.91	6.79	34.02	3.42
1991-92	37.33	6.37	22.82	12.59	20.69	21.88	15.33	35.15	3.83	24.02	2.64

Note: Marginal = upto one ha; Small = 1-2 ha; Semi-medium = 2-4 ha; Medium = 4-10 ha; Large =10 ha +

Source: Praveen K. Jha (2002 : 373).

most of them are landless. After independence under different schemes attempts were made to remove the problem of landlessness from among the SCs and STs. But because of different inhibiting factors like litigation, delay in transfer of land, and distribution of poor quality of land upto 1994 only 74,951 hectares of land could be distributed among SCs and STs. The Digvijay Singh government acquired 306150 acres of land and distributed 185624 acress (61%) among the landless upto March 1998 most of whom were SCs and STs but this development was also not free of problems. Although the government issued land documents to the poor among the SCs and STs but it did not ensure the possession of land to the allottees. Most of the beneficiaries encountered probems of lack of possesion, non-identification of location of land without any land maps, and manipulation of land records by Patwaris. Because of all these constraints even after allotment of land many SCs and STs households remained landless and poor (Chaudhary: 2006 and 2007).

Table 4.11: Landlessness in Madhya Pradesh

Sl. No.	*Region Name*	*Number of Landless Households*
1.	Mahakaushal	339318
2.	Bhopal	173435
3.	Malwa	478581
4.	Vindhya	236280
5.	Bundelkhand	225195
6.	Chambal	144515
	Total	**1597324**

Source: Commissioner of Rural and Panchayat Department, Bhopal & Situation on 1-5-2007.

Bhopal Declaration (2002:5) (BD) popularly known as 'Dalit Agenda' contains 21 points for giving land to the landless SCs and STs. The opening point of this declaration clearly states: "Ensure that each Dalit family will own enough cultivable land for socio-economic well-being. The government should pursue all possible measures including the distribution of surplus land, government revenue lands and temple lands within a specific timeframe. If the need be, the government should purchase cultivate land and distribute it among Dalits." People may have different views about the Bhopal Declaration and distribution of grazing land but it is beyond doubt that within 47 days (April 14 to May 31, 2002) about 5 lakh hectares of land were distributed among Scheduled Castes and Scheduled Tribes. In other words, of the total 5,23,645 hectares 3,01,356 hectares were distributed among both the categories of Scheduled Castes and Scheduled Tribes. Category one refers to landless families and category two stands for families which possess upto 2.5 acres of poor quality land. Since category two has more than 50 per cent dalit households, therefore, Charnoi land was distributed among category two households than among category one. This is clear from Table 4.12. Since sufficient amount of land was not available in all the villages for distribution, therefore, as per the desire of the Bhopal Declaration a significant amount was sanctioned by each district administrator to purchase land in the market and distribute it among the Dalits. For example, in Raisen district alone, in all the 7 development blocks Rs. 53,32,500 was sanctioned for both SC and ST population.

Table 4.12: Regionwise Distribution of Charnoi Land to SCs/STs

(*In hectares*)

Sl. No.	*Region Name*	*SC*	*ST*
1.	Mahakaushal	36127	65275
2.	Bhopal	25409	11095
3.	Malwa	60042	59937
4.	Vindhya	29981	50448
5.	Bundelkhand	23650	11637
6.	Chambal	18570	10694
	Total	193779	209086

Source: Obtained from the Office of Secretary to the Chief Minister, Government of M.P., dated 21-8-03.

Looking at the poor bargaining power of the new beneficiaries because of their poor economic conditions there is a general apprehension that beneficiaries at large may not avail the benefits arising out of this opportunity. Jha (2002) in another context had rightly apprehended that, "A land reform package has a chance to succeed only if there is a supportive macroeconomic policy framework for the intended beneficiaries of such reforms. Such a framework should include among others, provisions of production and consumption, credit for the peasantry, technical and marketing assistance for them and appropriate price policies." Without providing these conditions and opportunities provision was made by the Bhopal Declaration to provide them cash/kind inputs to help them improve land productivity without wage/economic loss. In the case of Sehore we found that 44 per cent of the beneficiaries did not receive any incentive, 33 per cent received economic support and 22 per cent received grain. Here it must be noted that large number of beneficiaries who received input support who were not supposed to improve their land because since long land was already under their control. This time only their ownership was legalized and over the time due to their own effort they had improved its quality. It would have been better had their input share been distributed among those who had received land for the first time and quality of land allotted to them was poor. Poor quality of allotted land and its encroachments, and corruption at different levels are reported from different parts of the state. For example, in Sehore (Chaudhary, 2007) it was found that 87 per cent beneficiaries did not face any problem while receiving possession of land. Majority of them were landless in the past. The role of Patwaris was crucial in these allotments. In several cases beneficiaries were forced to oblige Patwaris. More than 85 per cent beneficiaries received pattas within a couple of months of allotment. Quality of land was better in the case of land already encroached upon and under cultivation in comparison to the wasteland recently allotted. So far as encroachment of the allotted land by "others" is concerned, its number is small. For example, in 13 villages where the study was conducted, there are 1294 households of which 451 households are of the Scheduled Castes and only 219 SC households were allotted land and of which 13 beneficiaries' land is still encroached by others. Most of these "others" are from the backward castes of Meware, Khati, and Pawar living in the same village.

In the case of Raisen (Chaudhary, 2007) beneficiaries approached the functionaries of formal institutions like patwari, sarpanch and SDM for allotment of grazing lands; around 40 per cent obliged the patwari for land allotment. No serious case of encroachment of the allotted land was reported. At the district level 9,328 SC/ST households were allotted 8651.138 hectare of land upto 31st January, 2003 but only 78 beneficiaries were facing the problem of land encroachment which was successfully solved through "Operation Biswas" jointly organized by the police and the revenue department.

In this district also majority of the beneficiaries were landless. Majority of them received pattas in time and the beneficiaries at large did not face any problem while receiving land and land related papers except for bribing some patwaris. It is reported that in about 40 per cent cases bribe was paid to patwari to obtain land papers. But in other parts of the state like villages of Damoh and Panna districts it is said that the process of distribution of land was slow, land quality was poor, question of identification of landless dalit families for distribution of grazing land was informal, plot size of land was small, only partial help was extended by the government to cultivate the allotted land. In many cases measurement of allotted land was not made, in few cases there was opposition from the upper castes, there was indifference on the part of the state to solve problems of land disputes related to possession/encroachment, and delay in providing ownership papers (Kumar, 2007).

Agrarian social relations in Madhya Pradesh are tilted in favour of upper castes. However, due to institutional interventions after independence the situation is gradually changing. In recent past some specific efforts have been made to deal with the problem of landlessness especially among the marginalized. However, no efforts are in progress to enhance the contribution of agriculture to the national economy because of the shortage of irrigation facilities.

SCHEDULED CASTES AND TRIBES

The Scheduled Castes constitute about 16 per cent of the population in M.P. Among them the Chamar caste is the most powerful in comparison to the rest of the Scheduled Castes. Some of the important Scheduled Castes in the state are: Balahi/Balai, Balmiki, Basor, Bediya, Beldar, Khatik, Kotwal, Pardhi, Sansi, and Silawat. If we critically examine the social status of all these three caste groups, that is, upper castes, OBCs and SCs in the historical perspective we find that the Scheduled Castes are at the bottom in the caste hierarchy although their overall contribution for the development of Madhya Pradesh society in general and different social groups in particular is very significant and obvious. Historically, they are the victims of exclusion and marginalization. In order to include them within the social mainstream number of steps have been taken by the state and civil society in the past. The role of 'Satnami' Movement is obvious in this context in spite of the fact that the Scheduled Castes are the victims of untouchability and different forms of exploitation and marginalization. Not only this but over time different forms of crime committed against them has significantly increased and the reporting of such cases have also increased. For example, during 1996-97, 501 cases of all types of crime were reported, but its number increased upto 2746 in 2000-01 which further increased upto 4086 during 2003-04. This is clear from Table 4.13. It is very difficult to explain the specific reasons for rapid increase in cases of crime against Scheduled Castes in the recent past. Reasons may also differ from region to region. However, some of the broad and common causes leading to an increase in the crime rate may be lack of strong political and bureaucratic will to implement the existing laws honestly; constantly growing level of awareness among the *dalits* due to various reasons, increasing cases of reporting, misuse of untouchability laws by some sections of *dalit* population, emergence of neo-middle class among them and their relations with the higher castes have changed. For example, they have been refusing to do forced labour. Changes in the socio-political environment are slow and the process of transformation of caste hiearchy and social structure and related discriminatory practices is also slow. This state of affairs directly or indirectly contributes to crime against Scheduled Castes (Chaudhary, 2005).

Table 4.13: Crime against Scheduled Castes in Madhya Pradesh

Year	*Murder*	*Rape*	*Grievous Injury*	*Humiliation/ Torture*	*Others*	*Total*
1996-1997	111	171	95	58	66	501
1997-1998	108	352	59	21	237	777
1998-1999	82	290	11	698	229	1310
1999-2000	86	400	36	1529	69	2120
2000-2001	111	468	71	1993	103	2746
2001-2002	99	529	121	1776	145	3670
2002-2003	94	661	129	4457	1205	6546
2003-2004	95	414	150	2788	639	4086

Note: Upto 2001-02 there were 5 categories of crime, including "others". Its number increased upto 8 in 2002-03 and 9 in 2003-04. All these new categories were clubbed under "others" in the present study.

Source: Obtained from the Office of the Commissioner, Scheduled Castes Development, Bhopal, dated 16-12-2004.

Though the changes in the social hierarchy are slow the processes of raising the status of Scheduled Castes to the category of middle class is constantly going on and the rate is faster than that among the Scheduled Tribes. Today one can see thousands of *dalits* at all the three levels of panchayat bodies, both as members and as occupying the office of president. A significant number of *dalits* are today MLAs, MPs, bureaucrats, and social workers of repute. Traditionally, most of the Scheduled Caste members had affiliations with the Congress Party, but today they are found in all the three dominant political parties like Congress, BJP, and Bahujan Samaj Party. In the neighbouring district of Uttar Pradesh such as Datia, Bhind, Morena, Gawalior, Shivpuri, Chhatarpur, and Tikamgarh they are found in large numbers. And a significant number of them are the supporters of BSP but in the past they were the supporters of the Congress Party.

There are around forty five Scheduled Tribes in Madhya Pradesh. They are found in most of the districts of Madhya Pradesh and their number is above 25 per cent of the total population in districts— Shajapur, Ratlam, Sidhi, Umaria, Shadol, Seoni, Dindori, Mandla, Chhindwara, Barwni, Khargaon, Khandwa, Jhabua, Dhar, and Betul. The important tribes of M.P. are: Gond, Bhils, Korku, Saharia, Bharia and Baiga. Culturally each tribe has its own distinct culture, both material and non-material. Historically, there was symbiotic relationship between tribes and forests. Tribes perceived forest as an integral part of their life. They nurtured forests with the help of their culture and tradition. There are examples of tribal protest and movements in the interest of forest. And in return forests not only served as a source of their religion, civilization and culture but also provided them shelter, medicine, and food security. But with the coming of British-raj and the introduction of the capitalistic model of development and classification of forests under different categories and formation of forest acts and policies in favour of timber production the centuries old symbiotic relationship cracked. This question was addressed by the state with the help of environment friendly forest policy and Joint Forest Movement (JFM), Social Forestry, Environmental Forestry etc. were introduced after independence but these interventions could not address the trend initiated by the British-raj. It could not change the mind set of the people benefiting from timber trade. As a result of the interplay of all these negative forces tribals became rootless. While in the past they were dependent on forests for all their day-to-day needs, today the forest is no longer the only or the most powerful source of their culture and livelihood. Forest based indigenous knowledge is becoming insignificant. Even today there are a large number of Non-Timber Forest Products (NTFP) in Madhya Pradesh forests but the tribals have neither control over them nor access to these resources. It is the middle man or now the agents of globalization who are making profit out of NTFP. Tribal arts and crafts are getting space in the drawing room of urban middle class, and the number of drawing rooms is rapidly increasing, but it has nothing to do with tribes. Empirical data shows that tribes are either dependent on agriculture or wage work or both for their livelihood. They are increasing their dependence on agriculture and at the national level the importance of agriculture is decreasing day by day in national economy and hence on this basis we can simply think about the future of tribes and their economy. By making them dependent on wage work again the mistake is being made to make them prone to dependence and we are forcing them to experience corruption and exploitation by the local bureaucracy.

Of course, a number of development projects are going on for tribal development, but it is difficult to see the impact of such interventions in a positive way. For example, there are three primitive tribes in M.P. These are Baiga of Baga Chak of old Mandla district, Bharia of Patalkot of Chhindwara district and Saharia of Shivpuri district. If we see the amount spent for their development both by the state and the NGOs one can say that would it have been better had these tribes been handed over the money directly? Why is it that in spite of huge expenditure most of them are still poor and marginalized? This questions the transparency in the implementation, and delivery of development projects. In some areas especially in Malwa region in the name of development thousands of tribals have been displaced. Narmada Bachao Andolan is a social response to both the Mega development projects and the problems created by it. How and in what way these development projects are pro-tribal, to what extent are the rehabilitation policies pro-tribal needs to be explained.

In order to cope with adversity and to protect themselves from challenges, number of steps are being taken by tribals themselves and their spokespersons. Seasonal out-migration and the Naxalite movement are two among the many. Unfortunately these interventions and mechanisms have taken more and provided less to the tribals. There is cultural degeneration among the migrating tribes without showing improvements in their quality of life. Jhabua tribe is the best example. The rate of out-migration is highest in Jhabua and also the rate of illiteracy, indebtedness and poverty is also the highest in Jhabua. So far as the role of Naxalite movement is concerned it has created withdrawal syndrome among the change agents. Under violent situations the interventionists prefer to withdraw. The State has also spent huge amounts of money for the restoration of law and order which it could have spent for tribal development. Hence, it can be said that the group who requires more and more support from outside is unable to get the support and they are forced to live in poverty and deprivation. As a result of the failure of development programmes the problems of landlessness, poverty, illiteracy, and starvation continue among the trbals of Madhya Pradesh. The processes of accumulation of social capital and mobility into the middle class is almost absent among them. However, most of the tribes of Madhya Pradesh are free from malpractices such as dowry system, child marriages, *purdah* system, and untouchability.

ECONOMIC ACTIVITIES

In the state of Madhya Pradesh in general majority of the earning hands are engaged in primary sector of employment. For example, in Betul district 84.80 per cent, 4.70 per cent and 10.48 per cent are engaged in primary, secondary and tertiary sectors of employment respectively. In Jhabua 91 per cent are engaged in the primary sector of employment. In Bhopal the lowest proportion of population (24.9%) is engaged in the primary sector of employment and maximum (50.65%) in the tertiary sector.

Table 4.14: Districtwise Employment Status in Different Sectors, 1991

(in percentage)

Region Name	*Primary Sector*	*Secondary Sector*	*Tertiary Sector*
Bhopal	69.32	10.44	20.24
Chambal	76.03	6.84	17.13
Malwa	76.66	8.37	14.98
Mahakaushal	78.38	7.84	13.78
Vindhya	82.54	6.74	10.71
Bundelkhand	75.30	12.92	11.78

Source: Human Development Report, 2002.

Table 4.15 shows that as the society moves from agricultural to non-agricultural activities the number of people engaged in primary sector decrease and the number of people engaged in tertiary sector increase. Data from Bhopal region is a vivid example. Although agriculture and related activities are the main example of the primary sector of employment but in this field the situation is not upto the mark. A significant number of persons either do not own land or they own poor quality of land. Most of the villagers are marginal farmers. Their economic conditions are pitiable. Those who own more than 10 acres of land have also witnessed the deterioration of their economic conditions over time. Increasing costs of inputs, fragmentation of landholdings, poor availability of irrigation facilities and lack of modernization are some of the factors which have led to deterioration in the economic conditions of most of the farmers in this area.

Table 4.15: Production of Minerals in Madhya Pradesh during 1999-2000

Limestone	22.31 m.
Diamonds	40668 carats.
Iron-ore	92 thousands tonne.
Manganese ore	326 thousand tonne.
Bauxite	248 thousand tonne.
Copper ore	74 thousand tonne.
Rock-phosphate	155 thousand tonne.
Dolomite	103 thousand tonne.
Coal	43.0 m. tonnes.

Source: Statistical Summary of M.P. (2006), Directorate of Economics and Statistics, Bhopal, GOMP.

The state of Madhya Pradesh has also entered the era of high-tech industry such as electronics, telecommunications, and automobiles. The state is producing optical fibre for telecommunication. A large number of automobile industries have been established at Pithampur near Indore. Prominent industries in the public sector in the state are Bharat Heavy Electricals Ltd. at Bhopal, Security Paper Mill at Hoshangabad, Bank Note Press at Dewas, Newsprint Factory at Nepanagar and Alkaloid Factory at Neemuch. Over 81.13 million metre cloth in the handloom sector and 131.59 million metre cloth by power loom was manufactured in 1999-2000. The cement production touched 11.24 million tonnes during the period. An Air Cargo Complex, Indo-German Tool Room and an Inland Container Depot are being established at Pithampur. The Government of India has proposed setting up of a Special Economic Zone at Indore.

Madhya Pradesh is one of the leading states in the country in mineral production (Table 4.16). The state is also famous for its traditional handicrafts and handlooms in Chanderi and Maheshwar.

Table 4.16: Availability of NTFP

Region Name	*Forest land (in Per cent)*	*Major Non-Timber Forest Produce*
Bhopal	20.27	Tendu Leaves, Baheda, Aonla, Charota Seeds, Safed Musli, Chironji
Chambal	25.34	Tendu Leaves, Aonla, Baheda, Giloy, Bel, Arjun Bark, Katehri, Gudmar, Safed Musli, Malkangni, Gokhru, Nagarmotha, Adusa, Bhringraj, Palash Flower, Khair
Malwa	22.22	Tendu leaves, Harra, Sal seed, Salai Gum
Mahakaushal	37.91	Tendu Leaves, Baheda, Safed Musli, Achar Guthli, Nagarmotha, Harra, Bel, Aonla, Dhawai Flower, Imli, Mango Guthli, Charota Seeds, Vaividang, Kusum Seeds, Kosa Cotton, Bhilwa Seeds, Mahua Seeds, Karanj Seeds, Mahul leaves
Vindhya	33.99	Tendu Leaves, Aonla, Mahua flower, Mahua Guthli, Achar Guthli, Imli
Bundelkhand	32.12	Tendu Leaves, Ber, Mahua flower, Mahua Guthli, Charota Seeds, Nagarmotha, Palash Gum

Source: Districtwise data was available in the Third Human Development Report, Madhya Pradesh, 2003 and it has been arranged by us on regional basis.

Forestry Sector

Forest is the direct or indirect source of livelihood for most of the tribal populations since long. Historically they are engaged in a number of forest related activities. Of course, today the condition of forests has significantly deteriorated and in some of the districts its forests are now only on paper but still in most of the districts large number of Non-Timber Forest Produce (NTFPs) is still found. Many tribes are engaged in the collection of NTFPs, if not in the processing work. Districtwise details of the availability of NTFPs are given in Table 4.16.

Institutional Interventions for Workers

It is an established fact that economic conditions of the people engaged in the Primary Sector of employment is far from satisfactory, therefore, from time to time the government of Madhya Pradesh has taken a number of steps for their overall development. Creation of welfare board for the unorganized sector workers in both rural and urban areas is an example. In other words, on the basis of the powers conferred by the Madhya Pradesh Unorganized Workers Welfare Act, 2003, the State Government laid down the Madhya Pradesh Unorganized Welfare Rules, 2005, relating to the constitution of Welfare Board, its functions and other matters. This Act is applicable to all categories of employees specified in the Schedule and covers agricultural and allied workers, quarry and brick kiln workers, manual workers engaged in loading and unloading in markets, public transport and food godowns, workers making *agarbattis*, embroidery items, ready-made garments, food products like pickles and *papads*, cooked food and toys, workers in the leather and footwear industries; those engaged in cleaning and scavenging, rag-picking and door-to-door collection of old newspapers, *raddi* and *kabadi*, motor transport workers under the Motor Transport Workers Act, 1961, workers plying cycle rickshaws, auto-rickshaws and taxis, workers in flour, rice and *dal* mills, private security services, plastic industries, wood works, utensil making, artisans, fireworks and match-making, and cartons and other packaging material. Two separate Welfare Boards for Unorganized Workers were constituted for the rural and urban areas in the State. Each of them consisted of the Minister for Labour as the Ex-officio Chairman, Secretary to the Labour Department and Finance Department, Labour Commissioner, six members appointed by the Government representing employers of the unorganized sector and six members representing unorganized workers, two of whom had to be women, and one each belonging to the Scheduled Castes (SCs), Scheduled Tribes (STs) and Backward Castes (OBCs). Two separate

Madhya Pradesh Unorganized Sector Welfare Funds were constituted for the rural and urban areas, which were to be administered by the Board. The benefits to be extended to all the members who have contributed to these Funds are: old age and family pension disability assistance, loans for purchase or construction of house, interest subsidies for housing loan taken from a housing finance institution, assistance for education like scholarships, loans, interest subsidies for education loans, cash award for meritorious students, loans for tools and small machines, interest subsidy for loans for supplementary income-generating activities, marriage assistance, medical assistance, maternity assistance, group insurance, assistance for payment of insurance premium, funeral assistance and *ex-gratia* payment in case of death. These benefits are normally credited into the bank account of the beneficiary member. There is also a provision for the registration of the establishments to which the Act applies and for the contribution of the employer based on the number of workers in the establishment. Similarly, there is also a provision for contributions by the workers. No amount has, however, been specified in the Act.

ANTI-POVERTY AND RURAL DEVELOPMENT PROGRAMMES

During the British period by introducing railways and other forms of communication, documentation of information related to land, new revenue system, expansion of bureaucracy and English education, process of reward and punishment without much delay by law courts an effort was made to promote development although in a very narrow sense. The main purpose of these development projects was to serve the British. This model of development was quite close to the capitalistic model of development in which there was neither space for local concerns nor for people's participation. It was highly centralized and target oriented in favour of the Raj. The reformative approach was not the dominant theme in those days; though examples of some independent reform movements like the Birsa Movement, Satnami Movement, and the peasant struggle all directed against the British Raj and for social and culture transformation abound in the state. Number of small movements also took place against the then education, revenue and forest policies and schemes. Permanent settlement introduced by the Raj in 1793 was perceived as a blow by large number of farmers in the *zamindari* areas and therefore, there were protests against it (Chaudhary, 1999). Of course, the freedom struggle had wider political implications at the national level but other reform or protest movements had limited impact in safeguarding the interests of the common people. The two ideologically antagonistic interventions had little or no impact on the social and economic health of the common people living in rural and tribal areas of this state and in fact had a very negative impact. The concerns and plight of common people pertaining to ignorance and illiteracy, exploitation and underemployment, food insecurity, epidemic, and high mortality rates, and landlessness did not get proper place in the development manifesto and action agenda of the British.

After independence, *zamindari* abolition, reservation policy, five-year plans and area specific target group development programmes were introduced. Subsequently through these policies and schemes the state attempted to come to the doorstep of common people. But there was no change in the capitalistic model of development introduced by the British. There was a general thinking among the agents of change operating at the macro level that fruits of development would gradually reach at the grassroots level. This experiment had wide social and economic impact on the people. By examining the role and impact of *zamindari* abolition law, one can see how land ownership shifted from the established upper segments to the emerging social groups from among the other backward classes. This development further impacted political, social and economic life of population at large irrespective of their social background. Mishra (1961) rightly discussed the emergence and expansion of middle classes in the light of new socio-economic formations. This process of development with support from a section of neo-middle class people along with the traditional dominant class became so dominant that it forced the issue of land reform, and implementation of land ceiling acts to the back seat in the development process. To be blunt, India rejected the Gandhian Philosophy of development even before accepting it and it tried to achieve socialistic goal with the capitalistic path of development. It is worthwhile to mention that Gandhian philosophy was rooted in its conviction in the tenets of truth, non-violence and goodness of human being. Being influenced by the ideas of Tolstoy, Ruskin and the teachings of *Geeta*, he placed more emphasis on moral and spiritual values than economic motives as a means of overall progress. His suggestions of self-sufficient village economy, decentralization, importance of Khadi and Village industries and implementation of these ideas and schemes with the help of Panchayati Raj, cooperatives, trusteeship and '*Nai Taleem*' (a new system of education) did not get proper place in policy formulation for rural development. Natural death of Sarvodaya Movement and goal deviation of Naxalite movement from the main economic agenda to the issue of retaliation, are also examples of near stagnation/failure of the reform movements.

Rural Development and Anti-Poverty Schemes

Major rural development schemes introduced in the post-independence era up to 1991 may be classified under 5 broad categories as given in Table 4.17. All these schemes were introduced for the development of both area and target groups. Since the approach for introduction of these schemes was capitalistic and since the constraints of development like corruption, and manipulation was not controlled therefore, concern for local aspirations, people's participation and the content of social justice and equity was either absent from these projects or it did not draw attention of the strong social and political will, although it was loudly claimed that such interventions will encourage self-help, self-reliance and self-imitation. As a result only few people availed benefits and majority were denied. Denial of land as the only or the most important source of livelihood of the rural masses by the state may be realised from the following citation: *"Till date 272 legislations regarding Land Reforms have been enacted. But except in Kerala and West Bengal, Land Reforms were successful in no other State......... As against the estimated 30 million hectares of available surplus land, only 75 lakh acres have been declared surplus so far. Out of this, it has taken the government 50 years to take possession of a mere 6.4 lakh acres and redistribute 5.2 lakh acres of it. And, still about 10 lakh acres remain in ineligible hands......... Since 1961, despite a host of land reforms, a great many Dalits lost even the little land they had and had no choice but to join the rank of landless agricultural laboureres. In 1961, 38 per cent of Dalits were cultivators, but today only 25 per cent Dalits are cultivators. Today over 86 per cent of Dalits/Scheduled Caste households are landless or near landless and 63 per cent are wage-labour households"* (Sharma, 2004:151-152; Mahajan, 2003: 51).

Table 4.17: Major Rural Development Schemes

1. Equity Welfare Oriented Strategy	1. Community Development Project. 2. Minimum Needs Programme. 3. Applied Nutrition Programme. 4. Mid Day Meals Programme.
2. Growth Oriented Strategy	1. Intensive Agriculture District Programme. 2. Intensive Cattle Development Programme. 3. High Yielding Varieties Programme.
3. Area and Group Specific Strategy	1. Small Farmer Development Agency. 2. Marginal Farmer and Agricultural Labourers Schemes. 3. Drought Prone Area Programme. 4. Tribal Area Development Programme. 5. Minimum Needs Programme. 6. Integrated Rural Development Programme.
4. People Centric Strategy	1. Operation Flood. 2. Joint Forest Management. 3. Participatory Irrigation Management. 4. Rural Credit and Thrift Programmes of Self Help Groups.
5. Integrated or Holistic Strategy	1. IRDP. 2. Rural Employment Programme. 3. Training of Rural Youth for Self-Employment.

Source: Chaudhary, S.N. (2005).

As a result, lopsided development took place and disparities increased. Social groups became heterogeneous and elite formation process took place among most of the social groups. Philosophically those who gained from the state sponsored projects directly or indirectly many of them became custodians of capitalistic model of development. They strongly developed faith in it. In every geographical area the supporters and opponents of development projects and its impact emerged. Within the same area some supported the mega development projects like hydro projects on Narmada river of M.P. and Gujarat which produce substantial amount of electricity for wider use but it has also displaced thousands of local people most of whom are poor and marginalized. Even after so many years the displaced were not rehabilitated in the proper sense. In its recent Press Release, the Jan Sangharsh Morcha, an affiliation of 15 mass organizations working among the tribals of M.P. and Chhattisgarh, has expressed its anguish over the state sponsored human rights violations against the innocent tribals of Madhya Pradesh in the following words:

"In the district of Burhanpur, Damoh and especially in Betul the forest, police and revenue officials enter in one or other tribal villages every other day in the dark cover of night. They beat tribal women, misbehave with them and often put them in overnight illegal confinement without the knowledge of their husbands. In Betul, on the intervening night of 4th and 5th July they razed Bhandarpaani, a tribal hamlet under Chopana police station. In the incident they took away 73 tribal women and men, including children in their illegal confinement. Many of the women were taken away in the absence of their husbands. The poor tribes lost everything but for the clothes on their body. In the evening of July 9th, Danwakheda village was destroyed and the forest department without the knowledge of their husbands took two tribal women away. Recently on 17th July a team of 50 police, forest and revenue personnel team entered Ghorpadmal village under Mohda police station. They dragged tribal women out of their house; misbehaved with them and later abused and terrorized the villagers. To cover up the incident the police has registered false cases of dacoity against 13 tribals." (Shramik Adivasi Sangathan, Betul, telephone 07141-233971).

New Development Schemes

With the realization that development schemes have been excluding thousands of marginalized from their benefits, the state government started a number of target group specific projects which were exclusively meant for physically challenged, destitute persons, senior citizens, poor, and victims of dropout and non-enrollment in schools. But in the course of formation and implementation of such schemes also the same capitalistic model with same spirit and limitations was followed and therefore, in spite of radical changes in the social background of politicians from urban to rural or from upper castes to lower castes at all the levels of administration and large number of bureaucrats from the lower castes, there were no substantial improvements in physical and social quality of life of the tribals, *dalits*, rural women, victims of development, and unorganized sector workers. Some benefits notionally reached the target population. Rural development schemes either did not reach the poor or only a few "poorer" or "chronically poor" could become "less poor" due to these schemes. Persons who were locally dominant availed the maximum part of the benefits. Hence, it is wrong to say that in practice rural development schemes introduced during the pre-reform period were necessarily pro-poor. This statement has specific meaning particularly when one says that during pre-reform days state was welfaristic and poor centric in the functional sense but during the reform period its welfare face has gone. My contention is that during the pre-reform phase also in the functional sense the state was half-heartedly pro-poor or pro-common people otherwise the problems of poor and the marginalized relating to their health, economic and educational development might have been significantly reduced if not eradicated. Hence, during the reform period before drawing any strong conclusions there is need to make content analysis and impact studies of the ongoing development schemes.

The year 1991 may be perceived as a cutting point in the economic history of India because the New Economic Policy (NEP) popularly known as globalization was introduced by the Government of India during this year. It places greater reliance on market forces and the integration of national economy within a global economy would reduce the problems of poverty and unemployment through speeding up the pace and level of economic growth. Broadly there are economic and non-economic features of globalization. Economic features refers to growth in trade, growth in FDI and capital flows, global production and consumption, global competition, trade and investment liberalization policies and so on. The non-economic features refer to loss of national sovereignty, standardization of values and cultures and so on. In other words, the major feature of globalization is the growing concentration and monopolization of economic resources and power by transnational corporations and by global financing firms and funds and globalization of national policies and policy making mechanisms. National policies (economic, social, cultural, environmental, technological, human rights etc.) that until recently were under the jurisdiction of states and people within a country have increasingly come under the influence of international agencies or big private corporations and economic/financial players. This process has affected Third World countries like India in many ways.

Sociologically NEP (New Economic Policy) in India stands for reinforcement of the ongoing modernization model of development which has western origin and now more and more American concentration and which is capitalistic in nature and spirit. The important macro agencies of NEP, are World Bank, WTO, IMF and so on. Such organizations have their own philosophy and projects which they intend to operate in cross-cultural situations in collaboration with the concerned countries and agencies like NGOs, information technologies, both print and electronic media, multinational corporations and so on. As a result of these interventions there is improvement in per capita income at the national level, improvement in share prize index, improvement in export, increase in foreign investment, modernization in transportation and communication network, number of high profiled health services have increased in the urban areas, within few years number of mobile phone connections have increased than the number of landline telephones and so on. Number of job opportunities have emerged and increased. Growing number of STD/PCO booths, Call Centres, postal services, private banks are some of the examples. Bhagwati (2004) perceives globalization as diverse forms of international integration such as foreign trade, multinational corporations' direct investment, movements of short term portfolio funds, technological diffusion and cross-border migration. He further added that economic globalization is an unambiguously good thing, with a few downsides that thought and effort can mitigate. To him there is no need to give a "human face" to globalization. Already it has a human face. Reddy (2000) also endorsed this notion in the light of the concerns of poor. He said: *"The major instrument for public action in favour of the poor in the framework of globalization would have to be through higher growth and through orientation of the pattern of growth to impart benefits of such growth to the poor."* Critically both these views suggest that justice to those who were denied could not be achieved only by the state. The forces of globalization are also creating opportunities for their development. But there is need to capacitate them in such a way that they can associate themselves with the process of globalization and can avail its benefits. And here lies the role of state, civil societies and others.

But this is one side of the phenomena. The other side of the coin is not praiseworthy. Actually as apprehended globalization has failed to address the basic problems of poverty, hunger and unemployment on the one hand and has contributed to alienation, dehumanization, resource exhaustion, environmental pollution, ecological threat, violence and war on the other hand. Singh (2005) rightly said that: *"Globalization is good for only a fraction of Indian society, may be top 20 per cent of people. The number of people who are likely to lose or already losing from globalization has been increasing, particularly in those poor countries which are outside North America, Europe and the Pacific Rim."* According to Dhanagare (2003) also globalization is the ideology of capitalist superpowers. He agrees with the viewpoint of Amin (1997) that globalization harbours a utopian vision of running the world like a market. A market-focused vision of globalization legitimises hierarchy. It is primarily an institutional mechanism meant for one-sided accumulation. It has no history of being very poor friendly. Its general tendency is to polarize societies in both relative and absolute terms. He remarked that there is adverse impact of market driven global integration on the weaker and marginalized sections in the poor countries.

Table 4.18: Classification of Rural/Urban Development Schemes by Social Groups

Sl. No.	*Social Groups*	*Number of Schemes/Sub-Schemes/Projects*
1.	Scheduled Castes	217
2.	Scheduled Tribes	185
3.	OBC	128
4.	Women	109
5.	Farmers	84
6.	Minorities	82
7.	Student	72
8.	Boys and Girls	61
9.	Youth	55
10.	Agriculture Land Owners	46
11.	Unemployed	41
12.	Slum Dwellers	37
13.	Weaver	28
14.	Domestication Work	26
15.	Homeless	25
16.	Aged	24
17.	Artisan	20
18.	Patient	19
19.	Physically Challenged	18
20.	Labour	17
21.	Dependent Population	9
22.	Fishermen	8
23.	Consumer	6
24.	People Engaged in the Collection of Tendu Patta	3
25.	Jail Inmates	2
	Total	**1322**

Source: Publication of Public Relations Department, Government of M.P. (2000), pp. I-XLVIII, Bhopal.

But for Singh (2004) globalization is a "Unique process", a product of science and technology which is completely new to human history. In his view it offers new opportunities to humankind as also pose many challenges. Its impacts are different from the earlier socio-economic and technological era of capitalism, so are its challenges. In case of India, Singh identifies challenges like inequalities, required changes in economic policy, strengthening democracy and civil society. An open market economy with unequal competition from strong economies exposes farmers, small-scale sector and/or unorganized sectors, leading to increased unemployment and socio-economic displacement. It reduces absolute poverty but increases relative inequalities, consciousness of which has the seeds of conflicts in society. However, an integrated policy response may tackle these challenges.

Some of the important rural development schemes working in Madhya Pradesh since last several years are given Table 4.18. Schemes for Scheduled Castes and Scheduled Tribes comprise 16 and 20 per cent of the population of the state have the highest number of development/welfare projects.

Looking to the large number of welfare and development projects during the pre-reform period and after reforms in 1991 it may be commented that both globalization and the state can continue to function as custodians of citizens. At least looking to the type and number of rural development schemes introduced during last fifteen years or so no one can say at least in principle that globalization and state induced development schemes cannot go hand in hand. In other words, the apprehension of some that with the expansion of globalization both as an ideology and as a process the state will become weak, do not hold valid particularly in the state like Madhya Pradesh. Presence and effective functioning of states in many countries which are champions of globalization also refute the above apprehension. In the case of M.P. with having large number of modern NGOs and branch offices of foreign agencies at the state capital to keep close eyes on the development projects funded by them support the view that state is visible and it is performing responsibly. In case in spite of presence of number of development projects the state is not properly performing there are number of historical and contextual factors responsible for it.

Functioning of Development Schemes

As it is argued that economic development, both at the macro and at the micro level cannot necessarily lead to social and cultural change in the same way the development projects in itself, no matter how honestly and powerfully formulated, cannot ensure its success in itself. Success depends on so many external and internal, historical and contextual factors. It is also determined by social and political will of the change agents and honesty on the part of even those who in principle are not entitled for such development benefits but who are otherwise important for both success and failure of projects. Following are some of the studies to examine levels of success of the rural development schemes introduced after 1991 in Madhya Pradesh. Many more such studies may make a valid generalization about relationship between globalization, state and development of common people living in villages and tribal areas in Madhya Pradesh.

Gram Panchayats

As a result of 73rd Constitutional Amendment thousands of SCs, STs and women representatives are found at all the three levels of panchayats. They are directly elected members. In many cases it seems that democracy has really reached the doorstep of many due to Panchayati Raj Institutions (Chaudhary, 2004: 715). Current evidence indicates that no state has gone for direct democracy at the local level to the extent that Madhya Pradesh has now done. But commenting contrarily Narayana (2005: 2829) said that in terms of devolution of powers, resources, functions and capacity building among the elected representatives the situation is not upto the mark. In M.P. Panchayats are perceived as agents of the State Government, representatives lack skills to plan for development because their level, capacity and autonomy is low. To quote Narayana (*op. cit.*) "little effort seems to have gone into development of capacity to plan and budget. So, they end up implementing works under different schemes/programmes as spelt out by the JP/ZP. The estimates are prepared by the officials and closely scrutinized and monitored by them. The men are able to work under such an environment largely because of their political experience. The women do not seem to have that advantage." According to Pai (2004) the then government of M.P. in its publications claimed that there was an increase in participation in gram sabhas by all sections. But many field based studies do not subscribe to this conclusion. Villagers at large, for example, do not know about the schemes, new powers and responsibilities given to the gram sabha. An important factor has been the lack of participation in the gram sabha (Singh, 2002). A study on the functioning of panchayats covering 12-13 gram panchayats in one district from each of the five geographical regions of the state during the period 1995 to 2000, points out that participation of women and Scheduled Castes, Scheduled Tribes is increasing, but at a very slow pace and participation in decision making still remains very low. While lack of local leadership is important a major reason is the caste hierarchy within the village, which is reinforced by the landowning structure (Samarthan, 2002).

Table 4.19: Region-wise Number of Panchayats

Sl. No.	*Region*	*No. of Z P*	*No. of G P*
1.	Bhopal	27	2263
2.	Chambal	40	3022
3.	Malwa	91	5828
4.	Mahakaushal	81	5194
5.	Vindhya	37	3134
6.	Bundelkhand	37	2588

Source: Information obtained from the office of the Director, Panchayat and Rural Development Department, Government of M.P., Bhopal dated 22-11-2002.

In order to ensure participation of *dalits* and tribals at all the three levels of panchayat not only effort was made to reserve seats in different districts in M.P. depending upon their population size, but also efforts were made to empower them through different means. As a result of the reservation facility at all the three levels currently there were 52,726 Scheduled Caste members, that is almost 16 per cent of the total (3,29,788) panchayat representatives. This percentage is similar at all the three levels. For example, out of 45 Zila Parishad presidents 7, of 729 ZP members 114, of 21,721 Sarpanches 3,172 and of 3,00,582 ZP Members 48,368 members are from the Scheduled Castes.

As stated earlier, besides the reservation facility which led to joining of thousands of *dalits* and tribals the ranks of Panchayati Raj

Table 4.20: Panchayat Representatives in Madhya Pradesh on the basis of Caste/Community (1999)[1]

Level	SC		ST		OBC		Unreserved		Total	
	No.	%	No.	%	No.	%	No.	%	No.	%
ZP Presidents	7	16	8	18	17	37	13	29	45	100
ZP Members	114	16	186	25	211	29	218	30	729	100
JP Presidents	40	13	115	36	80	26	77	25	312	100
JP Members	1025	16	1712	27	1706	26	1956	31	6399	100
GP Presidents	3172	15	7299	33	5222	24	6028	28	21721	100
GP Members	48368	16	81541	27	71793	24	98880	33	300582	100
Total	52726	16	90861	28	79029	24	107172	32	329788	100
Population size per cent[2]	—	14.05	—	26.62	—	42.55	—	12.88	4.80 (minority)	100

Source: 1. Information obtained from the office of the Director, Panchayat and Rural Development Department Government of M.P., Bhopal, dated 22-11-2002.

2. Census Report, 1931.

Institutions various efforts like training programmes for panchayat representatives, provision for no confidence motion on objective basis, as well as intervention of NGOs have been ensured for the empowerment of panchayat leaders particularly with reference to the *dalit* representatives. Also, during the last few years many provisions have been made to safeguard *dalit* representatives from any type of encroachment of their rights. However, the socio-economic environment in the villages is still particularistic and not necessarily in favour of the *dalit* empowerment. In fact there is conflict between democratic values and socio-cultural values. In such a situation how and to what extent dalit leaders in Panchayati Raj Institutions can feel empowered and take active interest in development is a moot question.

Buch, Jain and Chaudhary (1999) conducted a study of Women in Panchayats in Madhya Pradesh. The study was conducted in three distinct socio-cultural zones like Jhabua, Chhatarpur and Bilashpur (now in Chhattisgarh). While Jhabua and Bilashpur are dominated by STs and SCs' in Chhatarpur semi-feudalism still persists. Around 343 women working at all the three levels of PR were included in the study. Majority (307) of them were from the marginalized sections of society. Majority of the representatives were above the age of 25 years. Their economy was based on agriculture and most of them were poor. More than 50 per cent were illiterate had no affiliation with political parties. Many of them have discontinued labour work after becoming PRI leaders but even today 92 are engaged in agriculture. The study concluded that they are from lower socio-economic status and totally dependent on state for their functioning. Financial independence and autonomy is yet to be attained. Also, role of others particularly their husbands in their day-to-day functioning is paramount. While working on *dalit* and tribal leaders in Panchayats in M.P. Chaudhary (2004) reports that due to reservation policy there are thousands of *Dalit* and Tribal leaders in Panchayats at all the three levels. Some of them have done wonderful work. But many of them are the first generation entrants in politics; they are from lower socio-economic status groups and lack the capacity to understand their rights and duties. Therefore, for taking decisions and action they are dependent on others such as the panchayat secretary. As a result they are manipulated by others. They have done some work but most of this work relates to infrastructure development.

Panchayat representatives fail to generate resources at the local level because they think that villagers are not capable to give taxes and partly because of disintegration of their support base. Under this situation if the government grant is discontinued they cannot continue construction work.

Training has sharp but limited impact. Similar is the situation with the NGO interventions. In such a situation in order to empower *dalit* and tribal leadership and making the agenda of this segment such as, removal of untouchability in Sehore and lack of drinking water in Betul it is necessary to strengthen the *Gram Sabha* which if honestly addressed, and through training of *Gram Sabha* members, and other representatives of panchayats and secretaries continuously, then only the effective functioning of *dalit* and tribal leaders in the various panchayat bodies can be ensured. Narayana (2005) conducted study on Panchayat Raj Institutions to understand the functioning of local governance during the last 10 years in Madhya Pradesh, Tamil Nadu and Kerala. About Madhya Pradesh, he said that elected ward members show poor awareness of powers and responsibilities. PRIs are perceived as agents of state government. Panchayat presidents understand the legislation better but planning for development is a far cry as little effort seems to have gone into capacity building and devolution of powers and resources. To him, unless powers and resources are devolved and elected representatives are trained properly local government will be a dream. To quote Narayana (2005: 2829), "In conclusion it may be said that the sarpanches believe that they have the necessary powers to carry out works to fulfil the needs of the Panchayats, and the officials at all levels cooperate with them. Then, what is it that prevents them from developing plans and implementing? Little effort seems to have gone into developing the capacity to plan and budget. So, they end up implementing works under different schemes/programmes as spelt out by the JP/ZP. The estimates are prepared by the officials and closely scrutinized and monitored by them. The men are able to work under such an environment largely because of their political experience. The women do not seem to have that advantage."

In short, if we look into socio-economic situation in M.P. it is interesting to note that during last several years, efforts have been made by all the change agents to bring qualitative improvements in quality of life of people across the region. Some new experiments have also been done especially in the field of economy, education and health. The result is really praiseworthy. But in spite of all these efforts Madhya Pradesh is still one of the BIMARU states in the country. Barring Narmada Bachao Andolan, there is no other example of protest or demand from below. The process of social capital formation on the part of the masses is by and large invisible. Historical constraints such as poverty, illiteracy, functioning of some of the cultural practices which have a harmful effect on society and the manner and displacement of weaker sections from their social economic and cultural bases is still going on. People at large are forced to become or remain dependent on external forces for practical reasons. Under the given situation when there is no formation of the critical mass, the state implements its agenda for development in a routinized manner. Traditional local institutions are gradually disappearing. Though, some new initiatives for development have been made in the recent past by the state but it is doubtful that these changes would be sustainable. However, the process of social change is very fast today. It is assumed that gradually the state will come out of the stigma of a BIMARU state.

REFERENCES

Ambedkar, B.R. (1995): *Writings and Speeches*, Vol. 13:62, Education Deptt., Govt. of Maharashtra.

Bhagwat, S. and D. Chirmulay (1997): "Traditional Healing Practices in Rural Karnataka", *Man in India,* Vol. 77. No. 1, 71-82.

Buch, N.; Jain, U. and Chaudhary, S.N. (1999): *Women in Panchayati Raj in Madhya Pradesh,* (Mimeo), Bhopal: Mahila Chetna Manch.

Chaudhary, S.N. (1998): *Socio-Economic Impact of Community based Watershed Management in selected villages of Raisen district of M.P. (mimeo)*, Research Project Report, Bhopal: Government of Madhya Pradesh.

———, (2004): *Dalit and Tribal Leadership in Panchayats,* New Delhi: Concept Publishing Company.

———, (2005): "Globalization and the Changing Patterns of State Run Rural Development Schemes in Madhya Pradesh", *Madhya Pradesh Journal of Social Sciences*, Vol. 10, No. 1.

———, (2005): Untouchability: A Study of its Causes, Mechanisms and

Consequences: Case study of Selected Villages of Sehore and Gwalior Districts of M.P. (mimeo), New Delhi: Ministry of Social Justice and Empowerment, GOI.

———, (2006): *Tribes of Pachmarhi Biosphere Reserve and their Indigenous Knowledge*, Bhopal: Indira Gandhi National Museum of Men.

———, (2006): "Indigenous Knowledge in Health Management: Case Study of Gond, Korku and Bharia Tribes of Pachmarhi Biosphere Reserve" (with R.P. Singh), *Bulletin of Tribal Research Institute*, Bhopal, Vol. 45.

———, (2006): "Grazing Land to Dalits in Madhya Pradesh: Social Opportunity and Political Cost", *The Indian Journal of Social Work*, Vol. 66, Issue 3, 243-261.

———, (2007): *Dalit Agenda and Grazing Land to Scheduled Castes and Scheduled Tribes*, Delhi: Concept Publishing Company.

Dhanagare, D.N. (2003): "Globalization: Towards an Alternative View", *Sociological Bulletin*, Vol. 52, No. 1, March.

Gopalkrishna and Amita Sharma (1998): 'EGS in Madhya Pradesh: Innovative Step to Universalise Education", *Economic and Political Weekly*, Vol. 32 (39), 2546-54.

Grove, R.H., Damodaran V., and S. Sangwan (1998): *Nature and the Orient* (ed.), New Delhi: Oxford.

Gupta Shaibal (2005): "Socio-Economic base of Political Dynamics in Madhya Pradesh" *Economic and Political Weekly*, November 26, 5093-5100.

Gurumurthy, U. (1987): *Panchayati Raj and the Weaker Sections*, New Delhi: Ashish Publishing House, p. 168.

Hirway, I. (1986): "Panchayati Raj at crossroads", *Economic and Political Weekly*, July 22: 1663-1667.

Jaffrelot, Christophe (2003): *India's Silent Revolution: The Rise of the Low Castes in North Indian Politics*, New Delhi: Permanent Black, p. 478.

Jha, P.K. (ed.)(2002): *Land Reforms in India: Issues of Equity in Rural Madhya Pradesh*, New Delhi: Sage Publications.

Kumar, Y. and Neha Chaturvedi (2007): "Dalit Agenda and Charnoi Land Distribution among SCs and STs in Madhya Pradesh: Case Study of Dalits and Tribes of Bundelkhand Region", in (ed.) S.N. Chaudhary, *Dalit Agenda and Grazing Land to Scheduled Castes and Scheduled Tribes*, op. cit.

Lal Bhadur Shastri National Academy of Administration (1994): "A Report on Land Reforms in Madhya Pradesh: An Emprical Study (1998-1991)" in P.K. Jha (ed) *Land Reforms in India: Issues of Equity in Rural Madhya Pradesh*, New Delhi: Sage Publications.

Leclercq, F. (2003): "Education Gurantee Scheme and Primary Schooling in Madhya Pradesh" *Economic and Political Weekly.*

Madhya Pradesh (2002): *The Bhopal Declaration*, Bhopal. What is this?

Madhya Pradesh (2003): *The Task Force Report on Bhopal Declaration*, Bhopal.

Mahajan Ulka (2003): 'Dalits and Land" *Land, People Centred Advocacy Series, National Centre for Advocacy Studies.*

Mainstream (1972): Madhya Pradesh: Ceilings, Exemptions and Loopholes, volume 6, pp.17-19.

Maine, Henry (1876): *Village Communities in the East and the West, Palgrave, London,* p.7. place and name of publisher?

Manor, J. (2001): "Madhya Pradesh: Experiments with Direct Democracy", *Economic and Political Weekly*, 36 (9), 715-716.

Mishra, B.B. (1961): *The Indian Middle Classes: Their Growth in Modern Times*, London: Oxford University Press.

Narayana, D. (2005): "Local Governance without Capacity Building: Ten Years of Panchayati-Raj", *Economic and Political Weekly, Vol. No 86(4),* p. 2832.

Neale, W.C. (1907): Bengal District Gazetteers, Muzaffarpur quotes the view of District Collector, Muzaffarpur, pp. 85, 79-80.

Pai, S. (2004): "Dalit Question and Political Response: Comparative Study of Uttar Pradesh and Madhya Pradesh", *Economic and Political Weekly,* pp. 1141-1150.

Randhawa, N.S. (1996): "Panchayati-Raj System for Decentralized Planning—Myths and Realities", *Man and Development.* June, pp. 56-61.

Rawal, O. (1995): "Niyogi aur Jan Vikas Andolan" in *Isliye Rah Sangharsh Ki Hum Chune*; Swargiya Omprakash Rawal Smriti Nidhi, Indore.

Reddy, Y.V. (2000): "Pro-poor growth: New realities and emerging questions", *Reserve Bank of Indian Bulletin*, 54 (6) June pp. 561-569.

Roy, Dunu (1992): "Land Reforms, People's Movements and Protests" in *Land Reforms in India: Issues of Equity in Rural Madhya Pradesh*, New Delhi: Sage Publications.

Sail, Rajendra K. (1992): "People's Struggle for Land—A Case Study" in P.K. Jha (ed.) *Land Reforms in India: Issues of Equity in Rural Madhya Pradesh*, New Delhi: Sage Publications.

Samarthan (2002): *Madhya Pradesh me Panchayati Raj: Ek Adhyayan 1995-*

2000, report (in Hindi) Bhopal.

Sharma, M. (2004): *Unquiet Worlds: Dalit Voices and Visions*, New Delhi: Heinrich Boll Foundation India.

Singh, A. (2002): "The land Question in Chhattisgarh" in P.K. Jha (ed.) *Land Reforms in India: Issues of Equity in Rural Madhya Pradesh*, New Delhi: Sage Publications, pp. 51-59.

Singh, A.K. (1996): "Panchayati Raj Legislation in Selected States—A Comparative Study", *Man and Development*, September pp. 49-64.

Singh, Y. (2000): "Globalization and Local Culture" in edited Y. Singh *Culture Change in India*, Jaipur: Rawat.

Singh, Yatindra (2002): 'Decentralized Governance in Madhya Pradesh: Experiences of the Gram Sabha in Scheduled Areas", *Economic and Political Weekly, Vol. 37(40)*, pp. 4104.

Singh, S. and K.S. Sridhar (2005): 'Educational Outcome: DPEP or Catching Up?" *Economic and Political Weekly, Vol. XL, 35*, pp. 3863-3873.

Yadav, D.N. (2004): *Socio-Economic Impact of Watershed Mission on Rural Development: The Case of Raisen district* (Ph.D. Unpublished Thesis) Bhopal: Barkatullah University Library.

Index